The Pathology of
Rheumatoid Arthritis

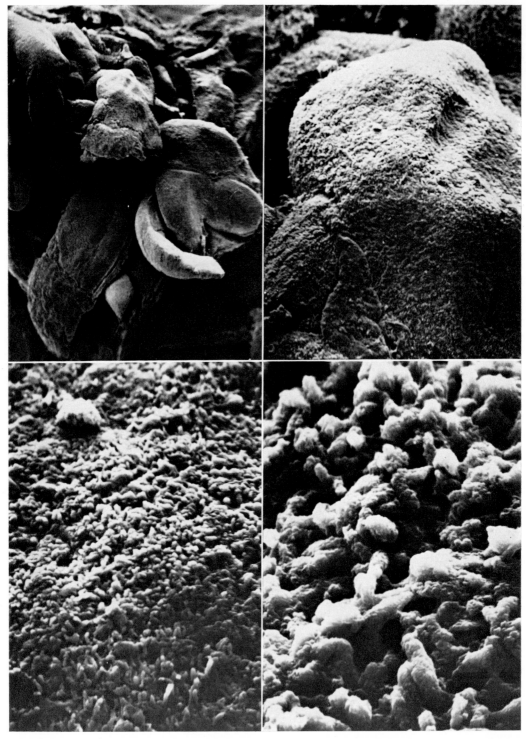

Frontispiece Synovial tissue from the subpatellar fat pad of a female patient with active rheumatoid arthritis. (*Top left*) Enlarged, prominent and irregular synovial villi. (*Top right*) Part of a single villus seen at higher magnification, and revealing the irregular synovial surface. (*Bottom left*) Part of the surface seen in the previous illustration, at higher magnification. (*Bottom right*) Selected portion of the centre of the previous Figure to show details of the surfaces of individual synovial cells. (*Top left* ×24; *right* ×120; *bottom left* ×580; *right* ×2416)

The
Pathology of Rheumatoid Arthritis

D. L. Gardner

M.A., M.D., Ph.D., F.R.C.P.(Ed.), M.R.C.P., M.R.C.Path.

Musgrave Professor of Pathology and Director of the Institute of Pathology, the Queen's University, Belfast. *Formerly* Director, and Head of the Division of Experimental Pathology, Kennedy Institute, London; Honorary Consultant Pathologist, Charing Cross Hospital Group; Senior Lecturer in Pathology, University of Edinburgh; Pathologist, Royal Infirmary, Edinburgh; Honorary Consultant Pathologist, South-East Region of Scotland.

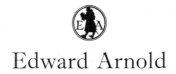

Edward Arnold

First published 1972

by Edward Arnold (Publishers) Ltd.,
25 Hill Street
London WIX 8LL.

ISBN: 0 7131 4194 8

To Helen, Rosalind, Iain,
Philip and Nicholas

Printed in Great Britain by
William Clowes & Sons, Limited
London, Beccles and Colchester

Preface

This slender volume reflects the present state of my understanding of the tissue changes in rheumatoid arthritis. The text is intended to guide pathologists, physicians and surgeons concerned with the rheumatic and connective tissue diseases, and postgraduate students of rheumatology and orthopaedic surgery; it is derived from a Honeyman–Gillespie lecture in the University of Edinburgh Medical School and from lectures given at the Royal Postgraduate Medical School, London, at the Institute of Orthopaedics, University of London, to the Medical Research Society and at the Nuffield Institute of Orthopaedics, Oxford. The views expressed are based upon an analysis of much biopsy material, upon a review of the relevant literature and upon a study of 146 cases of patients dying with rheumatoid arthritis.

No attempt has been made to survey the subject of experimental arthritis. Since 1960, when a comprehensive review was published,* the literature has grown so quickly that a separate volume would be necessary to do justice to this important field of enquiry. Historical aspects of rheumatoid arthritis have been deliberately curtailed; recent work and current debate are emphasised. Reports of the application to the tissues in rheumatoid arthritis of techniques such as immunofluorescence- and scanning electron-microscopy, and of tissue culture, microchemistry, and quantitative and qualitative histochemistry, have, however, been reviewed in some detail. These are the methods that appear most likely to determine our future understanding of the histological changes in this disease.

In the preparation of this review I have enjoyed the support of many colleagues. Drs. Helen Muir, J. Chayen, D. C. Dumonde and J. T. Scott who are, respectively, the Heads of the Divisions of Biochemistry, Cellular Biology, Immunology and Clinical Research at the Kennedy Institute, London, have allowed me liberal access to the results of their own research. The opportunity to discuss the problems of rheumatoid arthritis at meetings of the Heberden Society and of the Arthritis and Rheumatism Council for Research have been invaluable and I am particularly grateful to Professor J. J. R. Duthie, Professor E. G. L. Bywaters, Dr. L. E. Glynn and many other visitors who have taken part in Kennedy Institute meetings during the past 5 years, for their critical and freely expressed opinions. I am indebted to the Librarians of the Royal Society of Medicine (Mr. P. Wade), of the Royal College of Physicians of London (Mr. L. Payne), and of the Royal College of Physicians of Edinburgh (Miss J. P. S. Ferguson) for much help. Mr. Peter Marriott, my Chief Technician, has given unfailing support in the preparation of this work which has added substantially to his daily burden and my secretaries Mrs. Mei-Ling Foo, Mrs. Trudy Boarder and Miss Susan Nance have undertaken meticulous bibliographical investigation during the preparation of the manuscript.

My research at the Kennedy Institute, opened in 1966, would not have been possible without the unswerving aid of the Management Committee and, in particular, of the late Dr. W. S. C. Copeman, Chairman of the Institute Management Committee and a former Vice-President of

* Gardner, D. L. (1960). *Ann. rheum. Dis.*, **19**, 297–317.

the Royal College of Physicians of London, whose untiring efforts did so much to stimulate investigations in the rheumatic diseases. My scientific programmes have been dependent upon the extensive and magnanimous aid of the Arthritis and Rheumatism Council for Research and upon the generosity of the Trustees of the Mathilda and Terence Kennedy Charitable Trust, of the Wellcome Trust, of the Dan Mason Trust, and of the Nuffield Foundation. To Mr. Terence Kennedy I owe a particular debt for his enthusiastic encouragement. My investigations have also been aided by grants from the Government (Royal Society), the Sir James Reckitt Charity, Unilever Ltd., and May & Baker Ltd.

The compilation of this book was undertaken during the tenure of a Lectureship endowed by Sir Edward Lewis in memory of his late wife, Lady Lewis, herself a generous patron of the Kennedy Institute; its completion can be attributed to the eloquent persistence of Dr. Gordon Signy, Editor of the Journal of Clinical Pathology and Deputy Director of the British Post-graduate Medical Federation.

Finally, it is a pleasure to express my thanks to Miss Barbara Koster for her generous and expert guidance during the printing and publication of this volume. I am grateful to Mr. P. J. Price of Edward Arnold for his patience and understanding and to his colleagues for much technical advice.

D. L. GARDNER

April, 1972

Contents

CHAPTER 1

Introduction

Rheumatoid arthritis is 'a subacute or chronic, non-suppurative, inflammatory polyarthritis affecting mainly the peripheral synovial joints, normally in a symmetrical fashion, running a prolonged course of exacerbation and remission, and accompanied by signs of systemic disturbance such as anaemia, weight loss and a raised erythrocyte sedimentation rate' (Duthie *et al*, 1957, Duthie, 1969). The cause remains unknown. Remission is possible (Litwin *et al*, 1966). The incidence of rheumatoid arthritis is judged by subjective criteria that cannot be absolute. Thus, according to Cathcart and O'Sullivan (1970) a female incidence of 3·8% and a male incidence of 1·3% in a New England town, assessed by the 'American Rheumatism Association criteria' (Table 1.1), became 0·55% and 0·14% respectively when assessed by the stricter 'New York

TABLE 1.1. *American Rheumatism Association criteria for rheumatoid arthritis**

Point	Criterion
1	Morning stiffness
2	Joint tenderness or pain on motion
3	Soft-tissue swelling of 1 joint
4	Soft-tissue swelling of 2d joint (within 3 months)
5	Soft-tissue swelling of symmetrical joints (excluding distal interphalangeal)
6	Subcutaneous nodules
7	X-ray changes
8	Serum positive for rheumatoid factors

* 3 or 4 points indicate 'probable,' and ≥ 5 points 'definite' rheumatoid arthritis. (From Cathcart and O'Sullivan, 1970, *New Engl. J. Med.*)

clinical criteria' (Table 1.2). There is no single, certain diagnostic test (Sharp, Calkins and Cohen, 1964). With few exceptions, the synovial joints are the organs first affected; but immunological phenomena common in rheumatoid arthritis, such as the presence in the serum of rheumatoid factors, can be found in persons not clinically affected (Ragan, 1966). It is reasonable to assume that there is a latent or premonitory phase in which the joint tissues appear normal and in which biochemical and intracellular phenomena are not yet recognisable by any of the techniques at present in use to detect tissue changes in disease (Schoen, 1969). The absence of absolute diagnostic criteria has led to a suggestion that 'rheumatoid arthritis' is not a disease entity but a heterogeneous group of cases sharing selected, common features.

Histopathological studies on the tissues of patients with *very early* rheumatoid arthritis are seldom reported, partly because open surgical- and even needle-biopsy may be contraindicated in this phase of the disease, but largely because the majority of patients are seen for the first time after the disease has been present for many months or even years. Because of their high collagen content and of the frequent presence of zones of mineralisation, tissue samples in rheumatoid arthritis can be difficult to process technically. Advances in understanding the intimate details of the mechanisms of cell injury in synovial joints have been handicapped for this reason as well as by an insufficiency of material from early examples of the disease. The relatively small numbers

TABLE 1.2. *New York criteria for rheumatoid arthritis*

Point	Criterion
1	History of episode of 3 painful limb joints*
2	Swelling, limitation, subluxation or ankylosis of 3 limb joints:
	Must include hand, wrist or foot
	Must include symmetry of 1 joint pair
	Must exclude distal interphalangeal, 1st carpometacarpal, 1st metatarsophalangeal and hips
3	X-ray changes (erosions)
4	Serum positive for rheumatoid factors

* Each joint group, for example, proximal interphalangeal, counted as one joint, each side being scored separately. (From Cathcart and O'Sullivan, 1970, *New Engl. J. Med.*)

of cases of rheumatoid arthritis reported from *post mortem* enquiry even in the largest medical centres is a reflection first, of the fact that most patients with rheumatoid arthritis prefer to spend their remaining years at home and second, of the relatively slight interest that locomotor disease provokes in general pathological practice.

History (Figs. 1.1, 1.2, 1.3)

Rheumatoid arthritis was named by Sir Alfred Garrod, and distinguished from gout, at a time when he was assistant physician to the West London Hospital (1859). There had been constant clinical confusion between rheumatoid arthritis, gout and osteoarthritis and an entire dearth of pathological knowledge.

Rheumatoid arthritis is said to have been identified as a disease entity by Landré-Beauvais (1800) and recognised in practice by Haygarth (1805) but practically nothing was known of the morbid anatomical and histological features of the condition until the second half of the nineteenth century (Copeman, 1964). This appears strange since Scudamore (1816) dedicated his work *A Treatise on the Nature and Cure of Gout* to Matthew Baillie, John Hunter's nephew. Scudamore based his treatise on a series of one hundred patients with rheumatism whom he had observed and kept under review. Few were of 'rheumatoid' type but it might have been anticipated that the pathological changes in this disease would have been the subject of debate with his learned patron. Baillie had recently published the first textbook in the English language on Pathology (1793), a text accompanied by a beautiful atlas of engravings (1799–1802) derived from specimens in the Hunterian museum. There is no reference to rheumatoid arthritis in Baillie's *Morbid Anatomy* and no illustrations of the disease in the companion volume of engravings.

The anatomical features of rheumatoid arthritis did not appear to engage the interest of surgeons preoccupied with tuberculous and other forms of infective joint disease (Brodie, 1813). Brodie (1818) not only published a masterly description of gonococcal arthritis but clearly distinguished and delineated the first case of Reiter's (1916) syndrome. It seems very likely that the superficial similarities of the diseases, the frequency and age incidence of tuberculous arthritis and the low mean expectation of life in the years when Hunter, Brodie, Baillie and other great pioneers of morbid anatomy were at work (Morgagni, 1761; Cruveilhier, 1829–1842; Carswell, 1837; Rokitansky, 1842–1846), effectively disguised the problem of rheumatoid arthritis, a disorder much more conspicuous in ageing populations such as our own among whom infectious arthritis is now rare.

Drawings of the clinical deformities of the hands in rheumatoid arthritis are to be found in Charcot's doctoral thesis (Charcot, 1867) (Fig. 1.2) on the subject of *Rheumatisme Articulaire Chronique*, illustrations that anticipated by only four years the publication of what appear to be the first plates showing the morbid anatomy of the joint disorder (Adams, 1857 a,b). The bone and joint diseases which Adams depicts are not always easy to identify with certainty nor can they be interpreted invariably in modern diagnostic terms. However, figures illustrating what is

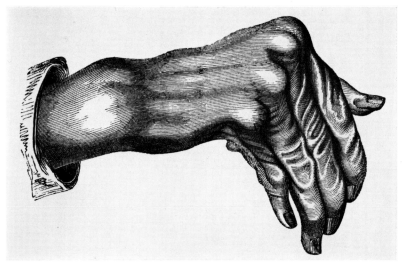

Fig. 1.1 Effects of chronic rheumatic arthritis on the right hand. The deformities illustrated typify those of advanced untreated rheumatoid arthritis as seen at the present time. (From a case described and illustrated in *A treatise on rheumatic gout or chronic rheumatic arthritis of all the joints*, Robert Adams, London, 1857.)

clearly rheumatoid arthritis are included (Fig. 1.3) and Adams can reasonably be regarded as the pioneer of the pathology of rheumatoid arthritis. As Copeman (1964) reminds us, Adams had exceptional opportunities for observing the features of rheumatoid arthritis among the Dublin poor and it was his astute clinical perception together with his interest in anatomy which led to his important studies of this disease. Adams recognised that rheumatoid disease was a polyarthritis, that it was inflammatory in nature and that bony ankylosis was rare. He admitted the possibility of clinical remission.

At the time at which Adams published his work, nothing was known of the cause and pathogenesis of rheumatoid arthritis. The clinical and anatomical features of the disease resembled those of infections such as tuberculosis but even the nature of tuberculosis was not understood and the identity of tuberculous arthritis, scrofula, Pott's disease and phthisis, for example, was not appreciated. It is therefore particularly interesting to observe that Garrod (1848) (quoted by Copeman, 1964) is said to have found the microscopic appearances of the rheumatoid joint synovium to be inflammatory in nature* and that he assumed that the disorder must be the result

* I have not been able to confirm this reference—Author.

of generalised infection. Nevertheless, the microscopic investigation of normal synovia and articular cartilage (Gardner and McGillivray, 1971*b*) was in its infancy and very little substantial data can have been obtained by the time at which Garrod wrote.

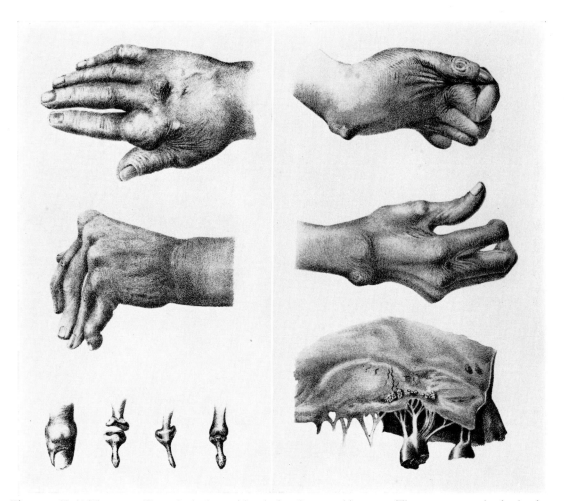

Fig. 1.2 (*Left*) The centre Figure is the 'gouty' hand of an 84-year-old woman. The appearances closely simulate those of chronic articular rheumatism and illustrate the difficulty in distinguishing the varieties of chronic inflammatory joint disease, in the absence of radiography and histopathology (from *Clinical lectures on the diseases of old age*, Jean Martin Charcot, translated by Leigh H. Hunt, London, 1882). (*Right*) The deformities of chronic articular rheumatism as delineated by Charcot are illustrated in the upper two Figures. The difficulties encountered in disentangling the French and German nomenclature of the rheumatic diseases during the latter part of the 19th century are excellently analysed and explained by Jaques Forestier (1963), *Ann. rheum. Dis.*, **22**, 63–70.

It seems most improbable that compound microscopes with achromatic objective lenses can have been used to study joint tissues before 1830. The emergence of the cell theory (Schleiden, 1838; Schwann, 1839) stimulated investigations of articular cartilage and of synovial tissue just as it provoked analyses of the other body tissues (Cameron, 1952; Singer and Underwood, 1962). By 1850, many reports of the structure of cartilage and of its cells had been published but, with few exceptions, attempts to define the microscopic features of rheumatoid arthritis were deferred until the 1860's and 1870's (Goodsir, 1868). By this time the implications of Virchow's *Cellular*

Pathology (1858) had been very widely recognised and the simple slices of tissue cut by the hand-held razor that sufficed for early nineteenth century microscopy had given way to more satis-factory preparations made with mechanical microtomes.

There is little doubt that understanding of the individual pathological identities of rheumatoid as opposed to infectious and osteo-arthritis was delayed because of Charcot's misconception (1889) that all forms of chronic arthritis other than gout were simply variants on a single theme, to be collectively described as 'rheumatisme articulaire'. Within this broad title Charcot em-braced rheumatic fever on the one hand and 'rheumatisme articulaire chronique' on the other.

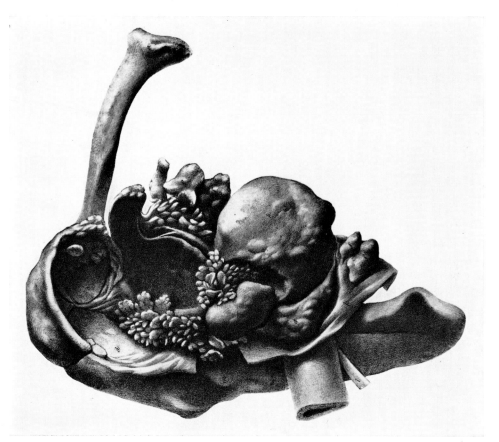

Fig. 1.3 Right shoulder joint. Drawing from a preparation preserved in the Museum of the Royal College of Surgeons of Ireland and exhibiting the effects of chronic rheumatic arthritis in a man aged 65. (From *Illustrations of the effects of gout on chronic rheumatic arthritis*, Robert Adams, London, 1857.)

One form of this latter disorder was 'progressif' and corresponded to rheumatoid arthritis. Char-cot's view was supported by Virchow who used the title 'arthritis deformans' to include all forms of chronic arthritis. The authority of these pioneers can be held responsible for the slow progress in analysing the pathology of rheumatoid arthritis which characterised the 1880's and 1890's. It was not until 1906 that Bannatyne, physician to the Royal Hospital at Bath, in the fourth edition of an excellent and readable monograph, differentiated the pathological features of rheuma-toid arthritis from those of osteoarthritis.

Bannatyne, whose text (1896) was the first to contain an X-ray plate (Copeman, 1964), supported the view prevalent between 1880 and 1930 that rheumatoid arthritis was a generalised microbial disease. His pathological observations were shortly followed by those of Hoffa and Wollenberg (1908) and of Nichols and Richardson (1909), who, in important papers, paved the way for systematic surveys of the histology of rheumatoid arthritis. Meanwhile, Strangeways (1905) had established a small laboratory in two Cambridge houses that he had purchased to found a hospital for the rheumatic and other diseases 'the pathology and treatment of which are as yet undetermined'. The discoveries of Pasteur, Lister and Koch and the rise of bacteriology dominated medical thought and Strangeways was able to satisfy himself that rheumatoid polyarthritis could result from general infective processes such as scarlet fever, gonorrhoea and dysentery. His work, which coincided with the epic studies of Poynton and Paine on the microbiological origin of rheumatic fever (Poynton and Paine, 1913) tended to favour a bacterial origin for rheumatoid arthritis, a view now again prevalent.

Although arthritis had long been known as a clinical characteristic of serum sickness, Friedberger (1913) obtained the first evidence to show that arthritis could be produced experimentally by serological techniques. Modern interest in the role of immunological mechanisms in rheumatoid joint injury can be traced to this time. A radiological classification of rheumatoid and of osteoarthritis as 'atrophic' and 'hypertrophic' (Goldthwait, 1904) was followed by a revised pathological classification which emphasised the prominence of the synovia in rheumatoid arthritis (Nichols and Richardson, 1909). The latter disease was termed 'proliferative arthritis' by these authors; osteoarthritis was named 'degenerative arthritis'. Subsequently, Stockman (1920) formulated clear views on the pathology of rheumatoid arthritis and very much of what is now known of the light microscopy of the joints in this disorder was clearly described and illustrated both by Stockman (1920) and by Fisher (1929). Klinge (1933, 1934) wrote definitive accounts of the pathology of this and of many other of the connective tissue diseases and his extensive 1933 monograph set the seal on the descriptive microscopy of rheumatoid synovitis. Collin's (1949) valuable work supplemented Klinge's views but, unfortunately, appeared almost immediately before the techniques of electron microscopy (Pease, 1969; Sjostrand, 1967) histochemistry (Pearse, 1953) and immunofluorescence microscopy (Coons and Kaplan, 1950) were introduced into the analytical histology of joint disease. Nevertheless, Collin's long account of the pathology of rheumatoid arthritis and the contribution by Sokoloff (1966) to Comroe's textbook are two of the most valuable descriptions of the pathological morphology of the disorder.

CHAPTER 2

Articular Tissues: Gross and Microscopic Pathology

In early rheumatoid arthritis, pain, redness, heat and swelling are localised, in varying distribution, to the small joints of the fingers and toes and to the synovial joints of the knees, elbows, wrists and hips. In individual cases, any of the 187 or so diarthrodial articulations found in the normal adult human may be affected although microscopic proof of disease of the synovial joints of the middle ear is not yet available (Friedman, 1971).* It is generally agreed that the first pathological evidence of rheumatoid arthritis takes the form of a synovitis which is sometimes fulminating and so severe as to suggest a pyogenic infection but is more commonly of a subacute character. The most notable feature is a proliferation of the synovial membrane. In the acute case, the membrane is a soft, oedematous, congested and papilliferous tissue filling the synovial pouches and encroaching upon the cartilages to which it adheres (Collins, 1949; Gardner, 1964).

The later pathological changes vary as widely in severity as in distribution but the microscopic evidence of the diverse nature and regional involvement of joints is very much more limited than is the clinical (Parker and Keefer, 1935). For example, 86% of the temporomandibular joints of one series of patients with rheumatoid arthritis appear to have been affected (Franks, 1969), 48% in another (Crum and Loiselle, 1970); by contrast, I have not yet found a single pathological description of the temporomandibular joint in this disease.

There is no histological evidence to show whether the inflammatory reaction is a response to a primary injury to cells of the synovial lining cell layer (Figs. 2.1–2.3) or whether the initial injury is to the underlying connective tissue with a secondary involvement of the surface cells. The early synovial inflammatory reaction is accompanied by hyperaemia (Whaley *et al.*, 1968; Dick, Neufeld *et al.*, 1970; Dick, Onge *et al.*, 1970; McCarty, Polcyn and Collins, 1970; McCarty, Polcyn, Collins and Gottschalk, 1970), oedema, cellular infiltration (Figs. 2.11–2.17) and fibrinous exudation. Isotopic labelling techniques have also confirmed that altered vascular permeability is a very early phenomenon in experimental joint inflammation (Soria–Herrera *et al.*, 1971). The synovial cells multiply. In clinical remission, these changes may subside; more usually, progression is followed or accompanied by a marginal proliferation of connective, granulation tissue which gradually replaces articular cartilage. This 'erosive' process, the nature of which is critical to an understanding of the pathogenesis of rheumatoid arthritis, has been termed an 'invasion' but more closely resembles a replacement fibrosis.

Among the young marginal vascular fibrous tissue that proliferates in this way are varying numbers of inflammatory cells. This granulation tissue is the material which, at surgical exploration or necropsy, is seen to comprise the macroscopic 'pannus'. Opposing joint surfaces, diminished by cartilage loss, become joined by fibrous ankylosis. Granulation tissue replaces bone at the margins of articulating surfaces and intraosseous 'pseudocysts' originate when the high

---

* Incudostapedial ankylosis is a common condition. Thirty examples were found among 1,000 tympanoplasties by Szpunar and Miszyke (1970) but the frequency of rheumatoid arthritis was not stated.

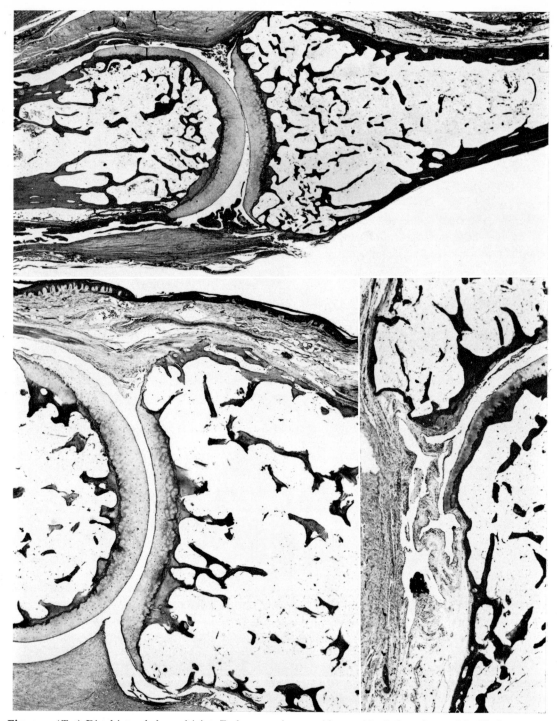

Fig. 2.1 (*Top*) Distal interphalangeal joint. Early acute rheumatoid synovitis. Inflamed synovial villi shown protruding into margins of joint. Intact articular cartilage. No evidence of osteoporosis. Inflamed synovia of tendon sheath seen in lower part of Figure. (*Bottom left*) For comparison with subsequent figures: normal proximal interphalangeal joint. Note cartilage structure, bony end plate and appearance of synovium. Moderate osteoporosis is present, a common finding in elderly women. (*Bottom right*) Proximal interphalangeal joint. More advanced rheumatoid synovitis with marginal cartilage loss. Note island of deep staining fibrin (fibrinoid) material near centre of Figure. Cartilage at margin of middle phalanx is partly lost due to associated osteoarthrosis. Moderately severe osteoporosis. (*Top* ×6½; *bottom left* ×14; *right* ×14)

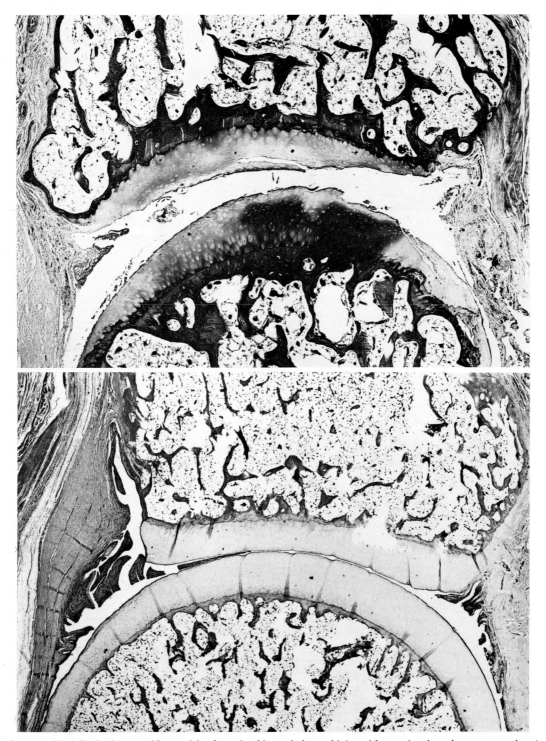

Fig. 2.2 (*Top*) Early rheumatoid synovitis of proximal interphalangeal joint with associated moderate osteoarthrosis. Note inflamed synovial villi (*left*) with intact synovial tissue at right. No osteoporosis but observe fibrillation of superficial cartilage surfaces. (*Bottom*) Proximal interphalangeal joint. Active and advancing rheumatoid synovitis. At both margins of the section of this proximal interphalangeal joint the rheumatoid synovial villi are deeply staining and appear black, or dark grey, due to the presence of numerous inflammatory cells. The villi interpose between and are adherent to articular cartilage surfaces which are, in other respects, intact. Mild osteoporosis.

(*Top* ×17; *bottom* ×10)

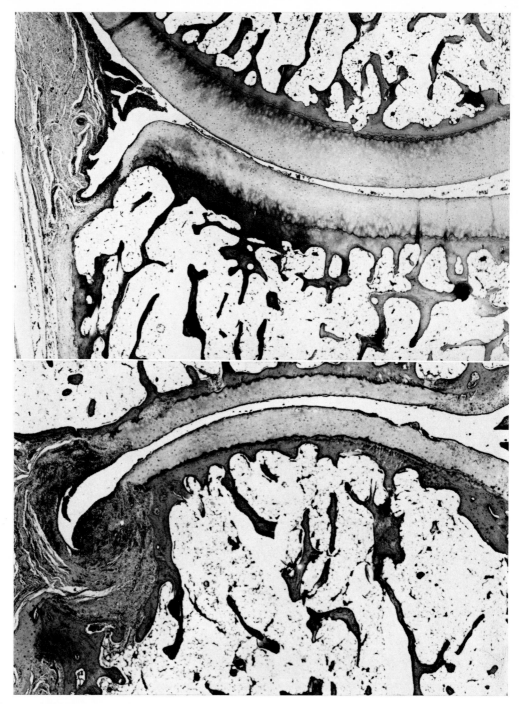

Fig. 2.3 (*Top*) Compare with Fig. 2.2 (*bottom*). Active synovitis is seen, synovial villi containing numerous inflammatory cells leading to a dark appearance in the photomicrograph. Note an intact synovial artery beneath the villus surface. At the margin (*left*) of the middle phalanx, inflammatory tissue extends into and is beginning to replace the margin of the articular cartilage. The remainder of the cartilage is intact. Mild osteoporosis. (*Bottom*) Metacarpophalangeal joint. Synovial inflammation has become widespread and normal synovial tissue is extensively replaced by granulation tissue that extends (*top and bottom*) to replace both marginal articular cartilage and subarticular bone. Appearances shown in this Figure correspond to the radiological 'erosion' that provides an early diagnostic feature for the disease clinically. This 'early' clinical feature therefore corresponds to an advanced histological lesion. Moderate osteoporosis. (*Top* ×14; *bottom* ×12)

pressures generated by joint movement force pannus and synovial fluid into nearby osteoporotic bone. The inflammatory process commonly extends to involve the joint capsule and adjacent supporting structures, weakening them, both because of direct destruction and perhaps on account of ischaemic and disuse atrophy. Where the zones of synovial inflammation adjoin soft tissues,

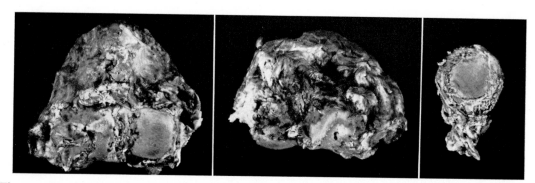

Fig. 2.4 Severe rheumatoid arthritis of the elbow joint in a woman aged 60 with disease of two years duration. (*Left*) Anterior surface of lower end of humerus. Rough irregular pannus covers the capitulum and the articular cartilage surface of the trochlear (*left*) is almost totally destroyed. (*Centre*) Posterior surface of lower end of humerus illustrating severe destruction of articular cartilage. (*Right*) Head of radius with rim of rheumatoid pannus replacing one half of the whole normal articular surface. Residual intact cartilage is present (*at the centre*). (From Gardner D. L., *Pathology of the Connective Tissue Diseases*, London: Arnold, 1965.)
$(\times \frac{2}{3})$

these also are hyperaemic, oedematous and infiltrated by inflammatory cells. In the case of laryngeal rheumatoid arthritis, for example, the disease process may extend posteriorly, producing pharyngeal ulceration as one consequence. In the untreated, or uncontrolled, advanced and irreversible case, subluxation and characteristic deformity are the common result (Figs. 2.4, 6.1 and 6.2).

(A) PATHOLOGICAL ANATOMY (Figs. 1.1–1.3, 2.4, 2.5)

Very little of significance has been added to knowledge of the gross changes in the synovial joints in rheumatoid arthritis since the descriptions of Stockman (1920), Fisher (1929), Klinge (1933, 1934) and Collins (1949) and the reader can do no better than to consult Collin's (1949) account and that of Sokoloff (1966) for formal descriptions of the anatomy of the disease. The present survey amplifies synopses given previously (Gardner, 1965, 1969).

At exploratory arthrotomy, in the earliest stage of the disease, the synovial tissues are found to be swollen and reddish-pink in colour and to protrude from the divided capsule as the joint is opened. The synovial fluid is in excess of normal in volume and is opalescent or turbid and thin in consistence. The detailed characteristics of the fluid are considered below (p. 84). With time, the congestion, redness, and swelling of the synovial tissues become more pronounced until, on arthrotomy, arthroscopy or at necropsy, a seaweed-like mass of hyperplastic tissue appears to occupy more than the normal joint space.

At this stage, and the progression of the disease ranges from low-grade through subacute (Rubens–Duval, 1966) to fulminating, the signs of two of the most characteristic and most destructive features of rheumatoid arthritis become evident. First, synovial villous processes are seen to be loosely adherent to marginal articular cartilaginous surfaces with which they apparently come in random contact. Adhesion to the cartilage margin is light and the adherent superficial

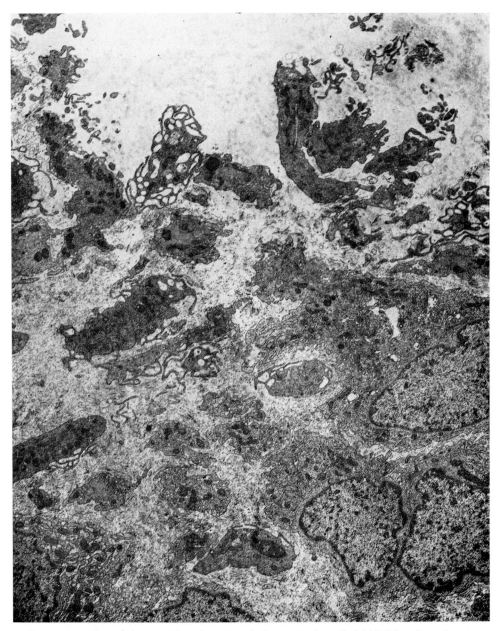

Fig. 2.5 Low power view of the many loosely textured phagocytic (so-called 'A(M)') cells and more compact fibroblast-like (so-called 'B(F)') cells of the synovium in rheumatoid arthritis. As with the light microscopic structure, none of the individual cellular changes is pathognomonic; the arrangement, frequency and form of these cells is, however, characteristic. (From a micrograph of Dr. J. A. Palfrey.)   (×6,000)

synovial villous processes can easily be raised from the articular surface. With time, the adhesions merge with, and become coextensive with the granulation tissue that comprises the 'pannus'. Second, at the peripheral cartilage margins where villous adhesions are most common the inflamed synovia extend onto and insidiously replace the edge of the articular cartilage. By a combination of this circumferential adhesion and replacement, the smooth margin of the cartilage comes to be transformed to a narrow but increasingly wide zone of synovial-like tissue that grows in continuity with the cartilage. The rough, dull, red-pink zone formed in this way is termed a 'pannus' (Latin: a cloth). It cannot be detached from the cartilage surfaces into which it extends actively.

In joints which have been inflamed for some weeks or months, and, typically in those that are most commonly affected—the finger, knee, hip, elbow and wrist—the opposing, roughened synovial and marginal cartilaginous surfaces are often seen to be loosely joined by strands of fibrin. In turn, these strands become organised, and more extensive and increasing volumes of the joint space are obliterated by the process of fibrous ankylosis. Subsequently, bony ankylosis may occur but this sequel, which is more usual as a result of other inflammatory joint diseases such as severely destructive bacterial joint infection, is quite uncommon in rheumatoid arthritis. Paradoxically, indeed, some residual joint movement may persist in spite of the total, structural replacement of the joint space by young fibrous tissue.

The inflammatory process, the severity of which can be measured clinically, begins in periarticular structures such as tendon sheaths and bursae at much the same time as it can first be detected in the synovial tissue of the diarthrodial joints. This extraarticular, peripheral oedema may contribute substantially towards the local limb or finger swelling that is an early feature of the disease. For reasons that are not fully understood, the entire early inflammatory process is accompanied by increasing laxity of the joint ligaments, by muscle wasting and by progressive osteoporosis that is disproportionately severe for the age and sex of the patient. The overlying skin becomes pale, tense and atrophic. A fluctuating course is common.

As the disease becomes more chronic and as the acute inflammation of early rheumatoid synovitis subsides, the rough granular and dull red surface of the synovial membrane is seen to be less swollen, the villous processes less prominent. A faint, orange-brown discolouration recalls the appearance of the florid synovial processes in villonodular synovitis or even of the synovia in haemosiderosis. A gradual atrophy follows in which synovial villi give way to a pale, thinned and fibrous membrane recalling that encountered after incomplete synovectomy (p. 179) but varying markedly in different areas on account of the range of severity of reaction encountered in different synovial zones. Collins (1949) remarks that a persistent, large synovial effusion seems to play some part in delaying or preventing the formation of adhesions. Morley (1971) postulates that, because of the strange relationship between the osmolarity of synovial fluid and that of the blood plasma, effusions, when formed, may be self-perpetuating. Effusions tend to become smaller with time, to be followed by partial, and sometimes complete fibrous ankylosis.

Clinical remission is common. The extent to which pathological remission can occur is less certain.

The factors that may contribute to the chronic nature of the inflammatory reaction are considered later (pp. 18 and 203). Rare instances of coexistent crystal arthritis are recorded (Olwen, Toone and Irby, 1966). Rest has been shown to be important in alleviating the symptoms and signs of inflammation. For obvious reasons, no exact morphological analysis has been possible of the influence of rest on the pathological features of the disease although analogous forms of experimental arthritis have provided corroborative experimental evidence on this point.

(B) LIGHT MICROSCOPY

Astonishingly few studies of the synovia in the *earliest* phase of the disease have been made (Moberg *et al.*, 1966). The most informative analysis of the early inflammatory changes in the joints of patients with rheumatoid arthritis is that of Kulka, Bocking, Ropes and Bauer (1955). These authors examined the knee joints and popliteal cysts of 8 patients who had the disease for less than one year: the earliest changes, it was estimated, had been present for 7 days, the latest 9 months. From this study a picture emerged of the relatively early lesions in rheumatoid arthritis. Even in this 'early' series, some patients appear to have had recurrent disease and, in one, 3 months elapsed between the time at which the joint lesion was diagnosed and the time at which biopsy was performed. The principal histological findings were first, an abundant lymphocytic, moderate polymorph and prolific plasma cell synovial infiltrate (3/10); second, much fibrin or fibrin-like material; third, synovial cell hypertrophy and hyperplasia; fourth, oedema and increased ground substance formation; fifth, slight or marked synovial tissue necrosis (5/10); and sixth, vascular narrowing (assessed on fixed material) (author's parentheses) (7/10).

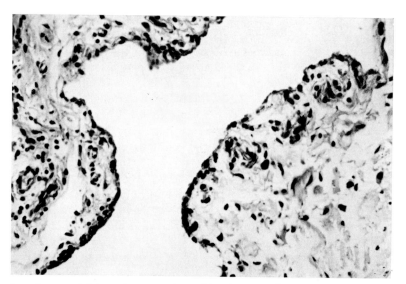

Fig. 2.6   Normal areolar synovial tissue for comparison with subsequent Figures. Note the narrow layer of single or reduplicated synovial cells bounding the surface and the numerous underlying capillaries and venules among the loose collagenous connective tissue.   (×400)

The account of Kulka *et al.* (1955) is supplemented by those of Nichols and Richardson (1909), Fisher (1929), Klinge (1933, 1934), Collins (1949), Castor (1960), Gardner (1965, 1969), Sokoloff (1966), Grimley and Sokoloff (1966), Wagner (1967) and Hamerman, Barland and Janis (1969). Collins (1949) stressed the coexistence of synovial inflammation and of inflammatory effusion in the joint space; he reiterated the views of Nichols and Richardson (1909). The latter interpreted the gross increase in amount of synovial tissue seen when the inflamed joint is opened as a 'proliferation'. It is generally accepted now that this enlargement of the synovia to form, typically, a congested, swollen mass of villous and papillary processes, protruding from the capsule of the opened joint and often loosely adherent to the marginal articular cartilaginous surface, is due mainly to vascular congestion, to inflammatory oedema and to inflammatory cellular infiltration. Microscopically, there is frequent evidence of hyperplasia of the synovial cells which cover the non-articulating surfaces of the joint; the normal single or double layer multiplies two- or three-fold in the course of the disease. The multiplication may be focal. It is, however, misleading to talk of synovial hypertrophy except in a general, descriptive sense: there is occasional evidence that the individual synovial cells or groups of cells become larger as the tissue increases in volume but the principal changes are modest synovial cell hyperplasia and pronounced subsynovial congestion, oedema and inflammatory cellular infiltration.

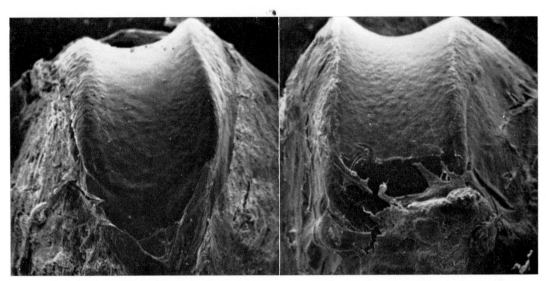

Fig. 2.7 Experimental arthritis. Arthritis was induced by intraarticular injection of turpentine into the rat knee joint. (*Left*) The appearances seen 24 hours after injection are depicted; there is no deposit of fibrin on the joint surface which appears intact. (*Right*) By contrast, 4 days after the injection the cartilage surface is becoming obscured by irregular deposits of fibrin that ultimately cover the articular surface. It is not yet known what changes take place in the surface structure of the articular cartilage lying beneath the fibrinous exudate. (*Left* ×17; *right* ×17)

Following the useful practice of Sokoloff (1966), the histological features of rheumatoid synovitis can be considered to show 3 main components: inflammatory exudation (Figs. 2.6–2.11), cellular infiltration (Figs. 2.12–2.17) and granulation tissue formation (Figs. 2.20–2.26).

(*a*) *Exudation* is particularly marked near the articular cartilaginous margins where the vascular loops terminate that are thought to supply the normal metabolic requirements of the avascular adult cartilage. In rheumatoid arthritis there must be some change in the normal lymphatic drainage of the joint (Bauer, Short and Bennett, 1933; Davies, 1946) but this has received little attention. There is, of course, evidence that in the young, and in some animal cartilages, nutrition is partly maintained by the subchondral vasculature. Congestion and oedema are accompanied, to a degree varying remarkably in different joints and even within different parts of a single joint (Bennett, Waine and Bauer, 1942; Cruickshank, 1952a; Wilkinson and Jones, 1963), by surface desquamation of synovial cells and focal superficial synovial tissue necrosis. The necrotic zones resemble small subcutaneous rheumatoid granulomata (p. 122). Eosinophilic material, predominantly fibrin and formerly termed fibrinoid, accumulates on the synovial surfaces (Fig. 2.10); it is assumed to have escaped from small blood vessels the permeability of which has increased during the early inflammatory response. Hageman factor (factor XII) may contribute to this process,

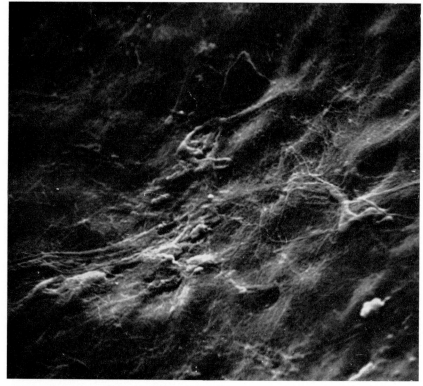

Fig. 2.8 Four hours after the intraarticular injection of turpentine, a fine meshwork of fibrin is seen deposited on the irregular, undulating surface of the articular cartilage. The undulating processes appear normal. The nature of the deposit has been determined by comparison with experimental studies of artificial coagulation where the 3-dimensional structure of fibrin strands has been defined.   ($\times$ 1080)

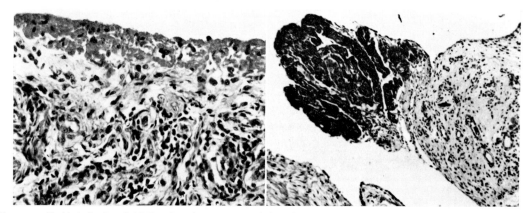

Fig. 2.9 (*Left*) A further field showing the presence of abundant eosinophilic fibrin at the synovial surface of an inflamed joint. Small blood vessels are numerous in the deeper tissue. They are surrounded by modest numbers of lymphocytes and plasma cells. Excessive capillary and venular permeability is assumed to be the cause of fibrinogen leakage and fibrin polymerisation in surface zones. (*Right*) A cap of polymerised, eosinophilic fibrin lying at the surface of the synovial villus. Note how synovial surface cells extend around, and probably cover, the exuded fibrin.
(*Left* $\times$ 310; *right* $\times$ 125)

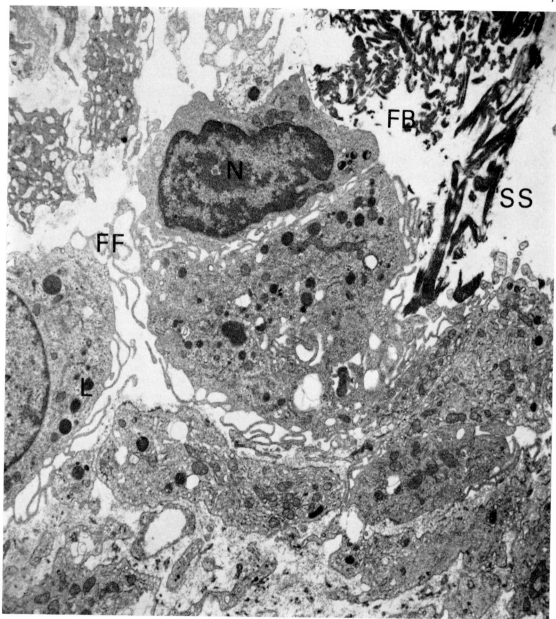

Fig. 2.10 Synovial surface showing loose arrangement, numerous filopodia and dense bodies of phagocytic A(M) cells. Note abundant electron-dense, fibrillar material resting on cell surface (*top right*) the appearance of which recalls that of fibrin. (From Davies, D.V. and Palfrey, A. J., 1971: *Modern Trends in Rheumatology*, ed. Hill, A. G. S., London: Butterworth, pp. 1–20.)

(× 3,600)

Key to this and subsequent electron micrographs

C = Collagen	G = Golgi complex
CD = Cell debris	GG = Grey globular bodies
CE = Cell	I = Intercellular space
CH = Calcium hydroxyapatite crystals	IM = Intercellular matrix
CS = Cartilage surface	L = Lysosome
DB = Electron-dense body	M = Mitochondria
ER = Endoplasmic reticulum	N = Nucleus
F = Unidentified fibres	PM = Pericellular matrix
FB = Fibrin	PS = Phagosome
FF = Filopodia	SS = Synovial space
FR = Fibroblast	V = Vesicle

first, because of its influence on vascular permeability which it increases directly or through the promotion of kinin activation, second, because of its role as an initiator of the coagulation cascade. Hageman factor attracted interest when it was shown to be activated by uric acid crystals in experimental urate arthritis. Considerable activity in rheumatoid synovial fluids has been demonstrated (Szpilmanowa and Stachurska, 1968). The activity has been found to be higher in synovial leucocyte suspensions than in supernates, an observation which raises the possibility that Hageman factor may originate within these cells or be adsorbed to their surfaces.

The reason for the persistence of fibrin within the chronically inflamed joints of rheumatoid arthritis is a matter of great interest. Continued vascular permeability and a deficient synovial fibrinolytic system are unlikely to be the entire explanation. Andersen and Gormsen (1970) for example, surveyed the fibrinolytic activity of synovial tissues in 20 cases of rheumatoid arthritis by the fibrinolysis autograph method and showed that activity was mainly concentrated in relation to blood vessels; where activity was low, vessels tended to be occluded by thrombi and to display white cell infiltration. Rheumatoid plasma had no inhibitory effect on fibrinolysis. The lowest plasminogen activator and highest fibrin-stabilising activity were found in rheumatoid arthritis.

The persistence of fibrin is considered by some authors to be of critical importance to the formation of the marginal granulation tissue of 'pannus' (Lack, 1962) and thus to the sequence of events that culminates in joint destruction. The presence of fibrin of altered antigenicity may also account for the chronicity of the rheumatoid inflammatory reaction (Riddle and Barnhart, 1964; Glynn, 1968) (p. 203). Failure of rheumatoid synovial tissue to remove fibrin by the fibrinolytic mechanism (readily activated in normal synovial tissue) may be due to defective fibrinolysis; alternatively, the change in fibrin structure that accounts for altered antigenicity may also, perhaps, contribute to an unusual resistance to physiological fibrinolytic mechanisms. In either case, morphologically identifiable fibrin can be recognised within rheumatoid synovial cells and rheumatoid synovial fluid polymorphs by electron- and by immunofluorescence microscopy; there appears to be no bar to the phagocytosis of the changed protein (Riddle, Bluhm and Barnhart, 1965).

Retention of the old term 'fibrinoid' may be a diagnostic convenience. It has, however, served to obscure thought on the difficult problem of the nature of tissue injury in systemic diseases of connective tissue such as rheumatoid arthritis. Since the term 'fibrinoid' was introduced (Neumann, 1880) it has gradually become clear that the eosinophilic material described at the base of peptic ulcers, in aneurysms and around placental villi, and which is commonplace in the lesions of systemic lupus erythematosus, systemic sclerosis (Klemperer, Pollack and Baehr, 1942), rheumatoid arthritis (Collins, 1949) and polyarteritis nodosa (Rich, 1947) is not a single, chemically homogeneous entity but a variety of substances (Janeway, Gitlin and Craig, 1956; Gitlin and Craig, 1957), derived from the blood plasma by insudation (Rössle, 1933) and varying in composition in different diseases while retaining identical staining characteristics with dyes of low chemical specificity (Movat and More, 1957; Gardner, 1965; Wagner, 1967; Maldyk, 1969a). The idea that the presence of 'fibrinoid' of similar staining properties might imply identity of origin was suggested by Klinge (1929, 1930a, b, c, 1933, 1934), on the basis of his work with rheumatic fever and with rabbit arthritis provoked by the injection of horse serum. This view was rejected many years ago (Klemperer, Pollack and Baehr, 1942), even before the heterogeneity of fibrinoid was established, and it can have little direct bearing now on hypotheses advanced to explain the pathogenesis of rheumatoid arthritis.

Within the articular space in rheumatoid arthritis it is not infrequent to find varying numbers of minute, ellipsoid 'rice bodies' the common name for which gives a ready guide to their shape, size and character. They were described in tuberculous arthritis (Riese, 1895) but have been encountered in rheumatoid arthritis (Albrecht, Marinette, Jacox and Vaughan, 1965). These authors give the typical appearance: intact rice bodies are 'small, soft, opaque, rather elastic round or oval particles measuring about 1·5 × 1·1 × 0·5 mm. They may freely float in joint fluid or may be attached to synovium.' Albrecht and his colleagues separated rice bodies from the knee joints of 2 rheumatoid patients at the time of synovectomy and studied the structure of the particles by light and electron microscopy. The rice body lipid, hexose and hexosamine, sialic acid and amino acid contents were measured and it was shown that only a relatively small part of the body was identical to fibrin, the bulk of the structure being composed of dense filamentous material lacking the usual 23 nm periodicity characteristic of fibrin. No hydroxyproline was detected but small amounts of lipid and neuraminic acid were demonstrable. The phospholipid pattern of these bodies was similar to that of cell lipid, an observation which suggested that they were not derived wholly from joint fluid. It seemed more likely that the bodies represented small detached portions of changed, degenerate synovium.

(b) Synovial and subsynovial tissues are found to be *infiltrated* by many neutrophil and occasional eosinophil polymorphs and by numerous lymphocytes and plasma cells (Figs. 2.11–2.17). There is

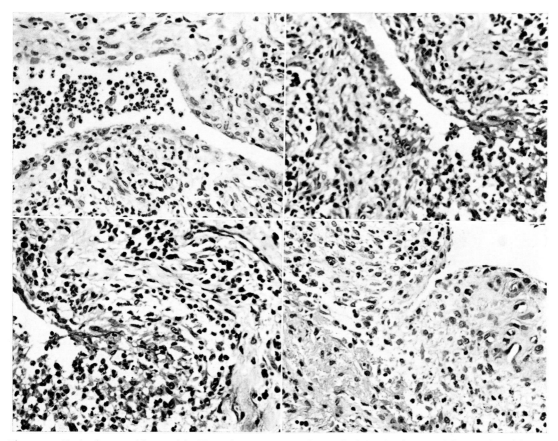

Fig. 2.11 Early rheumatoid synovitis. Note the numerous polymorphs lying in the synovial space (*top left*), the presence of similar cells within the synovial tissues, the increase in extent of the surface synovial cells (*top right*), and small numbers of plasma cells and lymphocytes (*bottom left*). An early feature is the presence of varying amounts of eosinophilic fibrin seen as pale grey material (*bottom right*), at and beneath the synovial surface.
(*Top right* × 310; *left* × 310; *bottom right* × 310; *left* × 310)

no evidence that the phagocytes aggregate in response to any of the known intracellular micro-organisms that have been shown to be present (Stewart, Alexander and Duthie, 1969). Indeed, corynebacteria isolated from rheumatoid joints depress leucocyte migration in culture (Maini, Stewart and Dumonde, 1970). The presence of so many polymorphs in the earliest phases of the synovitis invites speculation on the cause of the inflammation and emphasises that the lymphoid and plasma cell accumulations may be late, secondary consequences of an unknown, acute primary insult. The polymorphs, many of which escape into the synovial fluid, become particularly numerous when a secondary, pyogenic infection supervenes (Kellgren, Ball, Fairbrother and

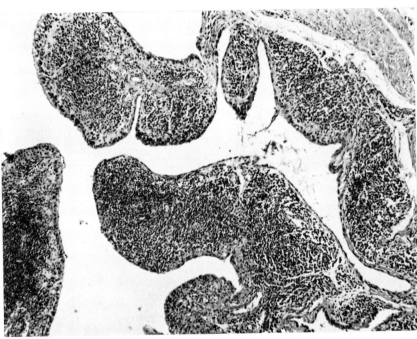

Fig. 2.12   A conspicuous feature of established rheumatoid synovitis at a stage commonly seen in biopsy material is an increase in the extent of synovial villi, a process frequently and misleadingly described as hypertrophy, due to the widespread infiltration of plasma cells, lymphocytes and histiocytes. Occasionally, lymphoid cells aggregate as follicles (*bottom left*). In this field, the surface synovial cells show only focal hyperplasia and reduplication. Fibrin, commonly seen within the synovial space and at the synovial surface, not visible in this illustration.   (×70)

Barnes, 1958); they reach the synovial fluid by penetrating the walls of synovial capillaries and venules. Contemporary views favour the importance of the latter rather than of the former in most forms of acute inflammation (Spector, 1964; Curran, 1967).

The possibility that cartilage degradation rather than an infective agent or the formation of synovial immune complexes (p. 97) may be the cause of leucocyte accumulations in rheumatoid joints has been raised by the observations of Chang and Houck (1970). These authors showed that a cutaneous collagenase degraded collagen to products which exerted an intense chemotactic activity via Millipore filters. Chemotaxis was evident at very low concentration and within 4 hours of testing. The macromolecular complexes demonstrated by Velican and Stroescu (1969) could have a similar role.

The metabolic characteristics of the polymorphs differ from normal: the recognised differences are presumed to be one consequence of the immunological reactions in which the polymorphs are engaged. Some evidence was obtained by Dimitrov, Stjernholm and Weir (1969) to show that the polymorphs of patients with rheumatoid arthritis differed from normal in terms of certain aspects of intermediary amino acid metabolism. Thus, less ^{14}C-proprionic acid was converted to products such as CO_2 and protein than normal, and rheumatoid white cells converted ^{14}C-proprionate to β-alanine rather than to aspartic and glutamic acids, the usual products identifiable in normal white cell metabolism. The difficulty in interpreting such results is considerable, particularly since the behaviour of polymorph metabolism in other comparable disease states such as systemic lupus erythematosus and osteoarthrosis is not known.

The microscopic picture usually seen in rheumatoid arthritis is the later widespread lymphocytic and plasma cell infiltration (Hoffa and Wollenberg, 1908): tissue is not often collected at the onset of the disease and the earliest changes are not well understood. Unlike the appearances in

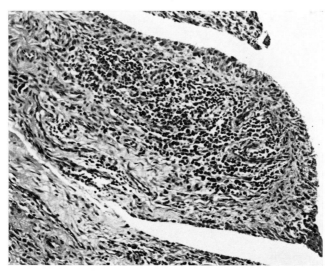

Fig. 2.13 Portion of corresponding field seen at higher magnification to show follicular arrangement of synovial lymphocytes. The loose texture of the surface synovial cells is shown. The presence of several arterioles and venules can be recognised. No surface fibrin.   ($\times 310$)

early rat adjuvant arthritis (Gryfe, Sanders and Gardner, 1971), mast cells are not abnormally prominent. Generally, the lymphocytic infiltrate is diffuse and varies from sparse to prolific; sometimes, in limited zones, lymphocytes multiply or aggregate in a follicular arrangement which does not display the framework of reticular fibres found in the primary follicles of normal lymph nodes (Hoffa and Wollenberg, 1908; Nichols and Richardson, 1909; Fisher, 1929). In exceptional cases, germinal centre formation is apparent. It is not clear whether this occasional presence of germinal centres indicates a basic immunological distinction from cases with only a diffuse synovial lymphocytosis or whether the presence of germinal centres simply reflects the pronounced lymphoreticular hyperactivity characteristic of severe rheumatoid arthritis and seen in its most advanced form in Felty's syndrome (p. 171). There is no proof that cases with synovial lymphoid germinal centres are those most actively engaged in the production, locally, of immunoglobulins including rheumatoid factor but this association is a reasonable assumption (p. 100): it can also be assumed that the formation of germinal centres is under thymic control.

It is probable that both T- and B-lymphocytes are present in rheumatoid synovia (Roitt *et al.*,

1969). The former, long-lived and susceptible to thymic control, could be those which, subjecting the surface antigens of synovial cells to incessant surveillance, 'recognise' antigenic changes induced in the synovia by whatever exogenous infective agent is responsible for the disease (p. 188). These T-cells may transform to blast cells which perpetuate a vicious circle of synovial cell injury through cytotoxic mechanisms, exaggerating the local inflammatory response: they lead to germinal centre formation. The B- (bursa-equivalent) lymphocytes, independent of the thymus and short-lived, could be the parents of the numerous effector cells of the plasma cell series which populate the synovial tissue so widely in rheumatoid arthritis. It will be of great

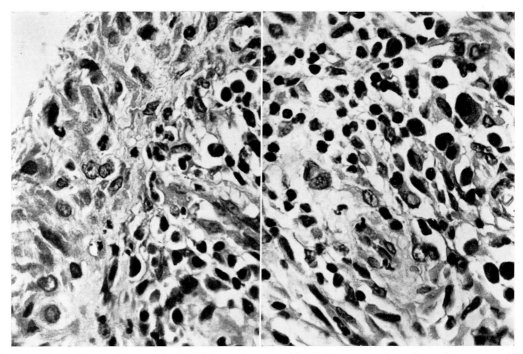

Fig. 2.14   Early rheumatoid synovitis. (*Left*) The surface synovial cells have assumed a variegated appearance. Their superficial margins are often entirely separated from one another and they appear increased in number. Occasional polymorphs lie among them but mitotic figures are rarely seen. (*Right*) More deeply, plasma cells begin to infiltrate the inflamed tissues and moderate numbers of histiocytes with reniform nuclei can be recognised. A venule (*lower corner of left part of figure*) shows no abnormality recognisable with the light microscope, but venulitis is frequent. (*Left* ×600; *right* ×600)

interest to observe whether the method described by Pompidou and Schramm (1971) will permit the thymic-dependent lymphocytes of rheumatoid synovia to be distinguished from the B-cells.

The lymphocytes, 'blast' cells and plasma cells of the rheumatoid synovia can all be termed 'immunocytes' (Burnet, 1969). It is by no means clear what part the individual cells play in the mechanism of rheumatoid synovitis or what relationship they bear to the injurious agent which first causes the synovitis. The plasma cells, derived from populations of B-lymphocytes, cannot be differentiated with certainty from early lymphoblasts simply on the basis of their usual pyroninophilia. This staining characteristic, an assumption of a violet-red cytoplasmic colour with the methyl green–pyronin technique by contrast with the green cytoplasm of lymphocytes, is a subjective index of the amount of cytoplasmic RNA present in the form of ribosomes, poly-ribosomes and rough endoplasmic reticulum. In transformed lymphocytes (lymphoblasts) pyroninophilia is attributed to numerous free ribosomes and polyribosomes. By contrast, plasma cells can be shown to have their RNA arranged as extensive rough endoplasmic reticulum, an organelle readily defined by electron microscopy. This technique consequently allows a distinction between the two cell forms.

The plasma cells of the rheumatoid synovia commonly contain immunoglobulin aggregates termed Russell bodies some of which may escape or be extruded and are seen lying in extra-cellular sites. The immunoglobulin aggregates can also be recognised by electron microscopy as the amorphous inclusions of Mott cells, inclusions that are presumably the precursors of the larger Russell body.

Synovial plasma cells in rheumatoid arthritis have been found to contain (Orlovskaya, Muldi-yarov and Kazakova, 1970), to be associated with, or to synthesise (Sliwinski and Zvaifler, 1970) immunoglobulins of classes IgG and IgM, including rheumatoid factors. The early evidence (Mellors, Nowoslawski, Korngold and Sengson, 1961) should be assessed critically. There are numerous technical pitfalls. Roitt et al. (1969) remind us, for example, that the demonstration of intracytoplasmic immunoglobulins in phytohaemagglutinin-stimulated blast cells can be due to an artefact encountered when *live* cells are stained in suspension by fluorescein-labelled anti-immunoglobulin sera. Sera may be of low specificity, contaminated with microorganisms and of low avidity. It is always possible that other artefacts may mask the precise localisation of immuno-globulins in rheumatoid synovial cells cut in cryostat section.

That the immunoglobulin-containing plasma cells of rheumatoid synovia are engaged in a local synovial tissue-damaging exercise in which they are secreting synoviotoxic antibody is not established. Because components of complement such as $C'3$ (β_1C) are also present it does seem reasonable to deduce however that an active immunological response is localised to the synovia and that the presence of immunoglobulin is not fortuitous (Townes and Soiva, 1970). It remains probable that this response is a *consequence* of primary synovial cell injury caused, for example, by activation of a latent viral infection, rather than that it is itself the agency provoking synovial injury. The latter view was at one time strongly supported by proponents of the autoallergic nature of the systemic connective tissue diseases (Glynn and Holborow, 1965) but the balance of present opinion favours a secondary role for the rheumatoid synovial immunological response (p. 195).

The lymphoreticular tissues (p. 148), the plasma proteins (p. 108) and the immunopathological changes (p. 90) in rheumatoid arthritis are considered more fully in later pages.

The presence of aggregates of free, extracellular, as well as of phagocytosed, intracellular haemosiderin is a common finding in the more superficial but not the surface synovial layers (Collins, 1949) (Fig. 2.14). Focal, microscopic haemorrhage from the congested synovial capillaries and venules is probably common: blood escapes into the inflamed tissues and the red cells liberated in this way, phagocytosed by histiocytes, are the source of haemosiderin. Newly formed, young vessels in granulation tissue are especially friable. When this intraarticular, surface bleeding occurs, and it may occasionally be substantial, synovial A(M) cells ingest the blood cells. Their content of ferritin, derived from haemosiderin by intracellular digestion, is readily shown by electron microscopy (Muirden, 1966) (Fig. 12.18).

Synovial iron, demonstrable by chemical analysis, by electron probe or activation analysis or by staining with the Prussian blue technique, must be distinguished from doubly-refractile materials that may be introduced into the joint therapeutically, from radioopaque contrast media and from deposits of therapeutic [198]Au or [90]Y.

A conspicuous but quite inconstant feature of the synovial cellular reaction in rheumatoid arthritis is the presence of multinucleated giant cells (Figs. 2.18, 2.19) distinct from the osteoclasts

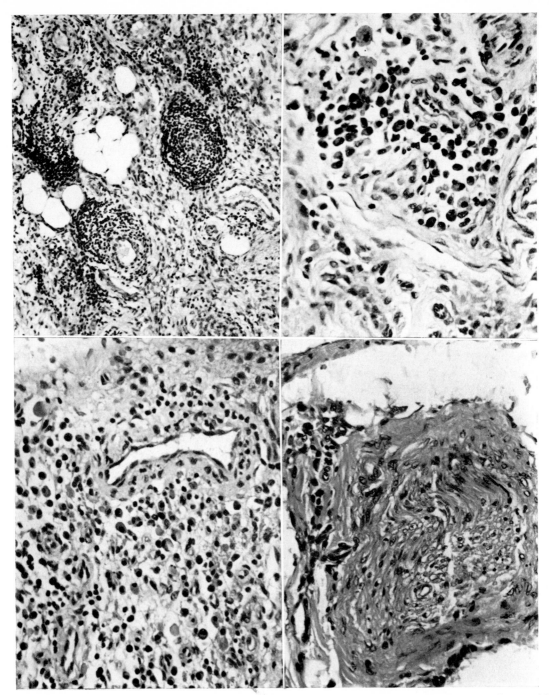

Fig. 2.15 This Figure illustrates representative zones of an established inflammatory synovial reaction in rheumatoid arthritis. (*Top left*) In areolar synovial tissue, lymphoid follicle formation with perivenular lymphocytic infiltration. Numerous histiocytes and fibroblasts extend among the fibro-fatty tissue. (*Top right*) An island of plasma cells, of varying size, lying near the venules and arranged in follicular formation. Whether some of these cells are transformed lymphocytes or lymphoblasts, cannot be determined in this photomicrograph. (*Bottom left*) Around and within the walls of a small vein are substantial numbers of plasma cells of varying size, lymphocytes and occasional histiocytes and polymorphs. Note further portions of the vessel (*lower left*). (*Bottom right*) Small nerve in deeper synovial tissue. *At left*, the venule adjoins the nerve and is surrounded and infiltrated by occasional polymorphs and plasma cells.
(*Top left* ×125; *right* ×310; *bottom left* ×310; *right* ×310)

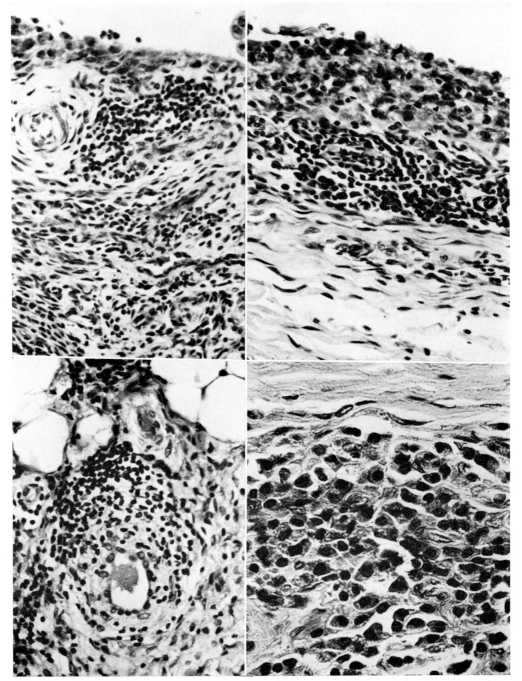

Fig. 2.16 In further representative fields in established rheumatoid arthritis, inflammatory cell infiltrates assume varying forms. (*Top left*) Note loose arrangement of surface synovial cells with polymorphs and nuclear debris adhering to the surface. Immediately beneath surface, arteriole adjoining follicular cluster of lymphocytes. More deeply, lymphocytes are sparse and lie related to walls of venules. (*Top right*) Cellular debris attached to surface the cells of which are infiltrated by polymorphs and lymphocytes. The latter assume a follicular form in the centre of the field, but more deeply an intact fibrovascular synovial structure is preserved. (*Bottom left*) The oedematous wall of a small synovial vein extensively infiltrated with lymphocytes and occasional polymorphs. At top, note small intact arteriole. (*Bottom right*) Arranged in a follicular cluster at the margin of the joint capsule, a cluster of lymphocytes, plasma cells and histiocytes. Similar islands of cells may extend (*centre*) for considerable distances from the synovial surfaces. Occasionally, as in the larynx and pharynx, synovitis may involve other nearby organs.

(*Top left* ×310; *right* ×310; *bottom left* ×310; *right* ×675)

that can often be seen at sites of marginal bone reabsorption and the foreign body giant cells occasionally seen in synovial tissue when material, introduced into the joint therapeutically, is being phagocytosed. Similar giant cells have been recognised in rheumatoid synovial cell culture (p. 39). These giant cells were described in tissue sections by Collins (1949) and subsequently by Grimley and Sokoloff (1966) (p. 47). The latter employed many special histological techniques including phase contrast and polarising microscopy in a detailed analysis of the cells' characteristics. The giant cells displayed strong acid phosphatase activity; the enzyme, it was suggested, was lysosomal.

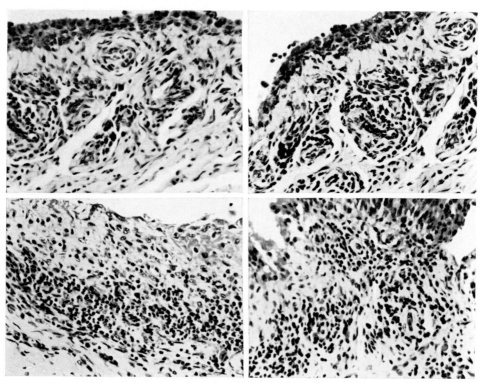

Fig. 2.17 Representative fields in active synovitis illustrating synovial cell changes, inflammatory cell infiltration and presence of surface fibrin. (*Top left*) Mild synovial cell hyperplasia. Note arteriole near surface with several underlying venules and lymphatics. (*Top right*) Comparable field with lymphocytes arranged as aggregates around surface synovial blood vessels. (*Bottom left*) Pale grey-appearing material in upper right portion of photomicrograph is surface fibrin incorporated beneath a thin synovial cell covering. Near centre of field, numerous lymphocytes and some polymorphs. (*Bottom right*) Nearby field showing palisaded arrangement of some surface synovial cells, appearance recalling that of the margin of the rheumatoid nodule, with moderate numbers of underlying lymphocytes and plasma cells. Small amount of pale grey-staining fibrin mingles with the synovial surface cells and lies between and above them.   (*Top left* × 310; *right* × 310); *bottom left* × 310; *right* × 310)

Others have confirmed the inconstant presence of giant cells in rheumatoid synovia (Donald and Kerr, 1968; Liso, Gillardi and Trizio, 1968); although a phagocytic activity is suspected on account of their content of ferritin (Muirden and Senator, 1968) they do not appear to contain any form of known microorganism and are distinct, for example, from the mulberry giant cells of virus synovitides such as measles. Erythrophagocytosis, occasionally seen in synovial macrophages in rheumatoid arthritis, is exceptional. Giant cells are not present in the synovia in bacterial arthritis, pigmented villonodular synovitis or osteoarthrosis (Donald and Kerr, 1968). Personal observation suggests that they arise from, or in close relation to, the hyperplastic synovial lining cell layer, are 40–50 μm in diameter and have 8–12 peripheral nuclei. In some cases they appear to form by the syncytial fusion of synovial surface cells. Considerable light has been thrown on their likely origin by the methods of tissue culture (p. 39).

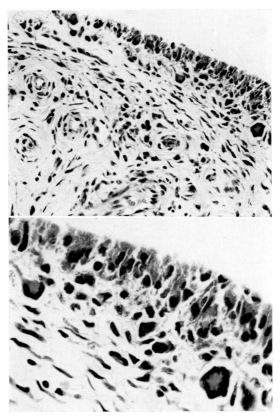

Fig. 2.18 The formation of synovial multinucleated giant cells, a process recognised by Collins (1949), is a common feature of rheumatoid synovitis. This illustration shows several typical giant cells of moderate size with 8, 10 or 12 peripheral nuclei, lying within and immediately beneath the synovial surface. (*Bottom*) All stages in the formation of the synovial giant cells can be traced in morphological continuity to the synovial cell surface. It seems reasonable to suppose that the giant cell is derived from defective division of the synovial cell, resulting in polyploidy.

(*Top* × 310; *bottom* × 675)

(*c*) *Granulation tissue formation* at the margin of joints affected by progressive rheumatoid arthritis is invariable and is generally regarded as a key to the peripheral, progressive destruction of articular cartilage that accounts for so many of the principal pathological features of the disease. The granulation tissue or *pannus*, extending centripetally (Figs. 2.20–2.26), takes the place of peripheral cartilage, and forms a dull, red-brown concentric vascular rim to the pale, translucent articular cartilage. The margin is in continuity with the inflamed synovial connective tissue and may provoke early marginal fibrous ankylosis.

Microscopically, there is a recognisable change in the staining characteristics of the cartilage matrix: decreased basophilia may be an indication of marginal loss of matrix proteoglycans but

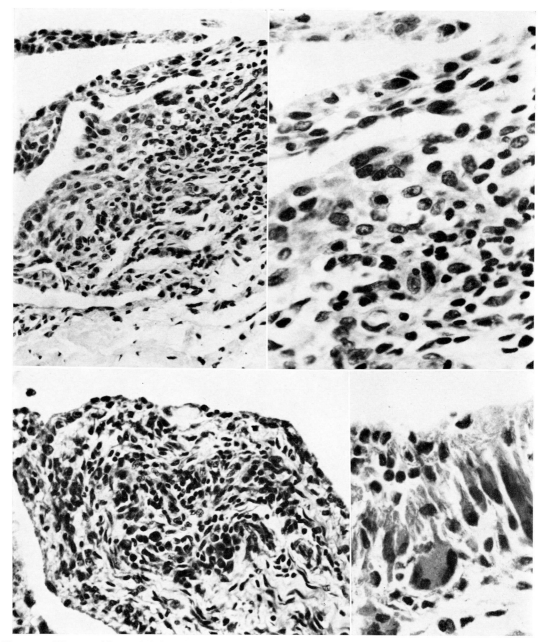

Fig. 2.19 Rheumatoid synovial giant cell formation. (*Top left*) In an area of active lymphocytic/plasma cell infiltration, a multinucleated giant cell (*top centre*) is seen lying at the surface of the synovial villus. (*Top right*) The giant cell, seen at higher magnification, has at least 6 peripheral ovoid nuclei the individual structure of which recalls that of nearby synovial cells. Note adjacent lymphocytes, plasma cells and histiocytes and varying numbers of capillaries. (*Bottom left*) Numerous capillaries extend into this synovial villus, which adjoins that, seen above, in which giant cell formation is prominent. (*Bottom right*) Multinucleated synovial giant cell seen, together with a number of separate but large synovial cells, at surface of zone of active rheumatoid synovitis. Cytoplasmic tails extend both from the multinucleated and from the other adjoining synovial cells and the morphological features of both the mononuclear and multinucleated cells have much in common. (*Top left* ×310; *right* ×675; *bottom left* ×310; *right* ×675)

whether the cartilage appears basophilic or eosinophilic is strongly influenced by the techniques and extent of decalcification during processing. The reduced content of sulphated glycosamino-glycans is detected by a loss of metachromasia on staining with dyes such as toluidine blue and can be shown by a diminished content of Alcian blue-positive material. These altered staining characteristics correspond morphologically with the situation of adjacent synovial cells and of the macrophages, polymorphs, lymphocytes and plasma cells of the synovial inflammatory exudate (Fig. 2.23). It has always seemed reasonable therefore to associate the changed quality of the marginal articular cartilage with the biological activities of the cellular exudate.

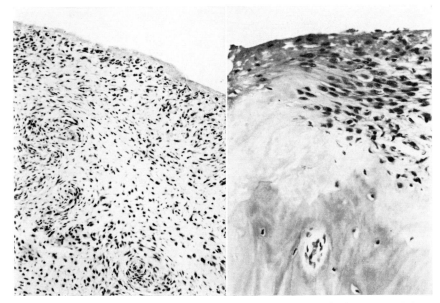

Fig. 2.20 Fibrin is abundant in the synovial spaces in rheumatoid synovitis. It is also commonly incorporated into the synovial surface as seen (*left*) in this Figure. There is no obvious relationship between fibrin incorporation and the severity of the underlying synovial cellular inflammatory reaction. (*Right*) An early stage in the formation of rheumatoid pannus (granulation tissue), is the appearance at the synovial margin of articular cartilage of a cellular tissue, in which eosinophilic fibrinous material is common. Note—fibrin (*top left*), lymphocytes, histiocytes and fibroblasts (*top right*), and cartilage and bone (*bottom*).   (*Left* ×125; *right* ×310)

Until recently, very few detailed studies had been made of the synovial/cartilage interphase in rheumatoid arthritis. Investigations of experimental arthritis are, however, now in progress by *in vivo* techniques, by scanning and by electron microscopy, that can be expected to shed light on this aspect of the human disease. One of the difficulties facing investigators at the present time is the lack of detailed knowledge of the *normal* synovio-cartilaginous junction. Much of the literature on normal cartilage fine structure (Figs. 5.1–5.5) is concerned with epiphyseal tissue; relatively few, controlled studies have been made of normal articular cartilage (Davies, 1969); and none, so far as I can determine, of the electron microscopic appearances of the cells and intercellular matrix in the 'no-man's-land' between cartilage and synovium. Scanning electron microscopy suggests that, even in the normal animal, there is a considerable zone at the margin of the articular surfaces of diarthrodial joints that has a surface structure that is neither cartilaginous nor synovial (Fig. 5.13). Transmission electron microscopic evidence is now beginning to accumulate that demonstrates that the cytological and matrix structures of this intermediate zone are distinctive.

Barrand (personal communication) believes that important early changes in experimental arthritis include the ingrowth of endothelial buds into altered marginal cartilage matrix and the extension of pseudopod-like cytoplasmic processes of adjacent synovial cells across the cartilage surface. It is here, in the complex interplay between cartilage and synovium, that an understanding of cartilage injury in rheumatoid arthritis is likely to emerge during the next five years.

X-ray studies throw very little light on the early joint changes. Radiologically, the replacement of marginal radioopaque bone by radiolucent granulation tissue causes the appearance of more or less sharply defined zones called 'erosions' at the margins of diseased joints. Cartilage changes cannot be detected. The phrase 'erosive rheumatoid arthritis', freely used clinically, signifies only that the extension of granulation tissue has led to focal loss of bone or to pseudocyst formation (p. 74).

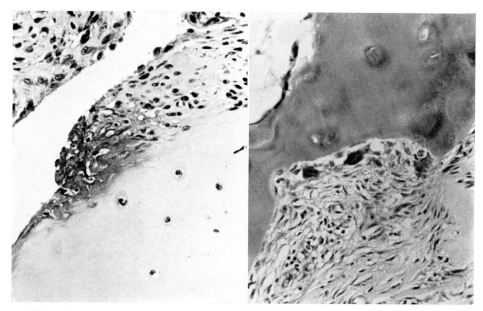

Fig. 2.21 (*Left*) Rheumatoid pannus formation, a critical feature in the evolution of the rheumatoid process, seen with a change in staining characteristics of the superficial, first effected, cartilage. The cartilage (*bottom*) is undergoing an unexplained series of changes in response to the extension of the granulation tissue (*top*). There is a loss of cartilaginous metachromasia at the junction between these two tissues, presumably a depolymerisation of proteoglycans and cartilage lysis with cell and matrix replacement by granulation tissue. (*Right*) Accompanying pannus formation, granulation tissue extends into and within subjacent bone. The reaction may be accompanied, as in this field, by osteoclastic bone reabsorption. This response appears to be a non-specific inflammatory reaction. It is commonplace in a variety of articular diseases.   (*Left* ×310; *right* ×310)

In considering the origin of marginal cartilage lysis in pannus formation we cannot, of course, be certain, in the absence of detailed measurements of the blood supply to the joint, that cartilage lysis is not simply an indirect consequence of an altered local circulation consequent on the early synovitis (Kulka, 1966). Changes in the microcirculation can, for example, be caused by cationic proteins extracted from lysosomes (Janoff and Zweifach, 1964). Perivascular cuffing of small arteries and arterioles by lymphocytes is not uncommon. Less frequently, there is plasmatic vasculosis similar to that seen in allograft rejection or in accelerated hypertension, or endarterial fibrosis. Venulitis is frequent and, as in other inflammatory reactions, the venule appears to be the site at which many of the cellular phenomena of inflammation such as leucocytic margination and emigration and red cell diapedesis are found. Electron microscopic evidence that the primary disturbance in rheumatoid arthritis is a synovial vasculitis (p. 150) has been obtained by Marin *et al.* (1969) although their published micrographs are difficult to interpret. Cartilage lysis does not, however, result from regional ischaemia alone (Collins, 1949) and morphological evidence of arterial occlusion in rheumatoid synovitis is exceptional. The view that cartilage lysis is determined by vascular disease is also difficult to reconcile with the suggestion (Sokoloff, 1966) that pannus formation is less pronounced in joints in which movement is maintained than in those kept at rest, unless it be assumed that the factors which digest cartilage and those which provoke the extension, into cartilage, of vascular granulation tissue, are different. Mechanical features are

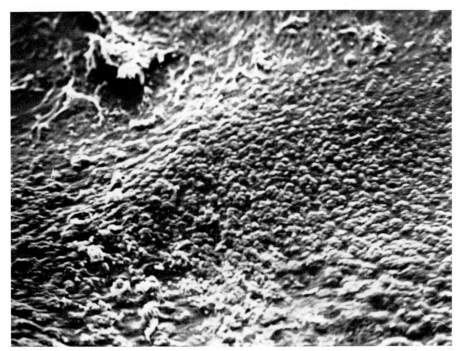

Fig. 2.22   Fourteen days after the induction of turpentine arthritis in a rat knee joint, the margin of a pannus progressively replacing articular cartilage can be seen extending diagonally across the field (*lower right*). (*Top left*) An irregular meshwork of fibrin adheres loosely to the joint surface.   (× 210)

important causes of microscopic connective tissue differentiation (Scapinelli and Little, 1970). Compression and rotation can promote the formation of typical rounded cartilage cells from elongated fibrocytes and analogous changes may provoke or modify pannus formation in rheumatoid arthritis; a similar process may account for Sokoloff's observations, which may not necessarily be relevant to interpretations of the role of small vessels in cartilage loss.

Considerable light has been shed on the ways in which altered joint blood flow could contribute to cartilage destruction by the observations of Sledge and Dingle (1965). These authors showed that hyperbaric oxygen supplied to cartilage rudiments in culture provoked lysis, apparently by altering lysosomal membrane permeability (p. 113). Similar observations were made on macrophage lysosomes. Extrapolating from Sledge and Dingle's (1965) evidence, it would seem possible that the hyperaemia of active rheumatoid synovitis could contribute to marginal articular cartilage lysis. That the explanation is less simple is suggested by the measurements by Falchuk, Goetzl and Kulka (1970) and by Lund–Olsen (1970) of gas tensions in rheumatoid synovial fluid (Table 2.1). It is clear that the more severe the rheumatoid arthritis, the lower the synovial fluid P_{O_2} and pH and the higher the P_{CO_2} and lactate. This is a metabolic situation in which cartilage cells might normally be expected to prosper and is the converse of that suggested by the results obtained from *in vitro* studies of embryonic cartilage. However, the observations agree with measurements of vascular diameter and tortuosity that have been made in experimental allergic arthritis (Bakowska and Gardner, 1971) (p. 203) and which reveal an important phase of diminished synovial blood flow in the early stages of the animal disease.

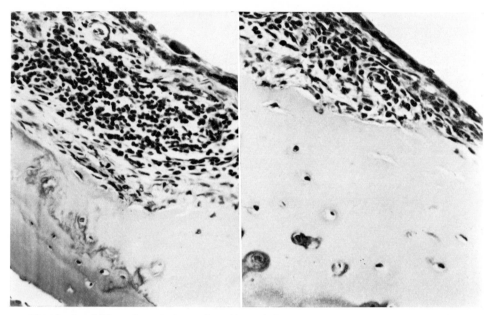

Fig. 2.23 Two further fields to show the extension of granulation tissue at an articular cartilage margin. The field (*left*) includes a surface synovial giant cell and a follicular cluster of lymphocytes. It lies in continuity with the second field (*right*) where the remarkably sharp margin between granulation tissue and intact cartilage can be observed. At this margin, cartilage matrix loss appears to precede cell lysis.   (*Left* × 310; *right* × 310)

It is still debated (Sokoloff, 1966), whether cartilage loss precedes replacement by granulation tissue, whether the changes are simultaneous as in metaplasia or whether granulation tissue invades the avascular cartilage, an older view (p. 30). The process is analogous to the widespread injury to cartilage which is common to the majority of the inflammatory synovial joint diseases. In searching for an explanation for the curious circumferential cartilage destruction that is so constant in rheumatoid arthritis, it is necessary to invoke some agent or process derived from the synovial inflammatory reaction which heralds the disease. Marginal cartilage injury in rheumatoid arthritis may be caused *directly* or *indirectly*. *Direct* destruction could be provoked by the causative agent (Hamerman, 1969), it could result from a humoral factor derived from the inflamed synovia, or it could be mediated by the cells infiltrating this synovia. *Indirect* destruction could be determined, for example, by an altered vascular supply of metabolites to peripheral cartilage or to the influence of the circulatory changes upon the synthesis and secretion of components of cartilage such as the proteoglycans that are essential for its normal physical and mechanical properties and for its resistance to stress, strain and deformation.

One view of the process of cartilage loss is as follows. Hyaline articular cartilage in synovial joints is avascular and apparently derives the intermediary substances necessary for its active metabolism by diffusion from the synovial fluid and from the blood vessels of the circulus

TABLE 2.1. *Synovial fluid oxygen levels. Clinical diagnoses, physiological measurements and histological gradings (in terms of fixed cell hyperplasia, leucocytic infiltration, obliterative microangiopathy, microvascular thrombosis, focal cell/vascular ratios and fibrinoid) (from Falchuk, K. H., Goetzl, E. J. and Kulka, J. P. (1970): Amer. J. Med., 49, 223–231).*

P_{O_2}	$Q : V_{O_2}$	Histological class	Relative blood flow (calculated)	Clinical entities in each group
> 37	0·2–0·6	1	1	Traumatic effusion, osteo-arthritis, psoriasis, Reiter's syndrome
27–37	0·1–0·19	2		Psoriasis, ochronosis, mild rheumatoid arthritis
< 27	< 0·1	3	4	Only severe rheumatoid arthritis

vasculosus of the joint (Davies, 1969). An inflammatory reaction within the synovial tissue, whatever its cause, must alter the normal flow of metabolites to articular cartilage cells. The effects are first detected marginally and a gradual lysis of cartilaginous matrix, probably caused both by collagenases (p. 37) and by lysosomal proteases liberated by the influence of altered redox potentials on lysosomal membranes (p. 37), is followed by the impaired synthetic activity and by the death of chondrocytes. The marginal rim of cartilage adjacent to the synovial reflection is first damaged and then destroyed (Fig. 2.24); its place is taken by less fully differentiated mechanocytes, precursors of which persist in mature connective tissue. These cells grow in continuity from the inflamed synovia and synthesise new collagen and ground substance which is subsequently infiltrated by lymphocytes and plasma cells, similar to those present in the inflamed synovia, and by histiocytes. There is no reason to invoke the property of invasiveness to explain pannus formation; invasion, indeed, is a term best restricted to the characteristics of malignant tumour cells and to those of the cytotrophoblast.

Pannus formation, can be said to be a form of reparative metaplasia, taking place while inflammation continues. It is unlike wound healing—the process is destructive rather than reparative—but the established inflammatory cellular reactions recall those seen in ulcerative colitis and in autoimmune thyroiditis. They are quantitatively dissimilar from the much more destructive changes caused by bacterial or mycotic arthritis, by traumatic or by chemical injury; they bring to mind states of well-adjusted parasitism such as syphilis in which an exogenous microorganism efficiently utilises the metabolic pathways of host cells and in which the development of an immunological reaction to the parasite is shown locally by an accumulation of lymphocytes and plasma cells.

The changes described in the synovial tissues also recall, by reason of their cellular characteristics, delayed hypersensitivity reactions in response to unknown antigenic stimuli such as viral infection (p. 192). They may, of course, be associated with a comparable immunological reaction against a connective tissue component of cartilage itself. In this case, the metabolic lysis of cartilage due to synovial dysfunction could be accompanied by a cytotoxic dissolution due directly to the action of immunocytes sensitised to cartilage antigens. There is, as yet, little direct evidence to support this view. An alternative view which held support at one time was the suggestion that immunological reactions were directed against cartilage because of the presence of antigens shared with microbiological agents such as streptococci to which the patient had been sensitised.

Cartilage matrix protein-polysaccharides can be degraded by blood contained in the synovial cavity (Guicciardi and Little, 1967), an observation which may be relevant to the occasional cases of rheumatoid arthritis in which haemarthrosis is recognised at necropsy but which cannot explain the constant marginal destruction of cartilage by pannus. Plasmin and plasmin activators

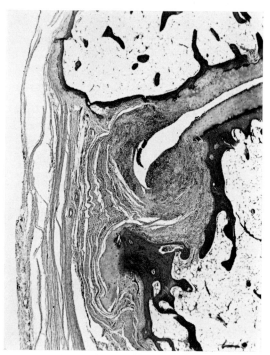

Fig. 2.24 The changes illustrated in the previous Figures culminate in the marginal process shown in this illustration. In continuity with the fibrovascular subsynovial connective tissue, abundant cellular granulation tissue extends into and replaces articular cartilage and nearby bone. The bone, osteoporotic and rarefied, is radioopaque, the granulation tissue radiotranslucent. Consequently, radiological study reveals marginal vacuities that are termed erosions in clinical usage.   (× 14)

have been invoked in the same way as causes of cartilage injury (Lack, 1959) and fibrinolytic systems have been tested as possible causes of experimental arthritis (Lack, 1969). Cartilage and bone fragments may break away from the articular surface, possibly as a result of proteolytic enzyme activity. They are readily recognised at biopsy and may provoke multinucleated foreign-body giant cell formation (Muirden, 1970b). The loss of cartilage is not accompanied by recognisable necrosis and is presumably due to the local release of cell-associated enzymes. In support of this view, there is good biochemical, electron microscopic and cell cultural evidence that synovial cells and synovial fluid enzymes can digest rheumatoid cartilage effectively in culture. Proteolytic digestion, it is assumed, is succeeded by increased local collagen and ground substance synthesis by dividing fibroblasts. The new fibrous, granulation tissue is then, in turn, infiltrated by the cells of the inflammatory reaction in which it is inexorably involved. There has been a continual effort, during the past 15 years, to identify the enzyme systems which could cause the localised tissue loss.

Enzymic activities in rheumatoid synovitis (see p. 113)

The synovial fluid in rheumatoid arthritis contains numerous polymorphs and there is a high activity of lysosomal enzymes such as acid phosphatase, naphthylamidase* and β-glucuronidase,

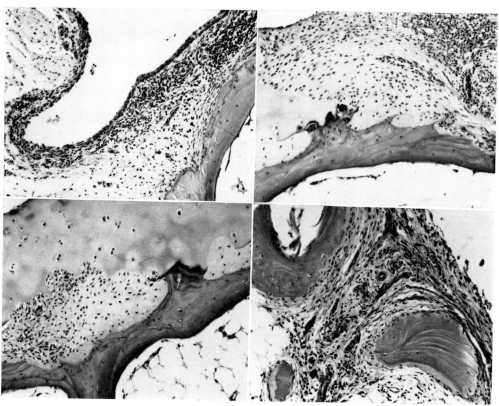

Fig. 2.25   Formation of rheumatoid pannus or granulation tissue represents extension of cellular inflammatory reaction in synovial tissue. (*Top left*) Lymphocytes, plasma cells and occasional polymorphs lie beneath synovial surface and extend to the margin of the cartilage, above bone, at margin of joint (*bottom right*). (*Top right*) A further field to show extension of synovial granulation tissue (*top right*), cartilage (*centre left*) and subjacent cortical bone (*bottom*). Note numerous small blood vessels in synovial tissue and the margin where cartilage and cellular marginal fibrous tissue adjoin. (*Bottom left*) A common feature of synovial granulation tissue formation is the extension of tissue beneath marginal articular cartilage as shown in this field. Two-dimensional sections give the impression of discrete islands of subarticular granulation tissue; it is probable that, in three dimensions, the granulation tissue represents a finger extending from nearby surface tissue. (*Bottom right*) The presence of vascular synovial granulation tissue within subarticular bone corresponds either to defects in the articular cartilage surface, as seen in this field, where cartilage (*top right*) has been lost or, as in the previous Figure, to an extension laterally from a nearby inflammatory zone.   (*Top left* ×125; *right* ×125; *bottom left* ×125; *right* ×125)

presumably derived from these cells (Jacox and Feldmahn, 1955). Ziff, Gribetz and LoSpalluto (1960) suggested that an endopeptidase obtained from the polymorph fraction of blood and rheumatoid synovial tissue could degrade cartilage, changing its physical properties. But if the

* See footnote on p. 115.

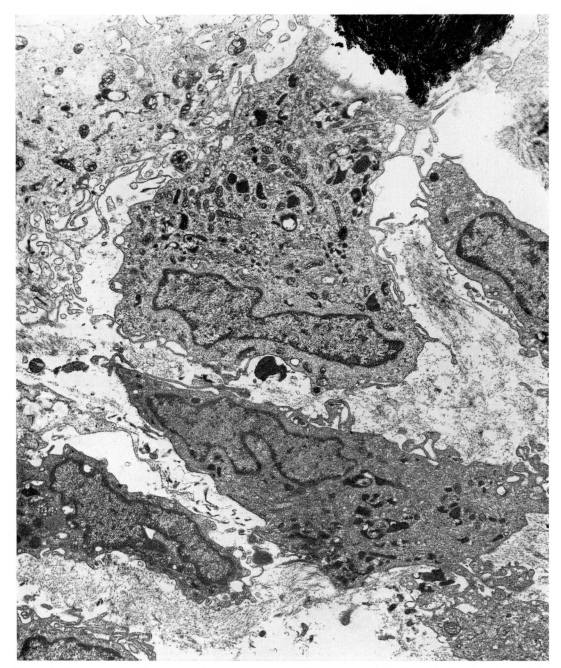

Fig. 2.26 Compare with Figure 2.10. Loose arrangement of surface synovial cells, with abundant intercellular matrix and fibrillary material, is characteristic. Note extracellular calcium hydroxyapatite crystalline aggregates (*top right*) a feature unlikely to be pathognomonic for rheumatoid arthritis in the synovia of which it is however a characteristic feature. Two of the cells seen in the present field display features recalling those of fibroblasts or smooth muscle cells; their presence is a constant reminder of the lack of absolutely distinctive features in both A(M) and B(F) synovial cells and of the many intermediary forms usually encountered in rheumatoid arthritis. (From a micrograph of Dr. A. J. Palfrey.)   ($\times$ 7,500)

activity of these acid hydrolases is held to account for cartilage injury *in vivo*, it would not be anticipated that cartilage destruction would be limited to the articular margin. Active synovial fluid enzymes would be expected to digest progressively the whole of the exposed intraarticular cartilaginous surface. The high activity of synovial fluid proteolytic enzymes which has been demonstrated therefore cannot readily account for the anatomical lesions observed, unless, of course, the articular margins are less susceptible to proteolytic digestion than the main, weight-bearing surfaces, a possibility suggested by the abundance of collagen in the latter situation, particularly in older persons. Any relevant enzyme activity restricted to the articular margins is likely therefore to be a property of the synovial or inflammatory cells that occupy the marginal synovial tissue. A further difficulty has been to identify hydrolytic and proteolytic enzymes active at the slightly alkaline pH characteristic of rheumatoid synovial fluid. Even if it is accepted that the redox potential of synovial cells is altered so that there is an intracellular accumulation of hydrogen ions (Chayen, Bitensky, Butcher and Poulter, 1969, Butcher and Chayen, 1971), it is difficult to see how activated synovial cell lysosomal enzymes can retain their activity extra-cellularly at suboptimum pH.

It is widely believed that extensive cartilage breakdown *in vivo* is likely to follow the destruction of the collagenous skeleton of the matrix. Evidence has now been obtained to show that rheumatoid synovial tissue is capable of producing collagenolytic enzyme(s) that can digest collagen *in vivo* at physiological pH. Cartilage extracts may contain significant levels of enzyme-like agents that depolymerise or degrade cartilage protein-polysaccharides (Fessel and Chrisman, 1964), thus altering the physical characteristics of the cartilage (Muir, 1971). Interest has, however, centred on the attempted demonstration of collagenases effective at physiological pH and not inactivated by body fluids or constituents.

Evanson, Jeffrey and Krane (1967) and Harris, DiBona and Krane (1969) reported the identification of collagenase(s) active at neutral pH and at 37°. They first showed that rheumatoid synovial tissue caused lysis of gels of reconstituted collagen fibrils in culture, the tissue releasing a soluble collagenase when cultured in a collagen-free medium. The collagenase was found to cleave collagen into $\frac{3}{4}$ and $\frac{1}{4}$ length fragments at 20° and 27°, while at 37° reconstituted collagen fibrils were degraded to low molecular weight polypeptides. Since this collagenase activity was not demonstrable at pH 5·0 and was not manifest by frozen-thawed preparations, Evanson and his colleagues believed that the enzyme activity was not of lysosomal origin. The further identification of 2 distinct collagenases in rheumatoid synovial fluid is discussed on p. 86 (Harris, Evanson, DiBona and Krane, 1970).

In comparable investigations Lazarus *et al.* (1968) investigated 24 rheumatoid arthritic patients and 8 patients with non-inflammatory synovial disease. Cells obtained from the two groups of patients were cultured and a collagenase recognised in the cells from the rheumatoid synovial tissue. The enzyme was shown to be effective at a physiological pH and to cleave the collagen molecule at a single site, a property shared with other vertebrate collagenases. The collagenolytic activity was found to correlate with the local and systemic disease activity in the rheumatoid arthritics from whom the synovial cells had been obtained. The collagenolytic activity of synovial fluid cells but not of 'R.A.' cells (p. 102) has been confirmed by Wegelius, Klockars and Vainio (1970).

The possibility that rheumatoid arthritis *begins* as an injury to hyaline articular cartilage has again been raised by Hamerman (1969). Articular cartilage is, however, avascular and aneural and not, by definition, susceptible to the classical microscopic phenomena of inflammation. 'Chondritis' is a misnomer. But, particularly under load (Maroudas and Muir, 1970), hyaline cartilage is relatively permeable to small molecules, including water; the products of cartilage cell or matrix injury, by whatever means they are produced, can in theory, therefore, reach the synovial and peri-articular tissues rapidly by the extracellular spaces and by synovial lymphatics. If these products of cell injury included molecules such as 5-hydroxytryptamine, kinin activators, nucleotides and lysosomal proteases capable of causing the phenomena of inflammation it might be possible for a primary cartilaginous insult to be followed by synovitis rather than *vice versa*. However, it seems much more probable that the synovia are first affected, then the vessels and finally the cartilage.

CHAPTER 3

Articular Tissues: Cell Culture

Tissue culture has been an accepted method for the study of synovial cells for more than 30 years (Vaubel, 1933; Stanfield, 1966) but, curiously, was not referred to by Willmer (1965). A huge literature on descriptive and evolutionary cytology (Willmer, 1970) attests to the growing understanding of mechanocytes in isolation, in cell and in maintenance (organ) culture by contrast with the cells of the developing (Gardner and O'Rahilly, 1968) and adult organism. The methods of tissue culture have been applied to the study of rheumatoid arthritis and have thrown light on the synthetic and secretory activities of the abnormal synovial cells, on their multiplication, on their metabolic characteristics and on their response to microbial infection (Castor, 1971; Palmer, 1970, 1971).

The morphological characteristics that distinguish rheumatoid synovial cells in culture from normal (Stanfield, 1966) have attracted particular attention. They have been the subject for considerable controversy. Multinucleated cells derived from synovial fluid fibroblasts and round cells were described by Lackington (1959): they were more frequent in rheumatoid than in normal cultures, an observation that was not confirmed, however, by Stanfield and Stephens (1963) in a survey of 75 rheumatoid and 113 non-rheumatoid synovia. Bartfield (1965) also drew attention to the presence of multinucleated giant cells, of bizarre nuclei, to wide variations in cell size and to coarse cytoplasm among his cultured rheumatoid synovial cells. Searching for an explanation of the features seen in his preparations, Bartfield (1965) failed to demonstrate rheumatoid factor (RhF) (p. 100) in or on cultured rheumatoid synovial cells but found that the cells proliferated earlier, formed multinucleate cells readily in the early and late stages of cultures (but not in the intermediate) and could not be maintained as long as normal synovial cells. Castor and Dorstewitz (1966) showed that the cells from rheumatoid synovia were more granular than normal and that there was more cell debris in the supernatant fluid. Multinucleated giant cells (p. 23) of the kind described by Lackington were present, as they were in cultured normal synovia, with nuclear budding and an increased number of nucleoli. Rheumatoid cells appeared to have an abbreviated life span and to take twice as long as normal synovial cells to generate. Palmer (1971), using resuspended synovial fluid cells, found epithelioid-like macrophages and polykaryocytes within 7 days of culture; but osteoarthrotic fluid cells gave a similar response and he was not able, therefore, to prove the observations of Lackington (1959) or of Castor and Dorstewitz (1966).

Castor (1957) confirmed the production of glycosaminoglycans (acid mucopolysaccharides) by synovial cells in culture, and Lever and Ford (1958) showed that there was simultaneous collagen synthesis (Castor, 1970). Although early observations (Hedberg and Moritz, 1959) suggested that the intrinsic viscosity of the hyaluronic acid synthesised in culture by rheumatoid cells was not changed by the addition of rheumatoid serum, it has been found more recently that sensitive techniques do show quantitative alterations in hyaluronate and collagen synthesis (Castor, 1971) and in the intrinsic viscosity of the material formed. The abnormal synovial cells are less responsive to the suppressive effect of hydrocortisone than is normal synovial tissue

(Castor and Dorstewitz, 1966), the relative unresponsiveness to added hydrocortisone being expressed in terms of altered cell proliferation, mean cell volume and glycosaminoglycan synthesis. Simultaneously, rheumatoid cells in culture synthesise a diminished amount of a component immunologically related to cartilage proteinpolysaccharide (Janis, Sandson, Smith and Hamerman, 1967). There is increased lysosomal hydrolase activity (Goldfischer, Smith and Hamerman, 1968) (p. 113), an increased uptake of glucosamine and an ability to deplete cartilage matrix in culture (Hamerman, Janis and Smith, 1967).

The significance of these various changes remains very largely uncertain. The increased secretory and synthetic activities probably contribute to the altered metabolic activities of rheumatoid synovia that are known to persist for some years (p. 41). (Table 3.1)

TABLE 3.1. *Metabolic comparison of normal and rheumatoid tissue*
(Mean ± standard error of mean)

	Normal tissue	Rheumatoid tissue		
		Villous	Fibrotic villous	Membrane
Q_{O2} (N)	trace	27·5 ±1·2	11·5 ±0·7	4·7 ±0·7
Glucose utilisation (μg/hr/mg)	46·8 ±3·6	292·0 ±24·0	174·0 ±22·0	95·0 ±16·0
Lactate production (μg/hr/mg)	14·4 ±1·3	88·0 ±16·6	47·0 ±3·8	10·8 ±5·1
Glycogen utilisation (μg glucose equiv/hr/mg nitrogen)	—	9·0 ±0·9	—	2·7 ±0·6

(From Dingle and Page Thomas, 1956)

The metabolic characteristics of synovia and cartilage cells are relevant to their behaviour in culture. It was clear that variations in the metabolism of synovial tissue might be important in the genesis of rheumatoid arthritis. Bywaters (1939) had demonstrated that specimens of horse synovial villi have a high rate of glycolysis relative to oxidative metabolism, a rate comparable to that displayed by other connective tissue cells such as fibroblasts and osteoblasts. A respiratory quotient of 0·71–0·72 was recorded. The metabolic activity of synovia was regarded as of the same order as that of other non-articular tissues. Bywaters concluded that the normal oxygen requirements of joint tissues could be met by synovial fluid alone, provided this fluid was in equilibrium with the blood; he also obtained evidence to show that synovial fluid 'mucin' concentration varied in proportion to the glycolytic activity of the synovial fringes.

By contrast with synovia, the oxygen uptake of articular cartilage was small but could immediately be increased to a measurable quantity by the addition of redox dyes. Although the presence of dehydrogenase and indophenol oxidase activities had been shown in synovial tissue, the former activity was low in articular cartilage, the latter not detectable. (Table 3.2)

As we have seen, synovial cells were early recognised to possess a capacity for secreting and thus, by inference, for synthesising 'mucins' (Vaubel, 1933; Castor, 1957). Systematic comparisons were therefore made between the metabolic characteristics of rheumatoid and of normal synovial tissue (Page Thomas and Dingle, 1955; Dingle and Page Thomas, 1956) and it was not long before some of the properties of normal and of rheumatoid synovia were defined (Page Thomas and Dingle, 1958). Page Thomas and Dingle (1955) distinguished anatomically between synovial villi and synovial 'membrane': the villi were shown to have a higher oxygen uptake, a higher rate of glucose utilisation and a higher lactate production. The subsequent results of these authors confirmed that normal synovial tissue has a low rate of oxidative metabolism although glucose utilisation and aerobic and anaerobic glycolysis are considerable. In rheumatoid arthritis, by contrast, oxidative metabolism and glycolysis increase, changes most obvious in tissues where proliferation is most active.

Dingle and Page Thomas (1956) made the important point to which subsequent authors constantly return, that much of the increased metabolic activity of synovial tissue in rheumatoid arthritis might be due, not to the changed synovial cells, but to the underlying leucocytic infiltration that is so characteristic. However, they were able to show that, in a single case, rheumatoid tissue devoid of lymphocytes displayed an oxygen uptake and a rate of aerobic glycolysis similar to those of tissues with the more usual white cell infiltration.

TABLE 3.2. *Metabolic characteristics of synovial tissue*

	Normal	'Villous' rheumatoid
1. O_2 uptake (μl/hr/mg/dry wt.)	trace	2
2. Glucose used in O_2 (μg/hr/mg dry wt.)	4·3	27·1
3. Glucose used in N (μg/hr/mg dry wt.)	7·2	44·7
4. Lactic acid prod. in O_2 (μg/hr/mg dry wt.)	1·6	6
5. Lactic acid prod. in N (μg/hr/mg dry wt.)	2·8	7·7
6. % Pasteur effect $\left(\dfrac{5-4}{5} \times 100\right)$	43	22
7. Glucose used in O_2 (μg/hr/mg protein)	16·2	72
8. Glucose used in N (μg/hr/mg protein)	18	81
9. Lactic acid[+] prod. in O_2 (μg/hr/mg protein)	8·4	38·7
10. Lactic acid[+] prod. in N (μg/hr/mg protein)	13·5	48
11. % Pasteur effect	37	20

(From Schubert, M. and Hamerman, D. (1968), *A Primer on Connective Tissue Biochemistry*, p. 297. Philadelphia: Lea & Febiger)

Thus, the anaerobic metabolism of normal synovial tissue is at a low rate. When synovial tissue from a case of active rheumatoid arthritis is grown *in vitro*, by contrast, a high rate of anaerobic glycolysis and of lactate production (the Pasteur effect) is observed. The rates of anaerobic glycolysis are greatest in hyperplastic rheumatoid synovial *villi* (Page Thomas and Dingle, 1955), a situation in which Hamerman, Stephens and Barland (1961) have shown by histochemical techniques that lactate dehydrogenase and NADPH-diaphorase activities are high.

Evidence of altered hydrolytic enzyme activities in cultured rheumatoid synovial cells was obtained by Goldfischer, Smith and Hamerman* (1968); these enzymes are considered more fully on p. 113. They confirmed that rheumatoid cells displayed the enhanced and altered acid phosphatase, aryl sulphatase and glucosaminidase activities which had been detected previously and found that these properties, like the morphological changes described on p. 39, persisted for up to 4 months, through 7 subcultures.

It now appears therefore that some of the abnormal characteristics of rheumatoid synovial cells may persist through several generations of cells. This observation supports the concept that the new characteristics are due to genetic mutation(s) perhaps caused by virus genomes or to the persistence of viral material in a latent form in association with synovial cell nuclei. It seems less likely that they are provoked by transient environmental stimuli.

* It is interesting to record that Goldfischer and his colleagues used brief aldehyde fixation prior to their histochemical observations.

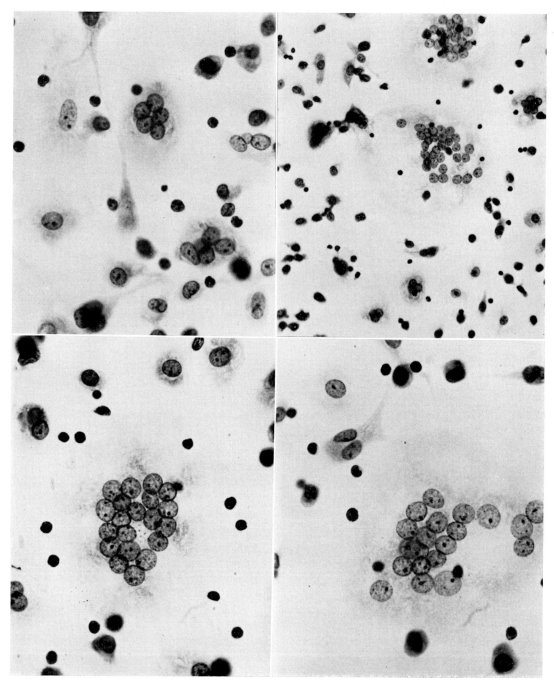

Fig. 3.1 Synovial cells in culture growing on a glass coverslip. (*Top left*) 4-day culture. A variegated cell population is seen. Macrophage-like cells are undergoing division and display polyploidy. The cytoplasmic processes of 2 fibroblast-type cells are seen. Lymphocytes, polymorphs and other unidentified cells are also present. (*Top right*) 10-day culture. Multinucleated cells are now more frequent. They predominate near the margins of the coverslip preparation. (*Bottom left*) Large multinucleate synovial cell seen at higher magnification. (*Bottom right*) A similar cell displaying well formed usually single nucleoli.   (From preparations of Dr. John McCormick)

(Giemsa: *top left* × 540; *top right* × 250; *bottom left* × 540; *bottom right* × 540)

Bartfield (1965) suspected the presence of a latent virus in rheumatoid synovia but, using acridine orange and ultraviolet microscopy, was unable to show the presence in his cultured cells of RNA or DNA inclusion bodies. Smith and Hamerman (1969) considered the apparently persistent differences, described above, that can be shown between rheumatoid and non-rheumatoid synovial cells in culture. They suggested the possibility that the observed differences may be due to viral survival and concluded, as had Bartfield, that the role of a slow virus in rheumatoid arthritis should be considered. The demonstration of resistance to superinfection could be held to provide support for this view. Some evidence of this nature has now been obtained. Rheumatoid synovial cells in culture can sometimes be shown to be resistant to infection with Newcastle disease virus (Ford and Oh, 1965). Resistance to infection by added rubella virus, however, is virtually complete (Grayzel and Beck, 1970) and is not due to an interferon-like mechanism (p. 194).

The intervention of a rheumatoid plasma factor, rather than the influence of a latent virus, would go some way to reconciling the differences, outlined above, in the morphological patterns of rheumatoid synovial cells in culture, as described by various authors. An entirely distinct application of the methods of cell culture was therefore devised by Fraser and Catt (1961). They employed trypsinised suspensions of human synovial cells to test for the presence of agent(s) in rheumatoid serum that would alter synovial cell behaviour. Using cell outgrowth, cell morphology and metabolic activity (assessed by changed pH) as guides, they demonstrated that rheumatoid but not control sera contained an agent, not destroyed by heat, that provoked morphological alterations in normal cultured synovial cells. The sera did not inhibit cell outgrowth but caused a fall in intracellular pH, shown by a colour change in an ingested dye.

The effects of added sera on synovial cell growth in cultures are, unfortunately, notoriously difficult to assess. Castor, Wright and Buckingham (1968) preferred therefore to base their conclusions on the measurement of hyaluronate synthesis which they showed was enhanced non-specifically by the addition of rheumatoid sera to their cultures. Using synovial cell 'fibroblasts', Castor et al. (1968) demonstrated that the rheumatoid sera depressed cell proliferation non-specifically, a finding at variance with that of Fraser and Catt (1961). Fraser and McCall (1966) had, however, modified their earlier views and now reported that the spreading of human synovial cells in culture was inhibited by rheumatoid sera to a greater degree than by normal sera, a finding that recalls the more recent observation of Palmer (1970) that heat-inactivation of rheumatoid serum added to cultures of synovial cells prepared by initial tryptic digestion, accelerated multinucleated cell formation (Fig. 3.1). The inhibitory component of the serum was heat-labile.

The methods of tissue culture of rheumatoid cells are referred to again in Chapters 11 and 17 (pp. 116 and 199).

CHAPTER 4

Articular Tissue: Electron Microscopy

A substantial number of studies have been published during the past ten years of the fine structure of synovial tissue in rheumatoid arthritis (Ghadially and Roy, 1967, 1969; Matsura, 1967; Davies and Palfrey, 1971). However, agreement on the details of the abnormalities revealed by this technique is less complete than is the case with the light microscopic investigation of this tissue. That this is so should not surprise anyone familiar with the pitfalls of electron microscopy. Six blocks of tissue taken from a single joint for paraffin sectioning could not be expected to show identical abnormalities by light microscopy (Cruickshank, 1952a). Certain areas may be severely affected, others normal. How much more then is it to be expected that electron microscopists will differ in their interpretation of random samples of patchily affected tissue in this variegated disease!* (Figs. 4.1–4.5)

When differences in technique are allowed for, and variations in fixation, it is perhaps surprising that any agreement is possible on the nature of the electron microscopic abnormalities recognisable in rheumatoid synovia. Critical information is often not available: for example, whether or not a tourniquet is used in preparing a joint for surgery during which blocks are to be taken, is often not stated in published papers.

Because there are very substantial descriptive differences in the literature on the electron microscopy of rheumatoid synovia, it is necessary to review the published data in some detail.

The two main forms of synovial cell identified by electron microscopy were designated A or M (macrophage-like in structure) and B or F (fibroblast-like in structure) by Barland, Novikoff and Hamerman (1964) and by Hirohata et al. (1963a, b) respectively. It is uncertain whether these cell types are absolutely distinctive or whether, as Davies and Palfrey (1971) suggest, a single cell type reveals misleadingly different appearances when cut in different planes: the A(M) and B(F) cells, they propose, may lie at opposite ends of a spectrum of continuous morphological variation. (Fig. 4.1)

Early studies of rheumatoid synovia were contained in the reports of Hirohata et al. (1963a, b), of Hirohata and Kobayashi, 1964, and of Barland et al. (1964). No single light microscopic feature of the rheumatoid synovium was diagnostic. The last group of authors drew attention to conspicuous differences between the A(M) cells of rheumatoid and of normal synovia. Thus, the rheumatoid cells often contain varying numbers of large, moderately dense vacuoles adjacent to a small Golgi apparatus. The A(M) cell lysosomes are larger and more numerous than normal

---

* An average block of tissue for light microscopy provides, say, 1 cm³ of material for study (ca. 5% of the total synovia of a diseased knee): if 10–10 μm sections each 1 cm² are surveyed in detail, 1% of this block will have been seen, or approximately 0·05% of the total synovial tissue of the diseased joint. The electron microscopist, however, investigating 5 large blocks each of say, 1 mm³ volume (ca. 5 × 0·005% of the total synovia), selects by this means 0·025% of the joint synovia for investigation. Given 20 sections each of 50 nm thickness for survey, his conclusions may be based on an analysis of no more than 0·002% of 0·005% of the total synovial tissue of the affected joint, i.e. 1×10^{-5}%. His chances of finding a specific abnormality, other things being equal, are approximately 50,000 times smaller than the light microscopist, his margin for error of interpretation, other factors being equal, 50,000 times greater.

It is, of course, now customary to select sections for electron microscopy on the basis of a preliminary survey of 0·5 or 1·0 μm sections of material embedded in a polymer suitable for ultramicrotomy. By this means the problems of selection are reduced.

(Fig. 4.2) and are readily identified by their high acid phosphatase activity. Complex granular cytoplasmic structures, termed residual bodies, show a variable content of electron-opaque material and measure 0·4–3·2 μm in diameter. The inclusions are probably of cytoplasmic origin and the dense bodies, which vary in frequency in different specimens, commonly lie in the perinuclear region. The B(F) cells, in these early studies, were not found to differ from normal.

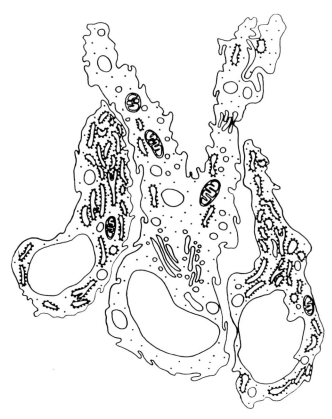

Fig. 4.1 A schematic drawing of type A(M) and type B(F) rheumatoid cells. In centre, a single A(M) cell extends processes towards the free synovial surface; there is an ovoid, basal nucleus, prominent Golgi apparatus (*centre*) one or two mitochondria and some cytoplasmic vacuoles. Endoplasmic reticulum is sparse, surface villous processes common. At either margin lies a type B(F) cell, rather smaller, with abundant endoplasmic reticulum, few cytoplasmic vacuoles and inconspicuous villous cytoplasmic processes (redrawn from Barland, Novikoff and Hamerman, 1962, *J. Cell Biol.*, **14**, 207–220).

Colloidal gold has been used as an electron-dense marker of the phagocytic properties of synovial cells (Norton and Ziff, 1964, 1966). Gold was injected into 30 synovial joints before surgery; electron microscopy was employed subsequently on material obtained at operation, to identify macrophages. The thickened synovia was found to have increased numbers of synovial cells resembling those of the normal joint. Both A(M) and B(F) cells were increased in number, but the increase of the former was generally greater. However, not surprisingly, different cells predominated in different areas. The older observation was confirmed, that lymphocytes and plasma cells were confined to the deeper (subsynovial) zones. The lack of a superficial, surface infiltrate and the absence of damage to surface cells suggested that the synovial cells themselves were not the 'target organ' in rheumatoid arthritis.

Rheumatoid A(M) cells contain many lysosomes and sporadic ferritin granules (Hirohata and Kobayashi, 1964). There is increased fibrillary material in the endothelial cells of synovial capillaries. The report of these authors was based on a survey of 41 joints and 3 tendon sheaths from 30 cases of rheumatoid arthritis, 16 in stage III and 9 in stage II; they drew attention to the wide range in cell morphology which can be seen within a small distance in the synovia. Hirohata and Kobayashi however stressed that changes were particularly common in the 10 μm of synovia

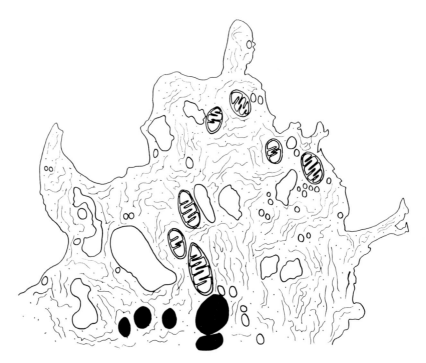

Fig. 4.2   An outline drawing of part of a typical type A(M) synovial cell in rheumatoid arthritis. At the lower margin are several dense electron-opaque bodies, probably of lysosomal origin. A number of cytoplasmic vacuoles are present and villous processes extend from the cell margin into the joint cavity. Endoplasmic reticulum is sparse. (From an electron micrograph supplied by Dr. A. J. Palfrey.)

immediately beneath the surface. Discussing the origin of fibrinoid, they explained that 'inflammatory changes in the superficial layers of the rheumatoid synovium were the result of a "degeneration" of collagen in the intercellular spaces'. They invoked this hypothetical process to account for what they termed 'secondary fibrinoid' in intercellular zones. The main role in secondary fibrinoid formation was played by changes in the intercellular substance; there was an increase in the height of synovial capillary endothelium, an observation that Ghadially and Roy (1967) could not confirm and which Brånemark, Ekholm and Goldie (1969) attributed, *inter alia*, to faulty technique and consequent artefact. Hirohata and Kobayashi (1964) recognised in addition, a primary synovial 'fibrinoid', drew attention to the mast cells in rheumatoid synovia (p. 21) where they were believed to be more numerous than normal, and described a synovial giant cell with 5–6 nuclei, an observation which confirmed Collin's (1949) description and anticipated the paper of Grimley and Sokoloff (1966).

Grimley and Sokoloff (1966) investigated 32 cases of rheumatoid arthritis, 25 normal synovia and 15 controls. In the synovia of 9 of 19 sero-positive cases but in none of 9 sero-negative, Grimley and Sokoloff found giant, ovoid, multinucleated cells approximately 40 μ in diameter, having up to 12 peripherally situated nuclei each of which resembled the nucleus of a mononuclear lining cell. They also showed, incidentally that some synovial cells were bound together by desmosomes. The presence of giant cells could not be explained by an association with intraarticular therapeutic injections. The giant cells lay deep to the surface and, by electron microscopy, were found to resemble the A(M) cells.

Like the majority of workers, Grimley and Sokoloff identified cytoplasmic granules in synovial cells: the granules were membrane-bounded, heterogeneous and apparently comprised lysosomal derivatives. There were no recognisable microorganisms. The surface cells displayed very high acid phosphatase activity, assessed subjectively. In capillary endothelial cells, rod-shaped bodies were present as Highton, Caughey and Rayns (1966) stated, but Grimley and Sokoloff believed that rod-shaped bodies were abundant in these endothelial cells in normal as well as in abnormal synovia, a view endorsed by Brånemark, Ekholm and Goldie (1969) in a study of 16 similar cases, mostly of longstanding origin, and by Ghadially and Roy (1969). The relationship of these observations to the progressive damage and obliteration of small blood vessels described by Bierther and Wegner (1971) is not clear.

Norton and Ziff (1966) made a full report of the synovial appearances in 19 definite cases of rheumatoid arthritis and in 3 of Still's disease. The former groups were all sero-positive and 3 were under treatment with corticosteroids. The cases of Still's disease were sero-negative and on corticosteroid therapy. Three of the 22 cases had been given intraarticular injections of gold before surgery. In adult rheumatoid arthritis, dense membrane-bound structures, probably lysosomes, were frequent in A(M) cells and these cells resembled macrophages. Both A(M) and B(F) cells contained much microfibrillar material. In different areas hyperplasia of one type or other tended to predominate. At the surface and in the underlying connective tissue, dense fibrin-like material was present; it rarely lay intravascularly. Polymorphs were rare and mononuclear cells very rare. Capillaries lay further from the synovial surface than normal and were fewer than normal. No infective agents were identified and no distinction between the synovial cells in adult and in juvenile rheumatoid arthritis was possible. In both, basement membranes became laminated in the deeper synovial tissues; in both mast cells were seen.

In a more limited survey of 6 cases of rheumatoid arthritis, the clinical details of which were not given, Ghadially and Roy (1967) spoke, by contrast with all other authors except Wyllie, Haust and More (1966), of a 'marked' increase in the type B(F) cells which showed increased endoplasmic reticulum material. Increased numbers of lysosomes and 'cytolysomes' were present. The description of 'many mitochondrial abnormalities' perhaps cast some doubt on the authors' techniques of preparation of the tissues. Ghadially and Roy emphasised the increased amount of microfibrillary material in synovial cells and in vascular endothelium, a change which tended to replace normal cell organelles (could this be amyloid?). Lipid droplets were more common in abnormal than in normal synovia and 'fibrinoid material', illustrated as an electron-dense, laminated material, was seen both on the joint surface in areas where the light microscopist commonly encounters fibrin, and in the intercellular matrix. No intraendothelial cell bodies (Highton, Caughey and Rayns, 1966) were identified.

The A(M) cells may correspond to macrophages in phagocytic potential and cytological organisation (Grimley, 1967). This author agrees with other investigators that Highton's intracellular bodies are not specific microbes but suggests that these bodies, common in endothelial cells, may play a part in blood coagulation. Grimley represents contemporary opinion when he

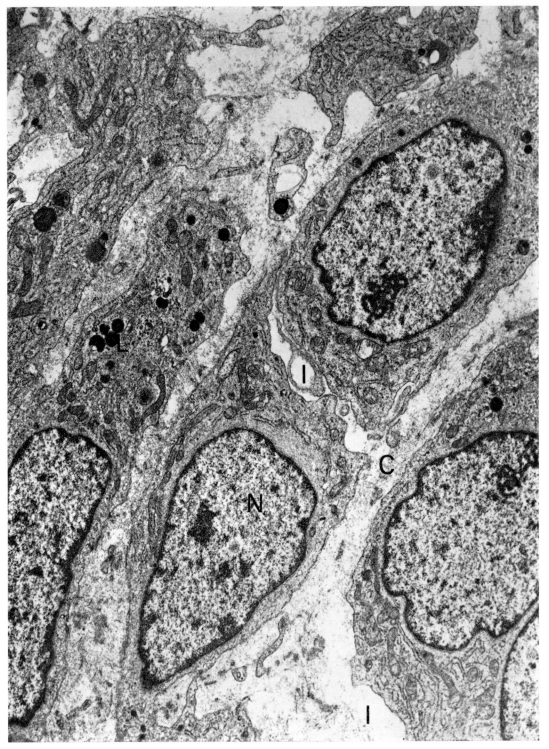

Fig. 4.3 Synovial surface cells. Abundant endoplasmic reticulum is present within the two central cells. Adjacent cells are separated by loose intercellular collagen bundles and electron-lucent proteoglycan matrix. In other cells (*left*) lysosomes are numerous. Mitochondria are abnormally frequent. The A(M) and B(F) surface cells and the many intermediary, indeterminate forms, are increased in size and number. Nuclei are prominent but mitotic figures are rarely seen. Lead citrate—uranium nitrate (From Davies, D. V. and Palfrey, A. J. *Modern Trends in Rheumatology* **2**, ed. Hill, A. G. S., London: Butterworths, 1971, pp. 1–20.)

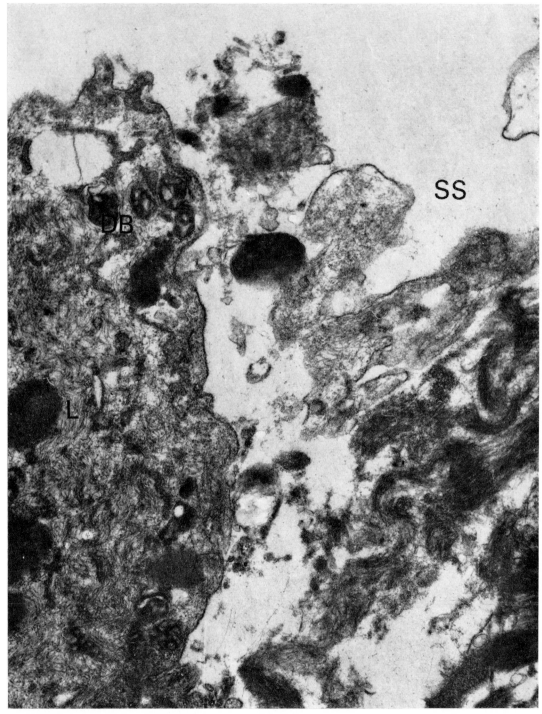

Fig. 4.4 Part of the surface of a synovial cell showing loose, almost fragmented structure of synovia seen at high magnification. Note intra- and extra-cellular fibrillary material, electron-lucent matrix, probably including much proteoglycan, and prominent, electron-dense bundles of fibrils with a recognisable periodic structure. (From a micrograph of Dr. A. J. Palfrey.) (× 30,000)

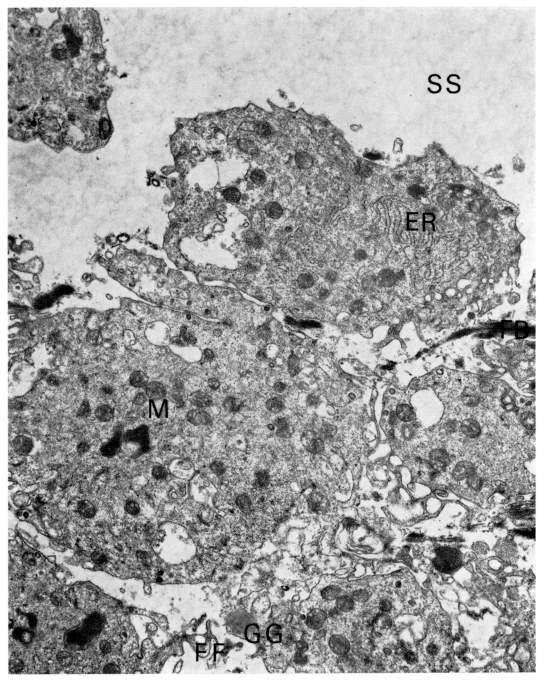

Fig. 4.5 Synovial surface cells for comparison with Figure 4.4. Filopodia are less numerous, cytoplasmic vacuoles and mitochondria very numerous. Occasional dense bodies may be seen: some are lysosomes. There is much apparent space between adjacent cells and the compact lamina densa occasionally seen in normal synovia are not evident. (From a micrograph of Dr. A. J. Palfrey.)   (× 12,000)

states that synovial tissue is relatively unspecialised and that synovial joints are not true serous structures, placing his emphasis on the absence of a basal lamina and the absence of complex intercellular attachments. This view accords with those who suggest an analogy between synovial tumours and mesothelioma of the pleura, and who raise the question of the possibility of inducing synovial sarcomata by the intraarticular injection of carcinogenic materials. Grimley (1967) accepts Norton and Ziff's (1966) view that the gaps between synovial cells recognised with the electron microscope are functionally significant. However, he cannot understand why the B(F) secretory and synthetic fibroblast-like cells of the synovia assimilate neutral lipid in rheumatoid arthritis and postulates that it might 'signify profound metabolic disturbances remotely analogous with the events in scurvy'. This view is not yet supported by any direct evidence.

The principal findings of Ghadially and Roy (1969), which were not always in precise confirmation of their early studies (1967), suggested an increased number of closely-packed A(M) cells from which they thought the Collins–Grimley–Sokoloff giant cells were derived, a view with which I agree. They quoted the well-marked increase in intermediate and B(F) cells described by Wyllie, Haust and More (1966) but did not reiterate their own views on the response of this cell type. Ghadially and Roy (1969) also analysed in detail the individual electron microscopic changes found in the membranous, cytoplasmic, nuclear and particulate structures in rheumatoid lining cells. Prominent filopodia and many micropinocytotic vesicles, increased endoplasmic reticulum, almost always with dilated cisternae, few or small Golgi complexes and swollen, altered mitochondria were described and lipid droplets similar to those seen in the normal cell were common. One of 'the most remarkable features' detected by Ghadially and Roy was the presence of abundant fine filamentous-material in synovial cells and in capillary endothelial cells, a feature also remarked by earlier writers. Lysosomes of very varied morphology were extremely numerous; there were many containing ingested endogenous organelle or membraneous remnants (cytolysomes) or exogenous material, sometimes fibrin (phagolysomes). The intercellular matrix between synovial cells was found to contain electron-dense material but, unlike other authors (Wyllie, Haust and More, 1966), Ghadially and Roy (1969) failed to identify in this material fibres with the 23 nm periodicity believed to be characteristic of fibrin.

The difficulties inherent in the use of electronmicroscopy to interpret abnormal synovial cell function are underlined by Ghadially and Roy's (1969) review. It is not sufficient to consider electron micrographs in isolation: the analyses must be linked to some form of measurable chemical, physiological or physical response.

A number of surveys of the fine structure of the synovial tissue regenerating after synovectomy have begun to be reported (Wassilev, 1971). The newly-formed cells appear higher than normal, and have rounded nuclei. The A(M) and B(F) cells reform and closely resemble those of the normal synovium, differing only in cytological details that suggest raised synthetic and phagocytic activities.

Electron microscopy in relation to synovial cell function

Although valuable information concerning the abnormal functions of the synovial cells in rheumatoid arthritis has come from the application of electron microscopy, these investigations have done little to show whether the synovial cell changes are primary, whether they are the result of cell injury by exogenous agents such as slow viruses, bacterial L forms, mycoplasmataceae or diphtheroids or whether they are the indirect result of disturbances initiated by such outside agencies but leading to the cytotoxic consequences of one or more immunological reactions.

The literature on the fine structure of normal synovia contains much evidence of the phagocytic capacity of A(M) cells. The ability of abnormal synovial A(M) cells to phagocytose foreign material has been confirmed by Muirden (1966). Muirden found ferritin scattered widely through the cytoplasm of A(M) cells but also within complex cytoplasmic granules and in lysosomes. (The presence of ferritin in lysosomes is, of course, an accepted feature of normal cells.) Muirden questions whether rheumatoid synovial ferritin comes from within the joint or from the blood (see Chapter 12; p. 157). A similar distribution in rabbit synovial tissue had been shown after the intraarticular injection of iron dextran and the capacity of normal synovial cells to synthesise apoferritin had been surmised. However, the quantity of iron in the rheumatoid joint attracted renewed attention and Muirden and Senator (1968) therefore made a systematic study of 27 joints from 23 patients with 'classical' or 'definite' disease. Prussian blue-positive material was present histologically in all save one. Haemosiderosis was seen in the sections in 15 of the 27 joints, and iron was present in the characteristic giant cells (Grimley and Sokoloff, 1966). Muirden and Senator concluded that synovial iron may come from a 'continued oozing of blood into the synovial cavity' and postulated that sequestration of a significant amount of iron in this way may be one causative factor in the origin of the curious hypochromic, normocytic anaemia of rheumatoid arthritis (p. 156). They placed their observations on a quantitative basis (Senator and Muirden, 1968), showing that the mean concentration of iron in 24 rheumatoid joints was 347 µg iron/g dry tissue compared to a normal of 15·2 µg/g, figures which were rather more striking than those of Mowat and Hothersall (1968) who found, by a different analytical technique which measured non-haemoglobin iron, 17·2 mg iron/100 g synovial tissue in rheumatoid arthritis compared wiith 2·8 mg iron/100 g in normal synovia. Muirden and his colleagues extended their analyses by the use of radioactive iron. More recently, Shannon and Graham (1971) adopted the intraarticular injection of peroxidases as a means of defining protein uptake by rabbit synovial cells. A(M) cells took up much protein by bulk incorporation and by pinocytosis; B(F) cells phagocytosed smaller amounts by pinocytosis. It is reasonable to assume similar mechanisms in human synovial cells. The increased bulk incorporation of protein with increasing molecular weight may influence both the synovial cell content of immunoglobulins and the composition of synovial fluid in rheumatoid arthritis.

Ishikawa (1967) demonstrated the presence of electron-opaque deposits, approximately 50 nm thick, on the surface of the plasma membranes of A(M) cells, a deposit analogous with those shown by Alcian blue staining techniques in light microscopy. In rheumatoid arthritis, he confirmed in A(M) cells that cytoplasmic vacuoles were numerous and small, and that $3 - 7$ µm electron-dense granules were common; in B(F) cells rough endoplasmic reticulum was increased in amount.

Perhaps the most provocative results obtained by the electron microscopic study of the pathological physiology of the synovia in rheumatoid arthritis have come from investigators who have attempted to link knowledge of cell injury, of phagocytosis and of immunoglobulin production with the structural changes suggested by electron micrographs. Zucker-Franklin (1966), for example, drew attention to existing knowledge of the toxic granules of polymorphs, to the inclusions described in the polymorphs of rheumatoid synovial fluid (p. 102) (Hollander *et al.*, 1965) and to the evidence that disruption of intracellular granules which contained γ-globulin might release rheumatoid factor (p. 100) (Rawson, Abelson and Hollander, 1965). Zucker–Franklin recalled that similar granules could be produced *in vitro* by incubating normal polymorphs with rheumatoid factor complexed with γ-globulin (Parker and Schmid, 1962) and proceeded to a survey of synovial fluid, thoracic duct and buffy coat white cells in 5 cases of classical rheumatoid arthritis. She concluded that the polymorphs of rheumatoid arthritis were replete with phagocytic vacuoles containing various elements, the larger of which corresponded to the inclusions seen by light microscopy (p. 102); some also contained organelles phagocytosed apparently from disintegrated leucocytes.

Synovial fluid and inflammatory cell phagosomes contained fibrin-like material, with amorphous protein and 'grey-globular' structures. The fibrin-like material constituted only a small fraction of the phagocytosed material and was unlikely to account for the chronicity of the disease as suggested by Riddle, Bluhm and Barnhart (1965) and, later, by Glynn (1968). The grey-globular structures were probably not RhF complexed with IgG since 20–30 times as many cells contained these structures as reacted with anti-γ-globulin in immunofluorescent tests. Further, the grey-globular bodies were present in normal synovial fluid and might, indeed, be hyaluronate-protein. Electron microscopy revealed no structures corresponding in frequency to the rheumatoid cell inclusions (p. 102) and the latter, Zucker-Franklin suggests, may therefore be large enough to be detectable by phase contrast microscopy but indistinguishable from other phagocytic vacuoles by electron microscopy.

Zucker-Franklin speculated, as had Hollander and his colleagues (1965), that the presence of so much phagocytosed material in rheumatoid synovia might lead to the release of lysosomal enzymes into the joint fluid, with secondary digestion of joint surfaces (p. 113). Zvaifler (1965) had followed a similar line of thought in his review and had suggested a sequence of injury in which (1) altered γ-globulin complexed with rheumatoid factor to (2) form an inclusion body that (3) was phagocytosed by synovial white cells, (4) releasing or activating hydrolytic enzymes which (5) damaged joint structures either directly, or (6) by activating kinins. In this thesis, Zvaifler believed that a specific initiating event was not necessary and suggested that any episode causing joint inflammation could lead to a self-perpetuating sequence. Ferritin incorporation, as revealed by Muirden, Zvaifler saw as only one step in a vicious circle of injury.

The changes in the fine structure of the main articulating surfaces in rheumatoid arthritis have recently been studied by Mitchell and Shepard (1970). Similar studies of joint surfaces in experimental arthritis are in process in my own laboratory. Comparing 20 rheumatoid with 10 control cartilages, and selecting areas devoid of macroscopic pannus, these authors recognised that cells resembling those of the synovium were growing across the articular surface and, in 6 cases, were penetrating the superficial cartilage layers. The deeper cartilage cells, they showed, were surrounded by 'moats' containing fibrillar material. There was recognisable cytoplasmic fat. Elongated chondrocyte cell processes were seen and cell death and degeneration were common.

It is not easy to interpret these unconfirmed electron microscopic studies. Generally, the integrity of wide areas of articular cartilage in rheumatoid arthritis (in the absence of incidental degenerative joint disease) is a conspicuous feature of surface structure and this is confirmed by conventional microscopy. If Mitchell and Shephard (1970) imply that submicroscopic injury to surface cartilage is relatively common (and they do not make this specific statement) then the argument (p. 35) that synovial fluid enzymic activity is irrelevant to rheumatoid cartilage injury loses much of its force. A reappraisal of the role of synovial fluid lysosomal activity and a reassessment of views on the pathogenesis of rheumatoid pannus formation would become necessary. However, I cannot yet accept this view. Mitchell and Shephard's (1970) evidence is incomplete, their electron microscopic interpretations difficult to understand and their experiments not yet confirmed.

CHAPTER 5

Articular Surfaces

(*a*) *Cartilage*. Until 1968, the nature of the surface of articular cartilage had attracted little attention. It was widely accepted that the surface was 'strikingly smooth' (Davies, 1969), a view which reiterated William Hunter's (1742–43) dogma and which had apparently only been questioned by Hammar (1894), by Weichselbaum (1877) and by Meyer (1931). The introduction of the scanning electron microscope led to a revolution in thought (McCall, 1968; Walker, 1969; Walker, Dowson, Longfield and Wright, 1968; Fujita, Kodama and Inoue, 1968; Gardner and Woodward, 1968, 1969; Longfield *et al.*, 1969; Walker *et al.*, 1969; Clarke, 1971*a, b*; Fujita, Tokunaga and Inoue, 1971) and a rejection of Hunter's (1742–43) views. Articular surfaces and their primary contours were shown to be covered first, by a series of secondary irregularities of the order of 0·4–0·5 mm in diameter, superimposed on which were large numbers of smaller tertiary undulations, approximately 20–30 μm in diameter. Comparable irregularities and undulations were detected in all mammalian and the single avian species examined. It became clear that articular cartilaginous surfaces were in no sense 'smooth'!*

The studies made with the scanning electron microscope are necessarily based on samples of excised human or animal cartilage that have been fixed in formaldehyde or glutaraldehyde, dried in air, coated with a thin layer of gold–palladium alloy or some similar protective and electrically conductive material, and that have been examined under high vacuum (Dowson, Wright and Longfield, 1969; Longfield, Dowson, Walker and Wright, 1969). Rapid freezing followed immediately by freeze-drying and coating *in situ* can be expected to diminish artefactual surface changes. A failure to retain proteoglycans could also be presumed, a difficulty that can perhaps be avoided by fixation with ruthenium (Highton and Donaldson, 1970) (p. 210). Considerable surface damage due to the electron beam can be anticipated however, whatever the preparative technique. Under these circumstances, it is not surprising that the criticism has been made that the surface irregularities and undulations detected with the scanning electron microscope, may be artefactual. It is almost impossible to believe that the irregularities had not been observed by transmission light or electron microscopy or by reflected light microscopy at an earlier date.

To meet these points, to overcome difficulties of orientation and preservation, and at the same time to amplify and confirm the information gained by scanning electron microscopy, a number of additional techniques have been adopted.

In the first place, two-stage collodion replicas of cartilage surfaces were prepared and viewed in the transmission electron microscope (Gardner and Woodward, 1969). The replicas revealed considerable surface detail but this detail proved difficult to correlate with that recognised in high resolution scanning electron micrographs. The replicas did, however, provide limited evidence that inflammatory diseases such as experimental hypersensitivity arthritis in guinea pigs, facilitated subsequent digestion by commercial preparations of hyaluronidase that were assumed to contain protease activity.

---

* Most authors use the term smooth to mean even, uniform and *not roughened in any way* (Chambers's Dictionary) (authors' italics); or (in accordance with the Concise Oxford Dictionary) to imply 'freedom from perceptible projections or lumps or indentations or roughness'.

In the second place, samples of articular cartilage excised, fixed, dried and coated as for scanning electron microscopy, were examined by incident light microscopy (Gardner and Woodward, 1969). The surface appearances closely resembled those seen at comparable magnifications ($\times$ 100–500) by scanning electron microscopy. To overcome the objection that fixation might distort surfaces, freshly excised material was also examined, intact or freeze-dried. The principal surface structures were unchanged and the presence of a system of secondary irregularities and tertiary undulations was confirmed.

Additional evidence for the presence of these surface structures was also obtained by placing very small samples of articular cartilage in the scanning electron microscope without preliminary drying, fixation or coating (Gardner, 1972). Measurement of the surface contours proved possible, furthermore, by reflected light interference microscopy in the rat; tertiary undulations appeared to be 1·2–2·6 μm in height.

Lastly, to answer the difficulty that excision of cartilage, with a consequent interruption to blood flow, might cause surface distortion, incident (reflected) light studies were made of the living articular cartilages of rabbits, guinea-pigs, rats, mice and turkeys. Foetal mice were similarly examined. Operating theatre surveys made also of the articulating surfaces of the knee joints of two male human patients aged 42 and 25. Internal, coaxial and external, oblique light sources were employed. The integrity of synovial blood flow in the anaesthetised animals was determined by direct observation of the marginal, synovial vasculature during the experiments. In all instances, series of minute 20–30 μm undulations were seen superimposed on coarser 0·5 mm irregularities. The latter were also noted on the living human joint surfaces.

These investigations appeared to establish unequivocally that normal adult, and adult and foetal animal articular cartilage surfaces are not smooth, that the lack of smoothness is a constant feature of the unloaded living surface, and that surface undulations are present on foetal surfaces before the joint can have been subjected to weight-bearing.

It seems probable that additional orders of irregularity will be revealed as images are surveyed at higher magnification.

In spite of the care with which these investigations were made, it is still necessary to reiterate that all forms of surface analysis must take account of the changes that occur when the living joint is opened, of the distortion that results from drying and of the alterations in surface structure that quickly follow the ending of blood flow. Preliminary studies show that 'ischaemic' alterations in cartilage surface appearance are identifiable within 14–17 minutes of the cessation of the circulation, very soon after blood flow through synovial vessels can no longer be recognised (Gardner and McGillivray, 1971a). Even in the living animal or patient, the exposed articular surface, opened with the utmost care, without touching or washing the articular cartilage or synovia, may, consequently, soon differ significantly from normal. The influence of surface-to-surface contact upon cartilage when normal loading takes place remains uncertain. Techniques are becoming available in which minute transducers incorporated into articular cartilage can be expected to give continuous traces of loading patterns during movements such as walking but there is, as yet, no possibility that these records can be gained from normal human joints. Naturally recordings from loaded articular cartilage in rheumatoid arthritis have not yet been made. Nevertheless, the opportunity exists for observing the exposed living cartilage in anaesthetised animals and, by means of a recently devised observation chamber (Gardner, 1972), it is anticipated that the reaction of these living surfaces to measured pressures will be recorded and photographed *in vivo* (Gardner, 1972).

The techniques described above are now being applied to the investigation of articular cartilaginous surfaces in rheumatoid arthritis (Gryfe, Woodward and Gardner, 1969; Inoue, Kodama and Fujita, 1969). It is natural to suppose that interest will concentrate on the zones in which cartilaginous and synovial boundaries merge, that is, the area in which synovial vascular branches and tributaries terminate and in which, in rheumatoid arthritis, the first evidence of rheumatoid

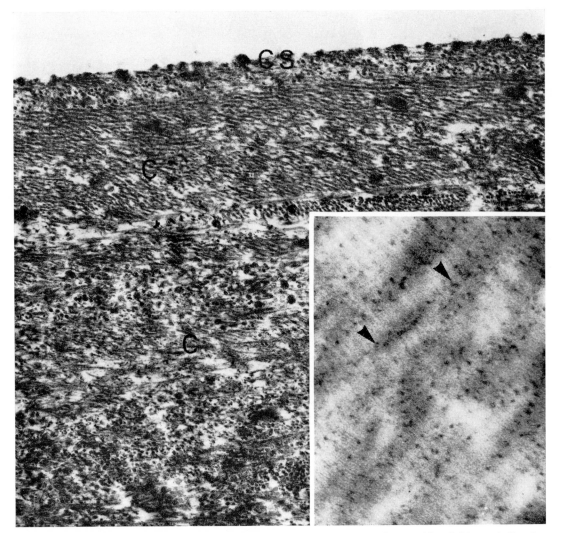

Fig. 5.1 The earliest degradative changes in articular cartilage structure in rheumatoid arthritis are believed to occur in the superficial, weight-bearing zones. Little is known of the nature of these early changes or of the origin of the enzymes believed to cause them. The Figure shows the characteristic broad laminae of coarse collagen bundles, arranged at varying angles to each other but parallel to the surface. (*Inset*) Ruthenium red, in the presence of osmic acid, fixes and stains glycosaminoglycans and can be used to elucidate the interfibrillar matrix proteoglycans. It may also delineate aggregates of polysaccharide-rich material arranged in register with the periodic cross-striations of cartilage collagen. The structures illustrated are believed to be destroyed at an early stage in rheumatoid arthritis.

(× 30,000; *inset* ×75,000)

Figures 5.1–5.10 are prepared from rat knee joint tissue

synovitis can be detected. The problems associated with the disturbed lubricating characteristics of the synovial fluid in rheumatoid arthritis are being examined in the same manner. An electrostatic mechanism has been considered as one explanation for the efficiency of synovial joint lubrication (Roberts, 1971). The role of surface proteoglycans (Radin, Swann and Weisser, 1970) and of fat (Freeman, Little and Swanson, 1970) in lubrication are being debated and it is clear that scanning electron-, transmission electron-, and incident light microscopy will be used to

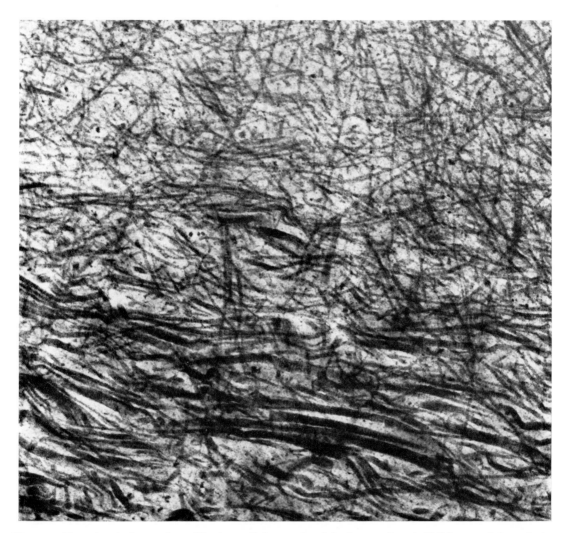

Fig. 5.2 Normal articular cartilage. The intercellular matrix of the intermediate (middle) zone of the articular cartilage from the femoral condyle of a 10 week male albino Wistar rat. The appearances simulate qualitatively those recognised in other mammals, including man. Note the finer beaded fibrils of the deeper cartilage (*top*), the thicker collagen fibrils of the more superficial cartilage (*bottom*). The structure of the articular surface comprises an interlacing meshwork of bundles of mature collagen fibrils: interfibrillar proteoglycans are sparse. Beneath the surface lamina, the beaded fibrils are arranged in a disorderly manner interspersed among an abundant matrix of protein polysaccharide and other, unidentified molecules. Degradation and loss of these structures in rheumatoid arthritis are attributed to enzyme action: there is no evidence of primary cartilage injury. (× 40,000)

examine the factors contributing to the abnormal lubrication in rheumatoid arthritis (Figs. 5.1– 5.10).

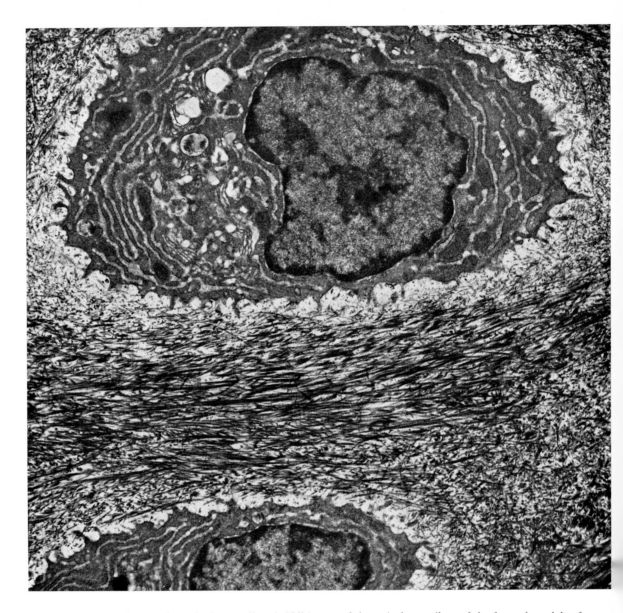

Fig. 5.3 Chondrocytes from the intermediate (middle) zone of the articular cartilage of the femoral condyle of a 10-week male Wistar rat. The appearances closely resemble qualitatively those encountered in the articular cartilage of other young mammals. Surrounding the cells which have ovoid, irregular nuclei and abundant endoplasmic reticulum, is a narrow rim of pericellular matrix containing relatively small numbers of fine, beaded fibrils. In this zone, Alcian blue-staining glycosaminoglycans are present in large amount; the van Gieson stain is negative. More prolific, coarser fibrils lie between the cells in the intercellular matrix. Here there is somewhat less metachromatic glycosaminoglycan than in the pericellular regions. Disorder and loss of the components shown in this Figure, in rheumatoid arthritis, are thought to be secondary to the enzymatic degradation of surface material.   (× 12,500)

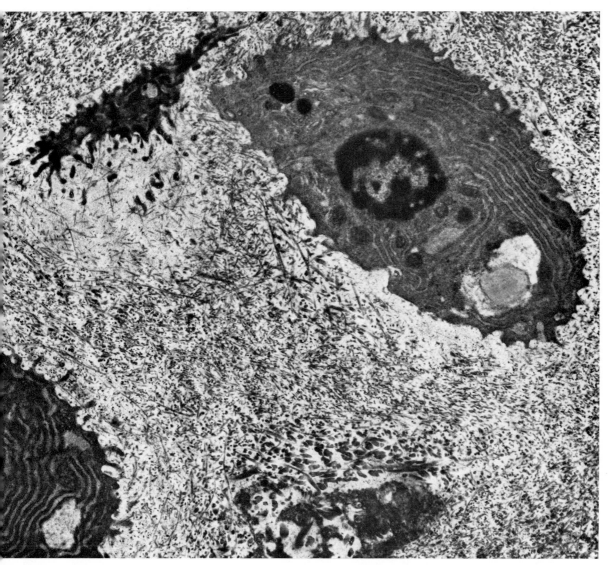

Fig. 5.4 Comparable view, at lower magnification, of lower intermediate zone of condylar cartilage. Two cells are cut near their centres, two peripherally. By comparison with the cells of the intermediate zone the deeper chondrocytes are smaller and more compact: they display intense alkaline phosphatase activity. In the rat, the chondrocytes of the superficial half of the articular cartilage show no such activity when examined in cryostat section. (× 13,500)

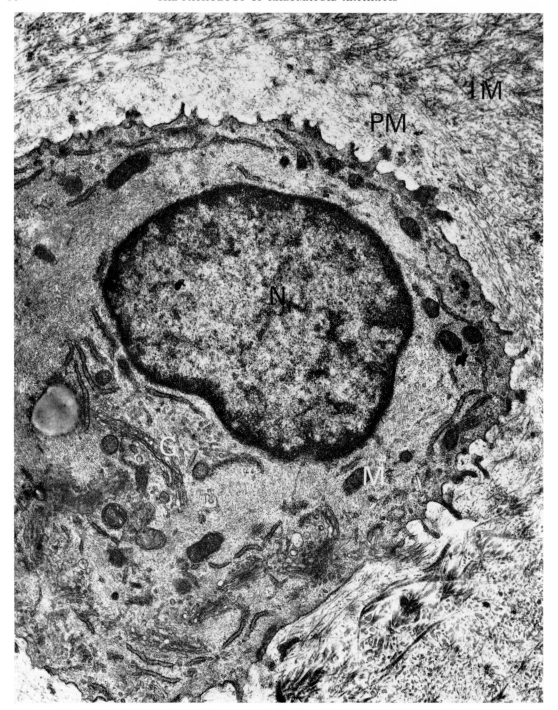

Fig. 5.5 Chondrocyte from the intermediate zone of the femoral condylar articular cartilage of a young male Wistar rat. The relative proportion of pericellular, and the abundant intercellular matrix are shown, together with the fine structural details of the cartilage cell. It is believed that these cells synthesise and secrete both the fibrillar and globular proteins of the matrix and the glycosaminoglycan moiety of proteoglycans. Mitotic activity is rarely seen but ^{3}H-thymidine incorporation can be detected by autoradiography.   ($\times$ 18,750)

(*b*) *Synovia*. Normal human and mammalian synovia have been examined in some detail by scanning electron microscopy (Fujita, Inoue and Kodama, 1968; Kodama, Takatori and Inoue, 1968; Woodward, Gryfe and Gardner, 1969.) The reports of Fujita, Inoue and Kodama (1968) and of Kodama, Takatori and Inoue (1968) are based on material washed with saline before formalin fixation, acetone dehydration, air-drying and gold coating. Those of Gardner and Woodward (1968, 1969), of Woodward, Gryfe and Gardner (1969), and of Gryfe, Woodward and

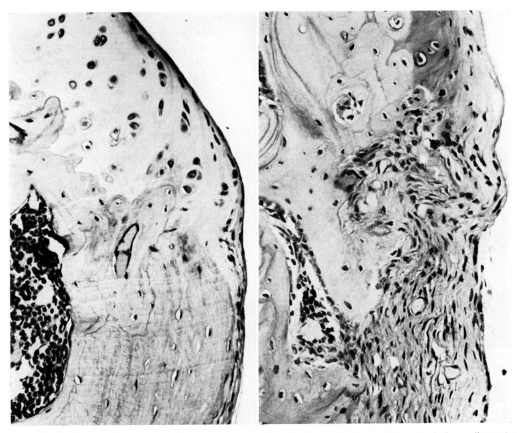

Fig. 5.6 (*Left*) Margin of normal rat femoral condyle. Note hyaline articular cartilage (*top*), bone (*bottom*) and intervening zone where reticular fibres merge with bone and periosteal margin appears to be in continuity with collagen lamina at cartilage surface. (*Right*) Identical site in rat 13 days after the induction of acute experimental turpentine arthritis (Gardner *et al.*, 1971, *Ann. rheum. Dis.*, **30**, 542–543). Vascular granulation tissue merges with and replaces calcified and non-calcified articular cartilage. There is a similar subperiosteal response, and remodelling of periarticular bone, with high osteoblastic activity, is evident. (*Left* ×300; *right* ×300)

Gardner (1969) were derived from material untouched after arthrotomy, plunged into cold buffered osmic acid, air-dried and gold/palladium coated. Even with this technique, there is considerable scope for the introduction of artefact and adequate studies of rapidly frozen, freeze-dried and coated material have not yet been reported.

With the incident (reflected) light microscope, the normal mammalian synovia of adipose type resembles the surface of a cluster of raspberries placed side-by-side (Woodward, Gryfe and Gardner, 1969). There are few species differences in intimate surface structure but wide differences in broad surface pattern. In the osmic acid fixed preparation, the clusters of secondary synovial processes, superimposed on the broad primary synovial folds or contours, are found to bear numerous smaller tertiary processes. The secondary processes are of the order of 40–50 μm in diameter, and are ususally hexagonal or pentagonal in outline. The tertiary processes, thought to be formed by the tips of individual protruding synovial cells, are no more than 3–5 μm in diameter.

Scanning electron microscopy confirms these general appearances and results gained with the two techniques are in mutual agreement. Adequate control of the investigation of synovial tissue by the simultaneous use of incident light microscopy is possible up to useful magnifications of × 400–500 but care is necessary in the interpretation of higher resolution images. Resolution and contrast in scanning electron microscopy tend to be mutually exclusive, partly negating the enormous advantages this technique offers in terms of depth of focus and in the very wide range of useful magnifications.

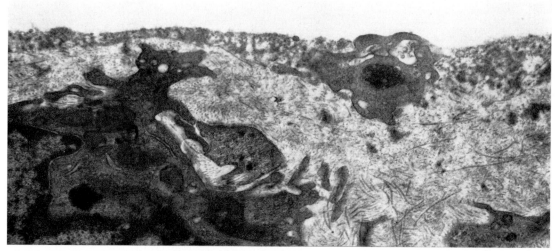

Fig. 5.7 Margin of femoral condylar articular cartilage of rat, 7 days after induction of acute turpentine arthritis. Cytoplasmic processes from polypoidal cells of marginal, vascular granulation tissue extend across and immediately beneath surface. These cells, probably fibroblasts, display a capacity for secreting collagen. They comprise the earliest cellular elements recognisable as a 'pannus' and are presumably similar to those encountered in the earliest stages of cartilage replacement in rheumatoid arthritis. Uranyl acetate—lead citrate.   (× 15,000)

In rheumatoid arthritis the first order synovial processes are large and complex and tend to be covered more or less completely by a fibrinous exudate in which red blood cells can be seen (Inoue, Kodama and Fujita, 1969; Woodward Gryfe and Gardner, 1969; Redler and Zimmy, 1970). The presence of these 'muddy' deposits lends a more homogeneous and smoother aspect to the second order projections and obscures those of the third. The appearances recognised in synovia which have regenerated after synovectomy and in which synovitis has recurred are similar (Inoue and Gardner, unpublished observations). No extensive systematic surveys of treated and untreated rheumatoid synovia have yet been published but it will prove of interest to attempt to correlate the pictures so obtained with those gained by arthroscopy (p. 208), at lower magnifications. Surface surveys of synovial margins of animals with experimental hypersensitivity—and with experimental turpentine-arthritis are in progress (Bakowska and Gardner, 1971; Soria-Herrera, Morley, Inoue and Gardner, 1971). In these disorders, as in active human rheumatoid arthritis, a conspicuous feature of the early inflammatory response has already proved to be the fibrin meshwork which clothes the cartilaginous surface, extending in continuity from the inflamed synovia. Red and white blood cells and platelets are trapped in the exudate rendering the cartilage surface difficult to observe (Soria-Herrera *et al.*, 1971). (Figs. 5.11–5.14)

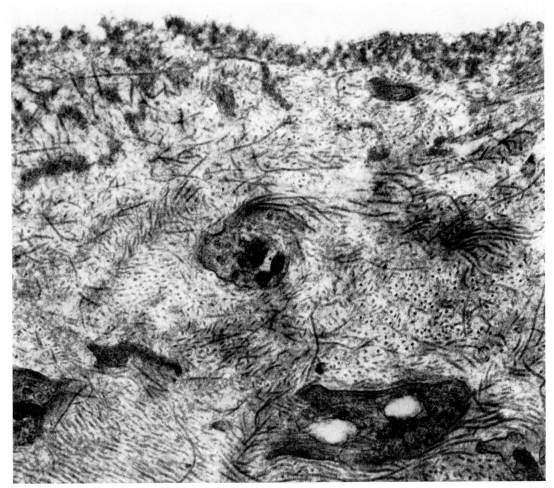

Fig. 5.8 Disorganised surface zone of marginal articular cartilage in rat femoral condyle, 7 days after induction of acute turpentine arthritis. Loss of orderly surface bundles of collagen (Fig. 5.1) is shown, with extension of cytoplasmic processes of fibroblast-like cells of pannus through surface zone. Note relatively orderly array of most superficial collagen. Uranyl acetate—lead citrate. (× 30,000)

Surface studies of the synovia and of articular cartilage in rheumatoid arthritis are in their infancy. In conjunction with techniques such as controlled enzymatic digestion of excised tissues it can be anticipated that much will be added to this existing knowledge within the next 2–3 years.

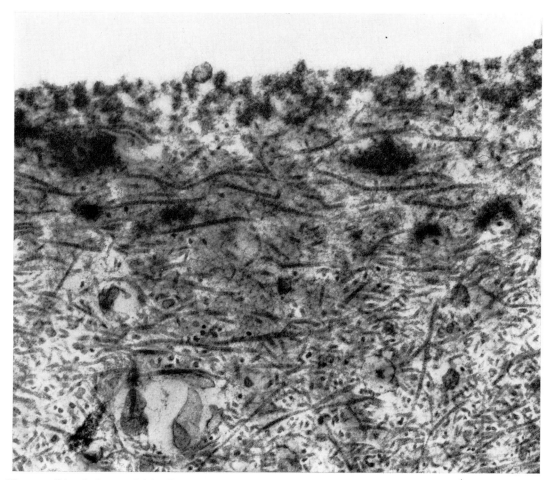

Fig. 5.9 Disorderly superficial collagenous lamina at margin of pannus on rat femoral condyle 7 days after onset of experimental turpentine arthritis. Observe that disorientated collagen displays normal periodicity: this collagen is believed to be an important component of the matrix of the pannus that replaces the surface of the hyaline cartilage as the acute phase of the disease evolves into granulation tissue formation. Uranyl acetate—lead citrate. (× 40,000)

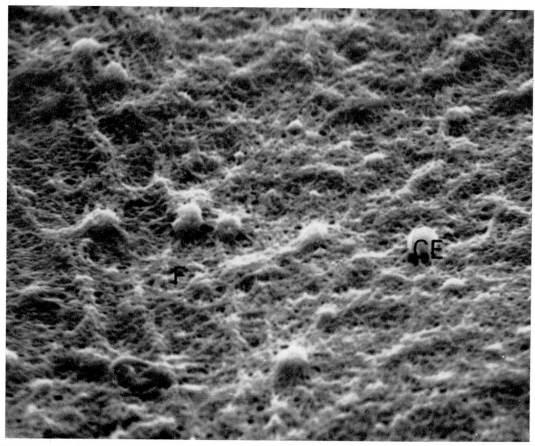

Fig. 5.10 Experimental arthritis induced 24 hours previously by intraarticular injection of turpentine into rat knee joint. Normal regular fibrillar structure of surface disturbed and partly obliterated. These changes are thought to be due to the degradative activity of synovial enzymes and their action may be analogous to early changes in rheumatoid arthritis.

(×2,100)

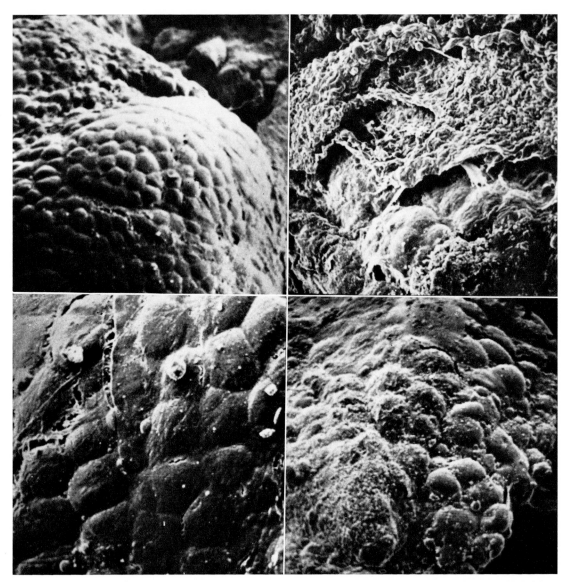

Fig. 5.11 (*Top left*) Surface of normal fatty areolar synovial tissue from intact part of rheumatoid knee joint. (*Bottom left*) Higher power view of part of field shown (*top left*). (*Top right*) Inflamed surface of rheumatoid synovium with fibrinous inflammatory exudate partially covering synovial villus. (*Bottom right*) Partial obliteration of synovial surface structure by inflammatory exudate. (From Gryfe, Woodward and Gardner, 1969. *Lancet*, **ii**, 156–157.

(*Top left* × 105; *right* × 335; *bottom left* × 335; *right* × 190)

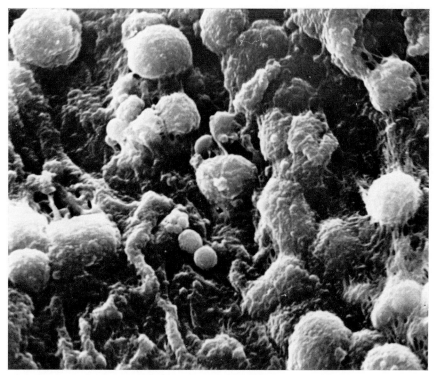

Fig. 5.12 Experimental arthritis. Synovial surface of rat knee joint tissue 3 days after the induction of turpentine arthritis. The many large, round or ovoid structures on the synovial surface are polymorphonuclear neutrophil leucocytes. The synovial surface is greatly disturbed and irregular. The nature of the smaller (*central*) round, smooth surfaced, bodies is uncertain; they may be lymphocytes, liberated nuclei or nuclear fragments. (×3,280)

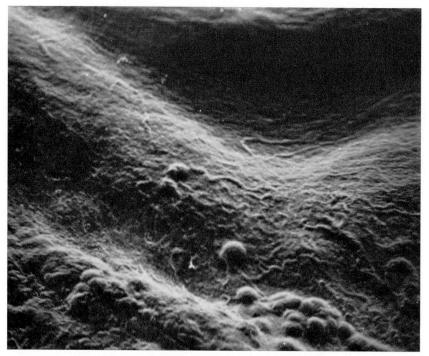

Fig. 5.13 Experimental arthritis. The earliest change detectable by surface study in the rat knee joint following the intraarticular injection of turpentine is a sparse accumulation of fibrin seen in the patellar recess 2 hours after the injection. In this field, the articular cartilage of the patellar surface of the femur is shown *at top*, adjoining adipose and areolar synovial tissue *at bottom*. The intervening zone, not previously recognised in periarticular tissues, has been termed the epichondrial surface. It is upon this surface that the first deposits of fibrinous strands are seen.

(×110)

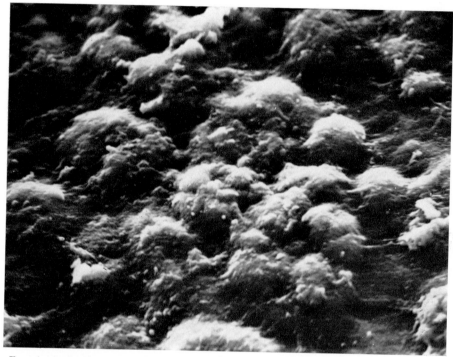

Fig. 5.14 Experimental arthritis. Fourteen days after the induction of acute turpentine arthritis in a rat knee joint, the synovial surface is greatly disorganised. The normal, fine, regular and repetitive structure of the secondary and tertiary processes is obscured by muddy deposits, first described in rheumatoid arthritis by Fujita and his colleagues, probably composed partly of fibrin, partly of other plasma-protein derivatives. (× 2,070)

CHAPTER 6

Physical Factors Contributing to Joint Disease

When rheumatoid arthritis is established as a result of the biological changes that have been outlined above, very many secondary factors come into play. They prolong the disease and cause it to extend, inducing secondary osteoarthrosis and leading to deformity and ankylosis (Kodama *et al.* 1966). Some of these contributory factors are exacerbated by the ageing process, some are the result of progressive mechanical disorders of wear or of pressure and some come from prolonged dietary imbalance and the chronic use of analgesic or anti-inflammatory drugs.

An idea of the complexity of the secondary mechanical factors can be gained by considering the important changes in the finger joints in the established disease (Figs. 6.1, 6.2).

The significance of the large flexion forces developed by the flexor tendons at the metacarpophalangeal joints during pinching and grasping movements has been discussed by Edwin Smith *et al.*, 1966. They believe that nearly all aspects of the basic deformity of the metacarpophalangeal joint in rheumatoid arthritis, including ulnar deviation and volar subluxation, can be explained by the forces transmitted by the flexor tendons, although they agree that ulnar dislocation of the extensor tendons is a contributory factor in some cases. They propose that the soft tissue changes such as periarticular fibrosis and intrinsic muscle contractures, result from rather than cause the initial deformity but that, once present, fibrosis and contracture accentuate deformity. In the case of the fifth digit Edwin Smith *et al.* (1966) believe that ulnar deviation results from the incompletely opposed pull of the hypothenar muscles.

A comparable study by R. J. Smith and Kaplan (1967) emphasises the widely accepted view that the metacarpal head, eroded by granulation tissue (p. 27) and softened by osteoporosis (p. 74), no longer effectively supports the base of the proximal phalanx. In this way the stability of the joint becomes more dependent on the integrity of the capsule, ligaments and tendons that surround it. However, the accessory collateral ligaments become stretched (Straub, 1960) and, due to replacement by granulation tissue, they degenerate. There is a simultaneous inflammatory injury to the flexor tendons; they may rupture (p. 73).

Smith and Kaplan summarise the numerous *normal* forces and anatomical relationships that may contribute to ulnar deviation of the fingers in rheumatoid arthritis and distinguish 6 changes which accentuate this process:

1. Osteoporosis, cortical erosion and resorption of subchondral bone at the metacarpal head and base of the proximal phalanx;

2. Attrition and stretching of the collateral ligaments leading to volar subluxation of the proximal phalanx;

3. Stretching of the accessory collateral ligaments secondary to metacarpophalangeal synovitis, causing ulnar and volar displacement of flexor tendons and their tunnel;

4. Flexor tendon sheath synovitis, stretching of the vaginal ligaments and ulnar and volar displacement of the flexor tendons within the widened tunnel;

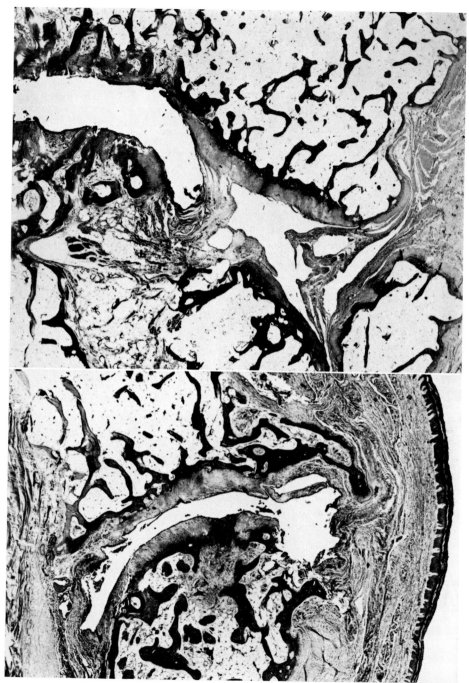

Fig. 6.1 (*Top*) Metacarpophalangeal joint. Longstanding rheumatoid synovitis with marginal cartilage destruction has culminated in extensive cartilage loss and secondary osteoarthrosis. Note loss of cartilage (*upper left*), a fibrous adhesion (*centre*), intra-osseous granulation tissue (*centre*) and some residual fibrous synovial tissue (*right*). An island of osteoporotic bone (*lower right*) is formed in the connective tissue adjoining the joint space. This is probably not a sesamoid bone but represents extraarticular, secondary bone formation. (*Bottom*) Advanced rheumatoid arthritis with extensive destruction of the distal interphalangeal joint by granulation tissue that extends (*top and bottom left*) to replace articular cartilage and (*right*) is associated with almost complete loss of this cartilage. At upper right centre, the proximal lip of the distal phalanx remains as a small process that appears like an osteophyte. No significant osteoporosis. Note, however, (*lower centre*) that granulation tissue can be seen extending into the bone of the middle phalanx, presumably in continuity with the synovial granulation tissue.

(*Top* ×10, bottom ×14)

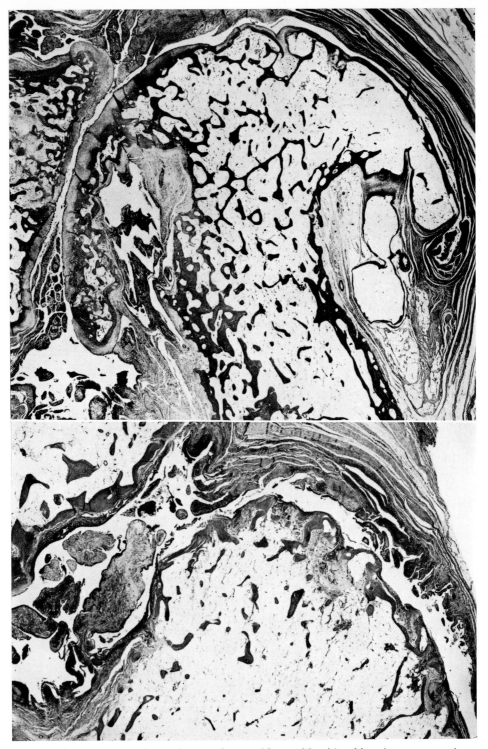

Fig. 6.2 (*Top*) Advanced longstanding and severe rheumatoid synovitis with subluxation, osteoporosis, secondary osteoarthrosis and continued inflammatory disease. Note deeply staining synovial villi (*bottom left*) extending into joint space. At each margin of the deformed middle phalanx osteophytic processes remain, that on the left being undermined by extensive rheumatoid granulation tissue. Inflamed synovial villi also seen (*top left*). Note partial loss of cartilage on both bone surfaces. (From Gardner D. L., *Pathology of the Connective Tissue Diseases*, London: Arnold, 1965.) (*Bottom*) Proximal interphalangeal joint. Compare with previous figure. Active continued disease is represented by the numerous large synovial villi lying within the joint space (*left*) staining deeply because of their content of inflammatory cells, and associated with comparable granulation tissue that extensively replaces and is incorporated in the bony surfaces. Note total absence of articular cartilage, subluxation of bone and severe osteoporosis. (*Right*) Synovitis of synovial recess extends to the tendon sheath. (*Top* ×8; *bottom* ×10)

5. Dislocation of the tendon of the common extensor digitorum at the metacarpophalangeal joint or rupture deep to the dorsal carpal ligament, causing volar subluxation and ulnar deviation of the proximal phalanx; and

6. Contracture of the interosseous muscles leading to volar subluxation of the proximal phalanx and ulnar deviation of the index finger.

Rheumatoid tendon and tendon sheath disease

A full description of the pathological changes in the tendons and tendon sheaths in rheumatoid arthritis was given by Kellgren and Ball (1950). These authors referred to the early views of Scudamore (1827) who described knotty, contracted tendons in rheumatism and to those of Stockman (1904) who spoke of 'tendinous rheumatism'.

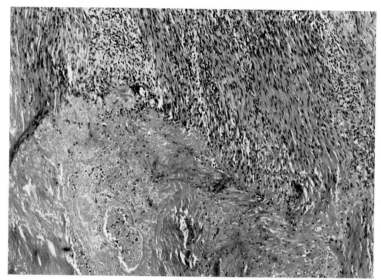

Fig. 6.3 Tendon necrosis in rheumatoid arthritis. A zone of necrotic material (*bottom left*) is separated from intact tendinous tissue (*top right*) by a remarkably sharp, and distinct, margin at which small numbers of lymphocytes are present. The necrotic zone distantly recalls the structure of a rheumatoid subcutaneous nodule. Tendon rupture may result. (From Gardner D. L., *Pathology of the Connective Tissue Diseases*, London: Arnold, 1965.)   (×65)

The incidence of tendon disease (Kellgren and Ball, 1950) was found to be 42%, a figure very similar to that of Edstrom (1945). In 37 of the 42 affected patients the tendons involved were those of the long flexors of the fingers. Histologically, 38 tendon biopsies and 15 tendon sheaths were investigated from 15 patients. The microscopic lesions were irregular in distribution. Occasionally (2/15) there was widespread replacement of the peritenon and mesotenon by granulation tissue among which were zones of 'fibrinoid' (p. 18) and of young fibroblasts, scanty polymorphs and lymphocytes. Inflammatory cells can be recognised by scanning electron microscopy on the tendon surfaces (Inoue, Julkunen and Vainio, 1970). Within the granulation tissue a structure may form indistinguishable from the rheumatoid nodule (Fig. 6.3).

The sequence of injury appeared to be first, an oedematous separation of the tendon fibres; second, the reduction of the compact tendon to a swollen, homogeneous, granular mass, at first containing reticular fibres but later afibrillar; and third, the onset of 'spontaneous' tendon rupture (Page, 1961; Vaughan–Jackson, 1966), of median nerve compression and of contracture and of weakening of support to adjacent joints. Rupture of the calcaneal tendon has been provoked by exogenous factors such as repeated local injections (Bedi and Ellis, 1970). The sequence of injury is, of course, an important determinant of the subluxation and deformity characteristic of the established disease, a contribution exaggerated by laxity of adjoining ligaments and of the joint capsule (Sokoloff, 1966).

Pseudocyst formation and bone

The bone adjoining affected joints in rheumatoid arthritis is frequently osteoporotic (McConkey, Fraser and Bligh, 1962; Duncan, Frost, Villanueva and Sigler, 1965; Saville and Kharmosh, 1967; Miller, Markheim and Towbin, 1967) and the bone end plate thinned. Smooth radiological outlines may mask active microscopic disease (Pazderka and Středa, 1965). Osteoporosis is particularly common in female patients of 50 years of age or more, whether treated with corticosteroids or not (Saville and Kharmosh, 1967). Synovial fluid or granulation tissue, part of the pannus, are probably forced directly into this osteoporotic bone during movement. The island of intraosseous granulation tissue formed in this way comprises a pear-shaped, radio-translucent pseudocyst (Maldyk, 1969b).

Since the demonstration of the very high pressures generated in large inflamed joints such as the knee by flexion movements in rheumatoid arthritis (Dixon and Grant, 1964; Jayson and Dixon, 1970a, b; Jayson, Rubinstein and Dixon, 1970) it has become easier to account for the origin of these subarticular 'pseudocysts' (Cruickshank, MacLeod and Shearer, 1954) or 'geodes'* (Jayson, Rubenstein and Dixon, 1970) which are such a common radiological feature of the disease. Dixon and Grant showed that 7 of 8 cadaver knee joint capsules, distended with fluid, ruptured at pressures below those found *in vivo* in patients with only modest rheumatoid effusions. In the latter disease, flexion pressures as high as 1,000 mm Hg were recorded. Jayson and Dixon (1970a) showed that the initial pressures and volumes recorded from rheumatoid knee joints were greater than those of controls, an observation which was handicapped by the author's inability to match their controls for age and sex. After the joints had been aspirated and redistended with fluid, higher pressures were again recorded in the rheumatoid patients. As the joints were progressively distended (Jayson and Dixon, 1970a) pulsations synchronous with the arterial pulse were recorded, suggesting that the increased pressure in rheumatoid knees could interfere with the synovial circulation. Curiously, no mention was made of the influence of intra-articular pressures on the venous circulation and the synovial lymphatics, the thin-walled vessels of which must surely be compressed during movement even in normal persons.

Pseudocyst formation may be encountered in any part of the joint surface. However, at the joint margins, bone involvement in rheumatoid arthritis seems less likely to be directly related to pressure, and the destruction of marginal periarticular cortical bone in the process of 'erosion' takes place both by osteoclastic bone reabsorption and by an insidious lysis. The relationship of this local change, which is of inflammatory origin, to the metabolic bone disturbance and defective bone synthesis shown in rheumatoid arthritis by Duncan et al. (1965) by the technique of fluorescence microscopy after tetracycline labelling, is uncertain. It is probable that the combination of local destruction with defective osteoid synthesis can account for the early and severe bone lesions in many patients and for the occurrence of stress fractures (Miller, Markheim and Towbin, 1967).

---

* *Geode*: this geological term has crept into rheumatology from Europe and is to be deprecated. Geodes are defined as 'large cavities in rocks lined with crystals that are free to grow inwards' or in mining, as 'rounded nodules of ironstone with a hollow interior' (Chamber's Technical Dictionary, 1958). Applied in a biomedical context the term could prove exceedingly misleading.

Spinal fractures have been recognised in 16% in one series of 164 patients (Saville and Kharmosh, 1967) but their occurrence differs little from the incidence in the normal adult female population. Osteolytic vertebral lesions are described (Lorber, Pearson and Rene, 1961). Rarely, bone necrosis has been encountered.

The parathyroid glands in rheumatoid arthritis appear normal. No studies of calcium metabolism or of thyrocalcitonin have yet been made. Serum mineral levels have been measured (p. 110) although the experimental evidence (Chiroff and Jowsey, 1970) suggests that porcine calcitonin does not influence immobilisation reabsorption in dogs. Where granulation tissue extends from the joint into the epiphyseal cartilage in young patients, defective long bone growth may result. This 'rheumatic dwarfism' (Sokoloff, 1966) must be distinguished in Still's disease (p. 173) from the dwarfism which may follow prolonged treatment with ACTH.

Considerable remodelling of bone adjoining affected joints may be encountered. Periosteal new bone formation is less marked than in infectious arthritis or in Reiter's syndrome and to explain the periostitis which is occasionally seen in rheumatoid arthritis, Sokoloff (1966) has drawn attention to the lengthy synovial recesses that extend proximally near the phalangeal bones, synovitis of which may cause periostitis locally. Why this periostitis does not provoke new bone synthesis is not clear: the reaction may, it is supposed, be retarded in aged persons with osteoporosis.

Ankylosis

The ultimate result of granulation tissue formation is ankylosis which is usually of a fibrous character; very exceptionally, ankylosis may become bony. Adjacent bones may be subluxated due to tendinous laxity and muscle atonia, bound together by fibrous adhesions, disfigured by marginal erosions and by periosteal new bone formation, impacted one into the other with resultant shortening, or fractured. The bone deformities may be particularly severe if there is a concomitant metabolic bone disease. They are compounded by the coexistence of senile or steroid-induced osteoporosis and by the dietary osteomalacia which is so common in elderly women (Chalmers, Conacher, Gardner and Scott, 1967).

Rheumatoid arthritis and paralysis

Paralysis, whether due to poliomyelitis or as part of a hemiplegia (Bland and Winston, 1968), prevents the clinical onset of rheumatoid arthritis in the immobilised joints of patients whose other limbs are affected. Presumably, the action is nonspecific and due to the influence of rest on inflammation. There is no reason to think that the agent(s) provoking rheumatoid arthritis spare the synovia of a paralysed limb. The pathological changes in human rheumatoid joints before and after paralysis have not been compared. However, Roy (1970), in a study by electron microscopy of immobilised rabbit joints, found that degenerative articular cartilaginous changes were detectable within 10 days of immobilisation. Necrosis resulted in superficial collagen fragmentation particularly in areas where opposing surfaces were in contact at the time of immobilisation. These results, substantiated by Sood (1971), suggest that not all the effects of immobilisation are beneficial.

Primary injury to connective tissue in rheumatoid arthritis

The interesting suggestion that systemic lupus erythematosus and systemic sclerosis were diffuse diseases of collagen (Klemperer, Pollack and Baehr, 1942) has never been substantiated; nor has adequate evidence ever been adduced to show that collagen, collagen-precursors or collagen-synthesising cells such as fibroblasts or chondroblasts, are directly and primarily injured in rheumatoid arthritis (Stŭdnička, 1934; Perez–Tamayo, 1961; Gardner, 1970). Fibroblast proliferation in culture and, presumably, collagen synthesis, may be depressed non-specifically by rheumatoid sera (Castor, Wright and Buckingham, 1968). Evidence, summarised by Cotzias *et al.* (1968), suggested that manganese metabolism in rheumatoid arthritis may be abnormal, a view related to the role of this element in activating enzymes in rheumatoid arthritis critical to protein-polysaccharide synthesis. Slow turnover rates were, indeed, demonstrated but, contrary to expectation, the cell manganese concentrations were elevated, arguing against classical manganese deficiency. Evidence that excess collagen-like protein and anti-collagen antibodies are present in the sera of rheumatoid arthritis continues to accumulate (Kriegel, Langness and Jahn, 1970; Kriegel, Langness, Jahn and Muller, 1970) and the hypothesis that rheumatoid arthritis is a form of autoallergy directed against collagen still attracts a small number of adherents (Steffen, 1970). The evidence relating to the antigenicity of connective tissue components has recently been reviewed (Hamerman and Sandson, 1970). The demonstration that certain collagenases may lead to the production of degradation products which are intensely chemotactic *in vitro* (Chang and Houck, 1970) is an interesting corollary to the evidence that has shown that collagenases capable of degrading collagen *in vivo* at neutral pH are present in rheumatoid synovial tissue (Davies, Krakauer and Weissman, 1970) (p. 37).

Taking the evidence as a whole, there is support for the view that collagen is directly injured and digested by one or more collagenases at some stage during the rheumatoid process and that one of the consequences of this injury may be the formation of antibodies to degraded collagen or to its breakdown products. There is insufficient evidence to show that a disturbance to collagen is a primary characteristic of any tissue in rheumatoid arthritis (Kellgren *et al.*, 1951; Lindner, 1968) and it is interesting to recall that foci of tissue damage such as the rheumatoid nodule often contain numerous morphologically intact collagen fibrils (Cochrane *et al.*, 1964). It is clear that dense collagenous tissues such as the sclera can be injured at sites where experimental antigen/antibody interactions take place (Mohos and Wagner, 1969) (p. 202) as well as by enzyme-catalysed reactions. Under these circumstances collagen is involved coincidentally, a mechanism that suggests that these responses occur as incidental secondary features in rheumatoid tissue injury (Fig. 6.4).

Synovial cysts

Bursae adjoin many normal joints; some communicate with the synovial cavity. Rheumatoid synovitis may cause bursal swelling and distension, and thickening of the bursal wall. One consequence is the formation of swellings, loosely termed 'cysts', recognised when they become inflamed. This sequence is the probable explanation for 'ganglia' at the wrists and for popliteal ('Baker's') cysts.

Rupture of popliteal cysts in rheumatoid arthritis (Dixon and Grant, 1964; Hollingsworth, 1968), with the escape of synovial fluid into nearby connective tissue planes, causes cellulitis that may not be easily distinguishable from thrombophlebitis (Perri, Rodnan and Mankin, 1968). Contrast arthrography has shown that these cysts may be extremely long, that they communicate with the knee joint and that a valve-like mechanism allows the passage of fluid from the joint to the cyst but not in the reverse direction. In this way, it is believed, the high pressures generated during joint flexion in rheumatoid arthritis (p. 74) can readily cause cyst enlargement and rupture.

Excised cysts have a dense, collagenous connective tissue wall, an inflamed synovial-like lining, and a cellular infiltrate of varying numbers of lymphocytes and plasma cells. The sterile content includes not only thin synovial fluid but much cellular debris. In a survey of the structure

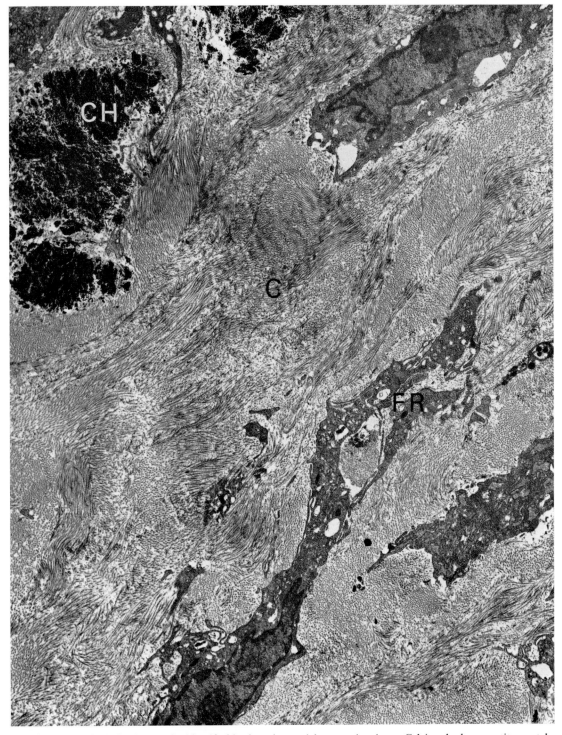

Fig. 6.4 Foci of calcification can be identified in the subsynovial connective tissue. Calcium hydroxyapatite crystals (*top left*) lie among broad, dense bundles of collagen: the presence of the bone mineral can be interpreted as a form of dystrophic calcification; its cause remains unknown. (From a micrograph of Dr. A. J. Palfrey.) (×4,500)

of 18 cysts from 14 rheumatoid arthritics Wagner and Abgarowicz (1970) found lymphoid follicles in only two. No Russell bodies were recognised and plasma cells were much fewer than in the rheumatoid synovium. A single specimen contained a multinucleated giant cell. The conclusion was reached that only the absence of villi distinguished the histological changes from those seen in the synovial joint. To the present writer, the cellular changes however appear distinctive.

CHAPTER 7

Regional Joint Disease

Rheumatoid arthritis, it is clear, can and often does affect any or all of the 187 synovial joints of the normal human. Every individual joint presents regional pathological problems of its own when affected by rheumatoid arthritis. Either by a direct disturbance of particular functions, as in the case of the larynx or mandible, or because of secondary pressure or space-occupying effects, as in the case of the cervical spine, the disease may come to have very far-reaching, possibly fatal, pathological consequences. It is only practicable to examine selected examples of these aspects of the late results of rheumatoid arthritis.

Aural arthritis

Both the incudostapedial joint, a ball-and-socket articulation, and the incudomalleal, a saddle-shaped union, are synovial in nature. Both, therefore, are susceptible to the ravages of rheumatoid arthritis. There is increasing awareness of the frequency of nerve deafness in rheumatoid arthritis, independent of the effects of salicylate therapy. Debate continues, however, on the question of synovitis of the synovial joints of the middle ear as a cause for deafness. I have encountered no reports in the literature of proof of such a causation but, through the courtesy of Professor I. Friedmann, I have had the opportunity of examining microscopic sections of the incudostapedial joints from two cases of rheumatoid arthritis. In one there was degenerative disease of articular cartilage. Residual synovial tissue was absent, so that the presence of synovitis could not be confirmed or disproved. However, granulation tissue of rather low cellularity extended beneath the articular cartilage of the lenticular process of the incus in a manner recalling the changes encountered commonly in larger synovial joints (p. 27) and the appearances strongly suggested therefore that rheumatoid arthritis was present.

Temporomandibular arthritis

Particular interest has concentrated upon the temporomandibular joints (Kayanjian, 1938; Dingman, 1944; Thoma, 1946; Cook, 1958). Temporomandibular rheumatoid arthritis is a gravely disabling condition; it may be a feature either of the adult or of the juvenile disease and, in its most advanced form, requires palliative orthopaedic surgery. In a survey of 100 cases of the adult disease, Franks (1969) found temporomandibular involvement clinically or on X-ray in 86% of patients. Occasionally, temporomandibular arthritis may be a terminal feature of the disease. There have been few pathological studies (Goodwill and Steggles, 1966).

Laryngeal arthritis (Figs. 7.1, 7.2)

Involvement of the cricoarytenoid joint was described by Copeman (1957, 1968) and Copeman, Elkin and Pearce (1959) although it had been known since the last century (Mackenzie, 1894) that the larynx was susceptible to 'rheumatism' (Polisar, 1959). The microscopic changes of laryngeal rheumatoid arthritis are very fully documented (Gresham and Kellaway, 1958; Gardner and Holmes, 1961; Bienenstock, Ehrlich and Freyberg, 1963; Montgomery, 1963; Smith and Shine,

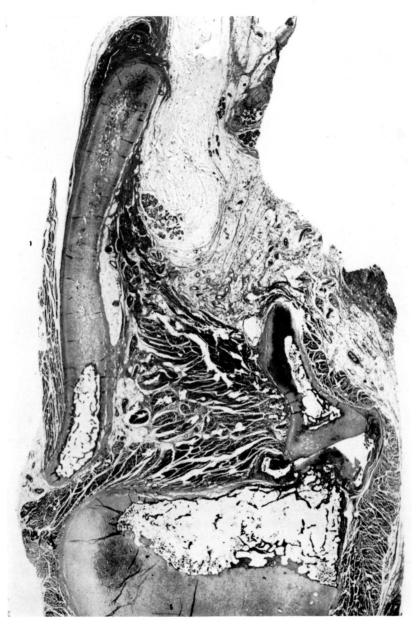

Fig. 7.1   Rheumatoid arthritis of larynx. Whole laryngeal section in the saggital plane, slightly off centre. The section bisects the thyroid, cricoid and arytenoid cartilages. Each cartilage contains islands of well-formed bone, a common feature in persons over the age of 30. Note at each lower edge of arytenoid cartilage, densely staining (grey-black) islands of synovial tissue at margins of cricoarytenoid joint. The changes are those of severe rheumatoid synovitis. Observe that new bone formed in laryngeal cartilage is osteoporotic.   ($\times 4\frac{1}{2}$)

1964; Pinals, 1966; and Vassallo, 1966) and the association of cricoarytenoid arthritis with postoperative pulmonary atelectasis and laryngeal ankylosis (Gardner and Holmes, 1961), with laryngeal ankylosis (Montgomery, Perone and Schall, 1955) and with rheumatoid pharyngitis (Gardner, 1968b) is recognised. There is a synovitis apparently similar to that characteristic of rheumatoid involvement of the larger joints. A marginal replacement of articular cartilage by granulation tissue infiltrated by lymphocytes and numerous plasma cells is accompanied by periathritis and, occasionally, laryngeal myositis, the muscles of the larynx being permeated by a

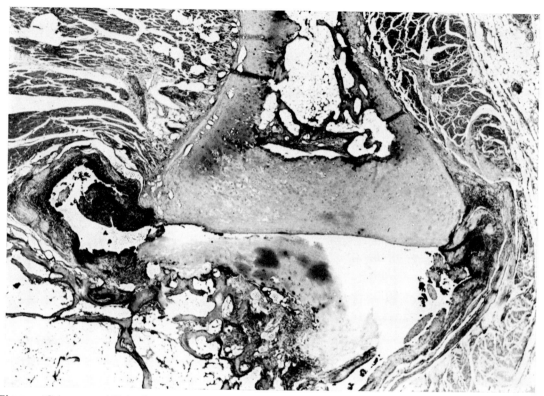

Fig. 7.2 Cricoarytenoid joint from previous illustration seen at higher magnification. Due to difficulty in sectioning, part of the surface of the cricoid cartilage (*lower centre right*) is missing. The synovial tissues (*left and right*) are extensively infiltrated with inflammatory cells and early pannus formation is seen, particularly at left. (×14)

similar cellular infiltrate. A suggestion has been made that the laryngeal dysfunction of rheumatoid arthritis could be explained by laryngeal neuropathy due to rheumatoid arteritis (Wolman, Darke and Young, 1965) but this view has not yet been confirmed.

Cervical arthritis

Involvement of the cervical spine has been recognised as a feature of juvenile rheumatoid arthritis since the time of Still (Still, 1896–97; Coss and Boots, 1946; Potter, Barkin and Stillman, 1946; Ziff, Brown, Badin and McEwen, 1954; Bland *et al.*, 1963; Bland, 1967; Martel, 1968). As Whaley and Dick (1969) point out in describing a single fatal case, it is only since the advent of radiological surveys made for epidemiological purposes (Kellgren, 1963, 1966; Lawrence 1966, 1969) that the prevalence of adult cervical spine disease has been fully appreciated. Cervical disease was known to accompany peripheral arthritis (Sharp, 1957) but was not thought to be common. The morphological characteristics of cervical rheumatoid arthritis are consequently not well documented, the majority of the published reports giving only clinical and radiological information (Whaley and Dick, 1969).

The pathological details of cervical rheumatoid arthritis have recently been surveyed by Ball and Sharp (1971) and by Ball (1971), and these investigations have done much to clarify this difficult field. Ball and Sharp give their own observations on 40 adult cervical spines among which the atlanto-axial joint was examined in 26. In 3 of these cases there was significant subaxial dislocation, in 9 a mobile atlanto-axial dislocation, and in 3, a fixed atlanto-axial luxation (Robinson, 1966).

The root of the problem in *subaxial dislocation* is apparently neurocentral and apophyseal synovitis with consequent erosion and replacement of the annulus fibrosus of the intervertebral disc. The absence of neurocentral joints from thoracic and lumbar spines and from children is held to account for the rarity of disc erosions in these sites and in this group of patients. Unlike the degenerative joint disease of the neurocentral joints described by Cave, Griffiths and Whiteley (1955) there is no new bone and osteophyte formation, a feature that may render dislocation more likely. Ossification of the disc margin, so common in ankylosing spondylitis, is very rare. Fibrous or bony ankylosis of apophyseal joints is, however, frequent and as Ball and Sharp emphasise, there is a tendency for the disorder to culminate in segmental cervical immobilisation. The spinous processes of the vertebrae are often atrophic.

In *atlanto-axial dislocation* the transverse ligament may remain intact; even if this ligament is torn or atrophic, severe displacement is not inevitable. Tendinous and ligamentous lesions are recognised similar to those encountered in peripheral joints. Osteoporosis may contribute to weakening of the atlanto-axial joint attachments and vertebral artery compression is a hazard. Occasionally there is cord compression but nerve root lesions are not well understood. Rarely, the lateral atlanto-axial joints may be destroyed by inflammatory disease with sudden subsequent death from medullary compression.

Rheumatoid arthritis of cervical discs and of the apophyseal joints may be complicated by disc degeneration, pyoarthrosis (p. 178), osteoporotic bone collapse and arteritis affecting muscles and nerves (Ball and Sharp, 1971).

Atlanto-axial displacement secondary to softening and stretching of the transverse ligament of the atlas occurs in up to 25% of patients with rheumatoid arthritis (Sharp and Purser, 1961; Mathews, 1969). Fourteen of Sharp and Purser's 74 cases and 25% of Mathews' 76 outpatients were found to have this complication. Martel and Bole (1968) commented on 3 cases. The process appeared to be relatively more common in males than in females but occurs regardless of age, being less frequent, however, in early cases.

Both atlanto-axial and subaxial displacements are usually asymptomatic but may cause neurological signs by compression of the spinal cord, of nerve roots or of adjacent blood vessels. Sometimes rheumatoid granulation tissue, presumably arising in relation to the synovia of the atlanto-occipital, atlanto-axial, or postero-lateral apophyseal joints, causes cord compression by narrowing of the spinal canal. However, there is limited pathological information on the distribution of the disease process in this region or on the microscopic features that distinguish rheumatoid from ankylosing spondylitis. Quadriplegia may develop (Martel, 1968). Mathews (1969) believes, and it is generally accepted, that atlanto-axial subluxation is a characteristic of severe, sero-positive, 'erosive' disease.

Subluxation of the upper cervical vertebrae below the axis is also quite common. Lower cervical subluxation with tetraplegia has been described (Hopkins, 1967).

Manubriosternal arthritis

The frequency of manubriosternal arthritis in rheumatoid arthritis, by contrast with its involvement in ankylosing spondylitis, has been underestimated. Thus, Kormano (1970) demonstrated radiological evidence of 'erosion' in 6 of 11 rheumatoid arthritics, 4 of whom displayed signs of active inflammation; 4 further cases showed the X-ray changes of fibrosis. Histologically, he found that the normal joint cavity was sometimes lined with synovial-like cells (9 of 20 cases) but such cells were only recognised in one rheumatoid arthritic in whom there was additional evidence of inflammatory disease. Kormano was at pains to emphasise that manubriosternal joints that are radiologically normal may show microscopic evidence of rheumatoid synovitis. Laitinen, Saksanen and Suoranta (1970) made a similar investigation and demonstrated, by X-ray, erosions, reactive sclerosis or ankylosis in 70% of 87 rheumatoid manubriosternal joints by comparison with 27% of 72 osteoarthrotic and normal joints.

Very limited biopsy data is available on the histological structure of these joints.

Lumbar arthritis

In radiological surveys, the incidence of rheumatoid arthritis of the lumbar spine in patients with clinical rheumatoid arthritis or positive tests for rheumatoid factor has been estimated at 5% in males and 3% in females. The apophyseal joints are affected, and Lawrence, Sharp, Ball and Bier (1964) included in their clinical survey of 19 males and 31 females in the 55–64 years age group, a brief synopsis of 4 patients in whom *post mortem* studies had been possible. The first case showed a minor degree of arthritis of the apophyseal joints with no disc involvement; the second also showed early apophyseal arthritis; the third osteoarthrotic changes only, with Schmorl node formation; the fourth displayed rheumatoid arthritis.

CHAPTER 8

Synovial Fluid

The characteristics of normal synovial fluid were summarised by Ropes and Bauer (1953) and are tabulated in the most recent edition of the Documenta Geigy Scientific Tables (Diem and Lentner, 1970) (Tables 8.1–8.4). (Fig. 8.1)

In rheumatoid arthritis, the volume of the fluid present in a knee joint, for example, is increased from the normal barely perceptible amount, perhaps 0·1–0·4 ml., up to volumes as large as 200–400 ml. The appearance of the fluid is often turbid but it may be clear and a fibrinous clot, or the presence of strands of fibrin, is usual. Depending on whether vascular injury is caused during aspiration, the number of red blood cells present is more or less raised but abundant red blood cells are indicative of superadded trauma. Very rarely the fluid is chylous (Newcombe and Cohen, 1965). Part of the lipid appears to be synthesised by synovial cells and lipid inclusions are commonly detectable within synovial fluid leucocytes. The number of white blood cells in the synovial fluid is markedly raised (Ropes and Bauer, 1953; Malinin, Pekin and Zvaifler, 1967) (Table 8.1) and there is a reversal of the normal differential cell count from a preponderance of mononuclear cells to an overwhelming abundance of polymorphs (Table 8.2).

The protein content of the synovial fluid in rheumatoid arthritis is usually considerably increased and approaches the values obtained for serum (Table 8.4; Fig. 9.3). Of a mean concentration of protein, estimated by the biuret reaction, of 4·5 g/l. (normal 1·8 g/l.: serum 7·0 g/l.) 45% was albumin, 5% α_1-globulin, 10% α_2-globulin, 14% β-globulin and 25% γ-globulin (Binette and Schmid, 1965) (Table 8.4). Ultracentrifugal analysis reveals a considerable increase in the 19S (4%) and 7S (24%) fractions. The diversity of proteins revealed by systematic assays and immunoelectrophoresis is, however, very great. Thus, many agents capable of influencing the coagulation mechanism are found. Among these proteins is abundant β-globulin; and much fibrin is present. Complement levels are characteristically low relative to other forms of inflammatory joint disease (Hedberg et al., 1964; Pekin and Zvaifler, 1964; Townes and Sowa, 1970) even in patients in whom blood complement levels are normal; but patients sero-positive for 'rheumatoid factor' usually display correspondingly high synovial fluid rheumatoid factor (IgM) levels as well as abundant synovial fluid IgG immunoglobulin. The possible contribution of synovial fluid IgM immunoglobulin to the pathogenesis of the disease is discussed on p. 100.

There are at least three possible sources for the lysosomal enzymes found in excess in the synovial fluid in rheumatoid arthritis and displaying high activity in rheumatoid synovial cells (p. 113). They may come from altered chondrocytes, from injured synovial cells or from the polymorphs that accumulate as part of the inflammatory reaction. The demonstration that the synovial fluid (Jasani, Katori and Lewis, 1969) and synovial cells (Weissman, 1967) in rheumatoid arthritis display abnormally high lysosomal enzyme activity and that both the fluid and cells are capable of digesting cartilage matrix in vitro (Hamerman, Janis and Smith, 1967), may mean no more than that these cells have themselves been injured by exogenous agents (p. 188) or that polymorph lysosomal enzymes have been liberated. The presence of activated lysosomal proteases

TABLE 8.1. *Synovial Fluid in Rheumatoid Arthritis*

Intraarticular pressure: in range 0–700 mm. fluid
Lactate 31 mg/100 cc. (sera: 22 mg/100 cc.)
pH 7·11–7·42 (mean 7·22; serum 7·45)
Freezing point de- −0·542°C (serum: −0·562°C)
pressions (2 cases) −0·551°C (serum: −0·606°C)

	Normal	Rheumatoid arthritis (definite, effusion under 6/52)	Rheumatoid arthritis (definite, effusion 6/52 –1 year)	Rheumatoid arthritis (definite, effusion over 1 year)	Rheumatoid arthritis (probable)
Appearance	clear	clear–turbid	clear–turbid	clear–turbid	clear–turbid
Clot	0	1·4	1·2	0·5	0·9
Red cells/cu. mm.	160	2,600	4,890	5,870	220
White cells/cu. mm.	63	13,790	14,210	16,780	8,150
% white cell types:					
polys	7%	63%	65%	66%	39%
lymphs	25%	11%	23%	17%	28%
monos	63%	24%	13%	15%	33%
Relative viscosity at 38°C	235	11·9	8·9	14·5	23
Sugar mg/cc.					
fluid	almost	78	65	58	88
serum	equal	95	95	91	98
Total protein (exclusive of mucin) g/100 ml.	1·72	4·75	4·69	5·24	4·14
Albumin g/100 ml.	1·02	3·11	2·71	2·67	2·65
Globulin g/100 ml.	0·05	1·79	1·93	2·71	1·60
Mucin nitrogen g/100 ml.	0·104	0·065	0·057	0·068	0·068
Mucin glucosamine g/100 ml.	0·087	0·048	0·034	0·043	0·048
Type of mucin pptate.	G	P	P	P	F

G: tight, ropy clump in a clear solution.
P: small friable masses in a cloudy solution.
F: soft mass in a clear or slightly cloudy solution.
(From Ropes and Bauer (1953), *Synovial Fluid Changes in Joint Disease*. Harvard University Press, Cambridge, Mass.)

TABLE 8.2. *Cell content of synovial fluid in rheumatoid arthritis*

Number of fluids examined:		77
Total nucleated cell count:		
	Average	19,170 per c. mm.
	Range	from 56,000 to 4,280 per c. mm.
Differential cell count:		
Polymorphs	Average	78%
	Range	from 95 to 26%
Lymphocytes:	Average	17%
	Range	from 68 to 3%
Monocytes:	Range	from 14 to 0·3%
Other macrophages	Range	from 7 to 0%
Synovial lining cells:	Range	from 18 to 0%

(From Collins, D. H. (1949), *The Pathology of Articular and Spinal Diseases*, Edward Arnold, London, by permission of the publishers.)

TABLE 8.3. *Composition of normal synovial fluid*

Physical data	Mean	95% range (extreme range in brackets)
Intrinsic viscosity (37°C)	46·3	26·9–65·7
pH value	7·434	(7·31–7·64)
Chloride (mEq/l.)	107·4	(87–138)
Calcium (mEq/l.)	—	(2·3–4·7)
Magnesium	...	...
Iron (µg/kg.)	43	(20–90)
Copper (µg/kg.)	210	(40–640)
Enzymes that have been shown to be present:		
lactate dehydrogenase	...	...
malate dehydrogenase	...	...
isocitrate dehydrogenase	...	...
glutathione reductase	...	...
aspartate aminotransferase	...	...
alanine aminotransferase	...	...
alkaline and acid phosphatase	...	...
β-glucuronidase	...	...
aminopeptidase	...	...
fructose diphosphate aldolase	...	...
glucose phosphate isomerase	...	...

(Reproduced from *Documenta Geigy Scientific Tables* (7th Edition), pp. 640–642, Diem K. and Lentner, C. (Editors), by permission of CIBA – Geigy Limited, Basle, 1970.)

cannot logically be held to support the suggestion that cartilage has sustained the first insult in rheumatoid arthritis (Hamerman, 1969) (p. 37).

Pruzanski, Saito and Ogryzlo (1970) have made a systematic study of the lysozyme (muramidase) activity of the serum from 120 cases of rheumatoid arthritis and of the synovial fluid from 67, demonstrating an increased enzyme activity in 35% of the former and in 55% of the latter. No correlation between enzyme activity and white blood cell counts in synovial fluid was detected in spite of suggestive evidence that cartilage lysozyme contributes to the matrix depletion that may be an early phase of rheumatoid joint destruction (p. 33). Kerby and Taylor (1967) obtained evidence that the synovial fluid supernate contains agents inhibitory to lysozyme.

The finding of two collagenases in rheumatoid arthritis synovial fluid, one inhibited by serum proteins, the other active *in vivo* and not so inhibited (Evanson, Jeffrey and Krane, 1967; Harris, DiBona and Krane, 1969) has lent support to the view that collagenase(s) as well as enzymes of the fibrinolytic system (Lack, 1959) or other proteases of non-lysosomal origin may be important causes of marginal cartilage and bone reabsorption (erosion) in rheumatoid arthritis. Harris, DiBona and Krane (1969) maintained cultures of rheumatoid synovium *in vitro*. The cultured cells were found to produce enzymes that degraded native collagen at neutral pH and which, therefore, could operate *in vivo* in the rheumatoid joint. There was no evidence of the presence of this collagenase in homogenates of fresh rheumatoid synovium. However, in occasional rheumatoid synovial fluids, 2 distinct collagenases were identified. The first, enzyme A, with a molecular weight of 40–50,000, was not inhibited by serum but, unlike the leucocyte collagenase which had been investigated by others, was capable of degrading collagen fibrils as well as collagen in solution. Enzyme B, inhibited by serum, resembled the collagenase obtained by synovial cell culture. Both enzyme A and enzyme B were shown to cleave the collagen molecule $\frac{3}{4}$ of the distance from the N-terminal end.

Although plasminogen and proactivator are found both in normal and in rheumatoid synovial

TABLE 8.4. *Protein fractions of synovial fluid*

| | Volume per knee joint ml. | Biuret reaction g. protein/l. | Paper electrophoresis at pH 8·6 | | | | | α_1-Globulin/ α_2-Globulin ratio | Ultracentrifuge | | | |
			Albumin %	α_1-Glob-ulins %	α_2-Glob-ulins %	β-Glob-ulins %	γ-Glob-ulins %		19S %	7S %	4S %	1S %
Synovial fluid												
Normal	0·2-0·4	18	63	7	7	9	14	1·0	—	—	—	—
Post mortem	7	18	50	9	7	12	23	1·3	2	12	83	3
Traumatic	10	26	55	5	8	11	21	0·7	3	8	88	1
Rheumatoid arthritis	—	45	45	5	10	14	26	0·5	4	24	72	0
Serum												
Normal	—	70	49	6	12	17	16	0·5	2	12	86	0

(From Binette and Schmid, 1965, modified, in the *Documenta Geigy Scientific Tables*, 1970, by permission of the publishers CIBA – Geigy Limited, Basle.)

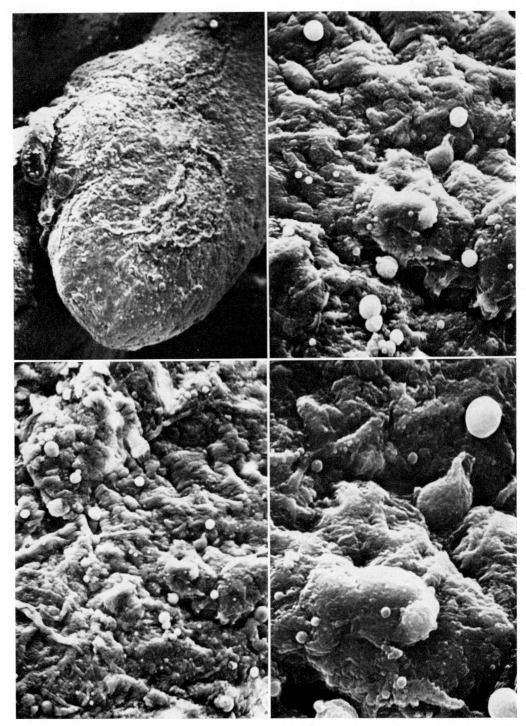

Fig. 8.1 A sequence of scanning electron microscopic views of the synovia from the intercondylar area of a female patient with active rheumatoid arthritis. (*Top left*) A single synovial villus showing the irregular surface partly covered by fibrin. (*Bottom left*) Red and white blood cells with cellular debris and unidentified material resting on the extremely irregular synovial surface. (*Top right*) Part of the surface seen (*bottom left*) at higher magnification. The synovial surface pattern is abnormally irregular and numerous cells of varying size rest upon the inflamed surface. (*Bottom right*) Part of the Figure at top right showing the surface structure of individual synovial cells and associated inflammatory cells in more detail. Some of the smaller round and ovoid structures resting upon the synovial surface are not identified. It is possible that they represent fat droplets, extruded nuclei, portions of individual cells or the processes of underlying synovial cells. (*Top left* ×120; *right* ×1,200; *bottom left* ×600; *right* ×2,400)

fluid, fibrinogen is detected only in inflamed joints in the synovial fluid of which it can reach concentrations approximately the same as those of the plasma (Caughey and Highton, 1967; Barnhart, Riddle, Bluhm and Quintana, 1967). The presence of fibrin is characteristic but not pathognomic of rheumatoid arthritis; fibrin clots form and fibrin lies as disorderly masses on or within the surface folds of the synovial tissue as it does in bacterial arthritides such as tuberculosis. Caughey and Highton suggest that the remarkable persistence of fibrin in rheumatoid arthritis may be due to repeated small intraarticular haemorrhages such as those that Muirden believes may explain the heavy concentration of haemosiderin and ferritin in rheumatoid synovial tissue (p. 157). The repetitive haemorrhages may 'overcome' (author's quotes: 'exhaust' might be a better term) the normal synovial fibrinolytic system. Alternatively they postulate a reduction in synovial fluid plasminogen or an excess of plasmin inhibitor. They state that the evidence does not support the presence of excess fibrin-stabilising factor. A further possibility is a combination of fibrin with a product of inflammation, making the conjugate resistant to the action of plasmin. Lack (1959) had shown the presence of plasmin inhibitors in normal synovial fluid. The persistence of fibrin has been held to contribute to the chronic nature of the rheumatoid inflammatory response (Riddle, Bluhm and Barnhart, 1965; Glynn, 1968) (p. 203) but it can be at least partly removed by the intraarticular injection of exogenous fibrinolytic systems. The role of intra-articular fibrin is referred to on pp. 18 and 108.

Desquamated cartilage fragments are encounterered from time to time embedded in synovial tissue (Muirden, 1970a, b). Kitridou et al. (1969) have shown that fibrils, distinguished from fibrin by electron- but not by phase contrast- or polarisation microscopy, may be present in osteoarthrotic synovial fluid. The fibrils can also be recognised in the synovial fluid in rheumatoid arthritis where, however, they tend to be obscured by the abundant fibrin.

The normal hyaluronate–protein macromolecular complexes of synovial fluid can be altered in rheumatoid arthritis in four possible ways. There may be separation of the protein and carbohydrate moieties, depolymerisation of the carbohydrate polyamino-sugar macromolecule, protein denaturation, or proteolysis. Ferguson, Boyle and Nuki (1969) adduce evidence from biophysical measurements, to show that the large protein–polysaccharide molecules that display increased polymerisation or are complexed in osteoarthrosis, are dissociated in rheumatoid arthritis, a change which causes the loss of the viscoelastic properties of synovial fluid in the latter disease and, perhaps, an alteration in the important contribution made by the protein moiety to surface lubrication (Radin, Swann and Weisser, 1970). These observations recall the changed viscosity of the hyaluronate synthesised by rheumatoid synovial cells in culture (p. 39).

It is virtually certain that the composition of rheumatoid synovial fluid will prove to be still more complex than has been supposed. Apart from the chemical and physical complexities of the protein-hyaluronate macromolecule the role of which in lubrication is actively debated (Radin, Swann and Weissen, 1970, show that the protein moiety, not the polysaccharide, is responsible for lubrication characteristics in vitro) a variety of pharmacological agents is present, the nature and properties of which are not yet fully understood. Many of course may be incidental products of the inflammatory disease. Thus, a histamime-releasing agent resembling an antigen/antibody complex and called rheumatoid biologically active factor (RBAF) has been described by Broder et al. (1969); the factor was identified with the aid of a biological system based on histamine release and was found in 33% of rheumatoid sera, but in 75% of rheumatoid synovial fluids.

The concentration of synovial fluid trace metals (Table 8.3; Niedermeier, Creity and Holley, 1962) has been studied in detail. There is no evidence of any disturbance characteristic of the disease but in view of the subtle changes detected in serum levels (p. 109), more extensive studies by modern techniques may be rewarding.

CHAPTER 9

Immunopathology

Surveys of the tissue and serological characteristics of rheumatoid arthritis show that signs of three of the four principal damaging aspects of the immunological response are commonly recognisable (Bollett, 1966; Medical Research Council Annual Report, 1968). There is direct or circumstantial evidence (1) of the cytotoxic reactions determined by circulating antibody; of (2) the disturbances caused by immune complexes; and of (3) the cell-mediated hypersensitivity response. The evidence, in brief, is provided (1) by the localisation of immunoglobulins, including autoantibodies, at sites of demonstrable tissue injury such as synovitis; (2) by the finding that immune complexes present in rheumatoid synovial cells and synovial fluid chemotactically attract and are phagocytosed by host white cells; and (3) by the lymphocytic and plasma cell infiltration of rheumatoid synovitis and by decreased lymphocyte responsiveness (Hoffa and Wollenberg, 1908; Allison and Ghormley, 1931; Collins, 1949; Christian, 1965; Glynn and Holborow, 1960, 1965; Nowoslawski and Brzosko, 1966, 1967a, b; McCormick, 1967; Ziff, 1968; Lightfoot and Christian, 1969).

It is now very generally agreed (Gell and Coombs, 1968) therefore that there is sufficient evidence to show that immunological phenomena are commonplace in the tissues in rheumatoid arthritis. It remains a matter of intense interest and concern to demonstrate whether these immunological phenomena are signs of a primary, autoallergic tissue-injuring reaction (Glynn and Holborow, 1965), whether they are characteristic and pathognomonic secondary effects of some other tissue-damaging mechanism such as viral infection, or whether they are coincidental and irrelevant to the pathogenesis of the disease.

Humoral antibody and rheumatoid synovitis (Figs. 9.1, 9.3, 9.5, 9.6)

The earliest suggestion that the lymphoreticular system, and hence, in contemporary terms, the immunological mechanism, might play a significant part in the genesis of rheumatoid arthritis was the description of the synovial lymphocytic foci (Hoffa and Wollenberg, 1908) (p. 21). The importance of the reticuloendothelial system to the pathogenesis of rheumatoid arthritis was implicit in the description of Felty's syndrome (Felty, 1924).

In 1931, Allison and Ghormley again drew attention to the widespread lymphocytic and plasma cell synovial infiltrates in rheumatoid arthritis which are so characteristic a part of the established disease (p. 23). The ratio of plasma cells to lymphocytes tends to increase with the duration of the disease (Julkunen, 1966). In his discussion on the nature and significance of these infiltrates, Collins (1949) quotes Allison and Ghormley (1931) who say 'Histologically, the tissue shows a definite picture, which is as clear cut as is that of tuberculosis, namely a proliferative change in the synovial membrane and marrow which is characterised by focal collections of lymphocytes. The microscopic picture will, we believe, be enough to establish the diagnosis of proliferative (rheumatoid)* arthritis and in our experience has been enough to predict the subsequent changes

---

* Author's parentheses.

in several instances where the tissues showed the characteristic changes in the early stages of the clinical disturbances.'

That the lymphoid foci and the plasma cell infiltrates of rheumatoid synovial tissue might be of more than purely diagnostic significance was suspected when Fagraeus (1948) established that plasma cells are the main source of circulating antibody. It appeared logical to suppose that synovial plasma cells might be engaged in secreting antibody protein and that this antibody might have a part to play in provoking or perpetuating local tissue injury. With the introduction of the fluorescein-conjugated antibody technique (Coons and Kaplan, 1950) it became possible to search directly for the presence of defined antigens and for immunoglobulins in rheumatoid tissues. Generally, it is necessary to employ cryostat sections for investigations of this nature. However, the presence of rheumatoid factors (p. 100), IgM anti-IgG macroglobulins whose nature

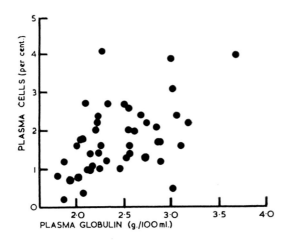

Fig. 9.1 The relationship between the plasma cell count in the bone marrow and the plasma globulin level is illustrated. (From Richmond *et al.*, 1956, *Ann. rheum. Dis.*, **15**, 217–226.)

is discussed below, has been successfully demonstrated in glutaraldehyde-fixed tissue embedded in paraffin (Ball, Bahgat and Taylor, 1964). More recently, new sensitive techniques for the detection of rheumatoid factor at the cellular level have also been devised (Bach and Delbarre, 1968; Bach, Delrieu and Delbarre, 1970*a*).

Some of the earliest observations made by the immunofluorescent method of Coons and Kaplan (1950) (Nairn, 1969) were those of Vazquez and Dixon (1957). These authors examined 7 rheumatoid subcutaneous nodules and found that a fluorescein-conjugated anti-human γ-globulin 'stained' the central areas of the nodules but not the marginal, pallisaded cells. The nearby connective tissue stained less strongly and control necrotic tissues, such as myocardial infarcts, not at all. In the same way, acutely inflamed, non-rheumatoid tissues such as those of the appendix gave greater immunofluorescent staining with anti-human serum albumin than with anti-human γ-globulin.

These early studies were extended and amplified by Mellors *et al.* (1959) who sought for the cellular origin of rheumatoid factor. Mellors *et al.* used a fluorescein-labelled aggregated human γ-globulin, reactive with rheumatoid sera in precipitin tests *in vitro*, as a reagent for localising rheumatoid factor (IgM anti-IgG macroglobulin) in cryostat sections of rheumatoid synovia, lymph nodes and subcutaneous nodules. They found that rheumatoid factor was present in the cytoplasm of synovial plasma cells in various stages of the disease. No rheumatoid factor was found in other cells and the appearance of the localised factor suggested that it was being secreted locally. Although many cells contained no γ-globulin, some contained 7S, others 19S γ-globulin. Immunofluorescent staining for rheumatoid factor could be blocked by prior treatment with

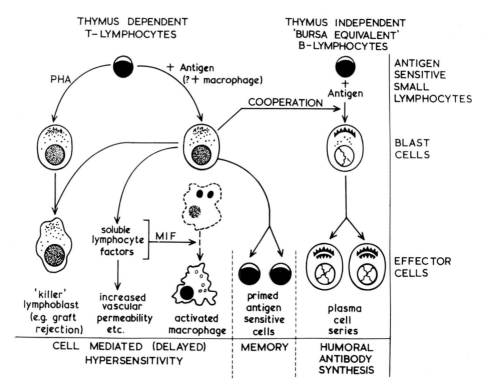

Fig. 9.2 A composite diagram illustrating how cell-mediated and humeral immunity are interrelated and defining the role of the T (thymus-dependent) and B (bursa-equivalent) lymphocytes. (From Roitt, Greaves, Torrigiani, Brostoff and Playfair, 1969, *Lancet*, **ii**, 367–371.)

unlabelled aggregated human γ-globulin or with rabbit anti-19S γ-globulin. Mellors *et al.* (1959) examined rheumatoid lymphoid cells in the same way and showed that rheumatoid factor could be identified in 1 of each 10 germinal centres as well as in internodular plasma cells. The localisation was confined to the cytoplasm of the plasma cells and to the characteristic protoplasmic processes of the germinal centre cells. In 8 of 10 germinal centres the γ-globulin identified was 7S and/or 19S. They subsequently suggested that the reactivity of two or more rheumatoid factors might be against different antigenic components of aggregated human gammaglobulin (Mellors *et al.*, 1961*a*) (Figs. 9.5, 9.6).

This work was extended and Mellors *et al.* (1961*b*) confirmed, by the same kind of analysis, that rheumatoid factor could be detected in some of the numerous plasma cells that abound in the synovial tissue of patients with active disease. Two 'reactants' were used: a fluorescein-conjugated antigen/rabbit antibody complex; and, as in the earlier work, a fluorescein conjugated aggregated human γ-globulin. Application of these 'reactants' to synovial, lymphoid germinal centre and internodular tissue confirmed that these were the sites of origin of (some) rheumatoid factor. Cells binding the immune complex were less common than those responding to the aggregated immunoglobulin. The macroglobulin of rheumatoid factor was found to be almost wholly cytoplasmic: this cellular origin suggested strongly its antibody nature. In a single case where a rheumatoid patient had died with amyloidosis (p. 164) precipitates that resembled antigen/antibody (IgG/IgM) complexes were found to be present in the amyloid deposits in the kidney and spleen. Opinion on the question as to whether the immunoglobulins in amyloid deposits are an integral part of the amyloid molecule remain conflicting (p. 164).

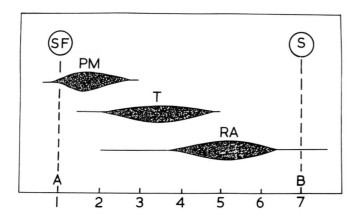

Fig. 9.3 Diagram indicating distribution of synovial fluid protein pattern by comparison with those of normal synovial fluid (SF) (position A) and normal serum (S) (position B). Total protein concentrations, relative concentration of α_2-acid glycoprotein, 19S α_2-glycoprotein and α_1/α_2 globulin ratios, are plotted in arbitrary units on the abscissa. Range of distribution, represented as a scattergram, is indicated by extension of corresponding areas in direction of abscissa (P.M.: post mortem non-traumatic; T: traumatic; R.A. rheumatoid arthritis). Width of figures in direction of ordinate gives rough measure of frequency of fluids at a given position. (Redrawn from Binette, J. P. and Schmid, K., 1965, *Arthr. and Rheum.*, **8**, 14–28, by permission of the authors.)

Further, very precise and critical studies of the site(s) of formation of rheumatoid factor in tissues were made by Kaplan (1963). Kaplan (1963) emphasised the differences between early and late findings, a distinction all too often neglected in the literature on rheumatoid arthritis. In the *early* disease, the evidence suggested that the presence in lymphoid tissue of aggregated γ-globulin might be the stimulus to rheumatoid factor (IgM) synthesis. Similarly, 7S but not 19S γ-globulin was deposited in the synovial and collagenous connective tissues in these early lesions at sites corresponding to the presence of fibrin. These results contrasted with those in the *late* disease where a massive distribution of 7S and 19S γ-globulins was found in the tissues of long-standing, sero-positive rheumatoid arthritis (Kaplan and Vaughan, 1962). Kaplan (1963) commented that the specificity of the γ-globulin accumulations in rheumatoid tissues should not be assumed. But, again, in rheumatoid nodules, as in rheumatoid synovia, 7S γ-globulin was present, closely associated with collagen, and in a manner suggesting an infiltration rather than an adsorption on cell surfaces. No 19S γ-globulin was detected.

Comparable investigations were reported by McCormick (1963). Rheumatoid factor was detected, both by fluorescent aggregated human gamma globulin and by normal or immune rabbit globulins, in lymph node and synovial plasma cells and in the intrinsic cells of reactive lymphoid follicles. McCormick considered that rheumatoid factor was of antibody nature and postulated that the factor might exert a protective action by complexing with anti-connective tissue auto-antibodies formed at another site.

During the past 5 years, efforts have concentrated on the analysis of the synovial tissues, searching for evidence locally not only of immunoglobulins that, as Kaplan (1963) pointed out, may accumulate nonspecifically, but also for identifiable components of complement. The presence, at a site of tissue injury, of fibrin, IgG and complement is generally regarded as adequate circumstantial evidence that cell damage at this site is of immunological origin. Fish *et al.*

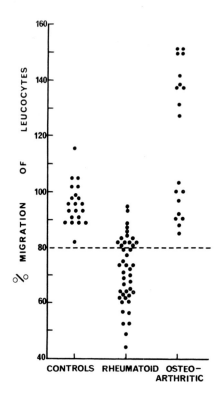

Fig. 9.4 Leucocyte migration in presence of preparations of membranes of *Mycoplasma fermentans*. White cells from rheumatoid, osteoarthritic and healthy, control patients are compared. In the presence of *M fermentans* membranes, rheumatoid leucocyte migration is inhibited. The positive test can be regarded as indicating a state of cell-mediated immunity to antigenic components of *M. fermentans*. By contrast, serological tests for circulating humoral anti-mycoplasma antibodies do not clearly differentiate rheumatoid from controls and patients with osteoarthritis. (From Williams, Brostoff and Roitt, 1970, *Lancet*, **ii**, 277–280.)

(1966), for example, studied the synovium of 8 children and of 7 adults, searching for evidence of the localisation of immunoglobulins and of complement (Tables 9.1 and 9.2). Three cases were found to have complement and immunoglobulins within the cytoplasm of synovial cells; 4 showed discrete localisation within the connective tissue stroma; and in the remaining 7 there were larger, weakly-staining collections spread more diffusely throughout the synovium. Ten of 11 control synovia displayed no immunoglobulin or complement localisation. Sliwinski and Zvaifler (1970) also established the synthesis of IgG by rheumatoid synovium. Nowoslawski and Brzosko (1967a) made comparable analyses, showing that all germinal centres in rheumatoid

TABLE 9.1. *Immunofluorescent studies of juvenile rheumatoid arthritis synovium*

Morphology	Case	Gamma G globulin	Beta 1C globulin	Rheuma-toid factor	Gamma M globulin	Gamma A globulin
Cellular deposits	1	1+	1+	o	tr	o
	2	1+	1–2+	—	o	o
Discrete noncellular deposits	3	1–2+	1–2+	—	—	—
Amorphous deposits	4	2+	2+	—	—	—
	5	tr	1–2+	tr	o	o
	6	o	2+	o	1+	o
	7	o	2–3+	o	tr–1+	o
Negative	8	o	o	o	o	o

(From Fish *et al.*, 1966, *Arthr. and Rheum.* **9**, 267–280.)

TABLE 9.2. *Immunofluorescent studies of rheumatoid arthritis synovium in adults*

Morphology	Case	Gamma G globulin	Beta IC globulin	Rheuma-toid factor	Gamma M globulin	Gamma A globulin
Cellular deposits	9	1+	tr	o	1+	o
Discrete noncellular deposits	10	2–3+	o	2+	1+	o
	11	2–3+	1+	tr–1+	tr–1+	o
	12	1–2+	o	1–2+	1+	o
Amorphous deposits	13	2+	2+	o	tr	o
	14	2+	1+	1+	tr	o
	15	2+	2+	tr	o	o

(From Fish *et al.*, 1966, *Arthr. and Rheum.* **9**, 267–280.)

synovial tissue contain and can be assumed to synthesise IgM and IgG immunoglobulins with rheumatoid factor specificity. Plasma cells producing IgM only were more common than those containing both IgM and IgG immunoglobulins. The number of cells forming IgG was roughly equivalent to the number producing rheumatoid factor: the majority reacted with aggregated human IgG, the remainder reacting only with a heterologous immune complex formed with rabbit antibody or simultaneously with both human aggregated immunoglobulin and heterologous complex.

Nowoslawski and Brzosko (1967a) concluded that the rheumatoid synovial inflammatory cell infiltrate may result from prolonged local antigenic stimulation, the source of the antigen being, apparently, from within the joint cavity. This view, they thought, would tend to favour the role of fibrin (p. 18) or of the other products of inflammation as initiators of the prolonged local inflammatory reaction rather than the activity of a synovial cell viral antigen. Nowoslawski and Brzosko (1967a) extended their observations to rheumatoid subcutaneous granulomata (p. 122) and deduced that the exudation and tissue destruction of these lesions are the consequences of an interaction between IgG as autoantigen and rheumatoid factor as autoantibody (Nowoslawski and Brzosko, 1967b).

Kazakova, Orlovskaya and Pavlov (1967) reached essentially the same conclusions as Nowoslawski and Brzosko (1967a). The intensity of rheumatoid factor deposition in synovial tissue varied, they found, with the local histological activity of the disease, and with the stage of the disease and was higher in cases of longer duration. Bonomo, Tursi and Gillardi (1968) examined synovial biopsies from 43 rheumatoid patients and identified anti-γ-globulin in three patterns which they termed (a) sparse; (b) lymphoid; and (c) vascular. These patterns and their terminology reflected the associated histological alterations. Anti-γ-globulin concentration was greatest in the main sites of inflammatory disease activity: i.e. in contrasting rheumatoid arthritis with other inflammatory states they found most anti-γ-globulin in the synovium in rheumatoid arthritis, in the liver in liver disease, in the bone marrow in macroglobulinaemia and in the polymorphs of the sputum in chronic bronchitis. They also observed that cells binding both

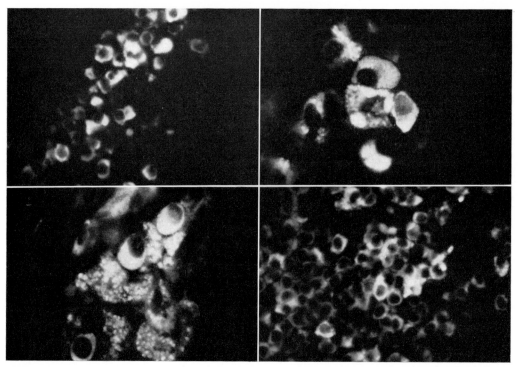

Fig. 9.5   Immunofluorescent localisation of immunoglobulins and rheumatoid factor in rheumatoid synovial tissue. (*Top left*) Rheumatoid factor in plasma cells. (*Top right*) IgM immunoglobulin in synovial plasma cells. Note autofluorescence of macrophage (*centre*). (*Bottom left*) Rheumatoid factor in plasma cells. Note granular autofluorescence of macrophages. (*Bottom right*) IgM immunoglobulin in plasma cells and plasmablasts. (From preparations of Dr. John McCormick.)

aggregated human γ-globulin and rabbit γ-globulin were detected in rheumatoid arthritis not only in the synovium but also in liver. Very similar conclusions were reached by Friis (1968, 1969) using synovial tissue that, like the preparations of Ball *et al.* (1963), had been fixed in alcohol.

There can be no serious doubt therefore that the synovial tissues of cases of active rheumatoid arthritis commonly contain cells that morphologically are 'plasma cells' but which may presumably be either plasmacytes or lymphoblasts; and that these cells contain, and are apparently secreting, anti-IgG immunoglobulins of IgM (rheumatoid factor) type. These observations, together with the investigations of synovial fluid leucocytes described on p. 102, establish that immune complexes commonly exist both in synovial fluid leucocytes and in relation to the immunologically competent cells infiltrating the synovia.

Studies of articular cartilage by immunofluorescence microscopy appear to have been restricted to the investigation of normal and of osteoarthrotic material (Barland, Janis and Sandson, 1966).

On the assumption that the focus for injury in rheumatoid arthritis is the lining, synovial cell layer (p. 38) (and this is not established unequivocally), it remains to prove that immune complexes capable of binding complement and thus of attracting polymorphs and activating or perpetuating inflammation, are present in relation to these synovial cells. Evidence that strongly supports this hypothesis has been obtained by a number of authors including Kinsella, Baum and Ziff (1969). Using synovial tissue obtained by needle biopsy and digested with trypsin, cell

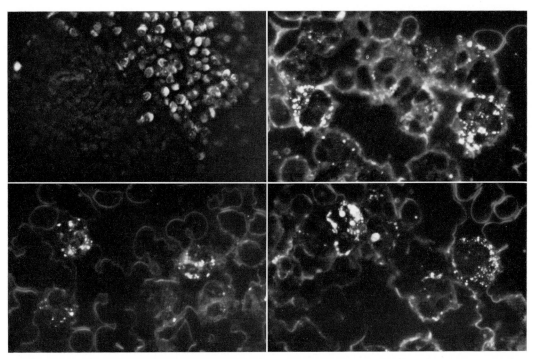

Fig. 9.6 Immunofluorescent localisation of immunoglobulins, of complement and of rheumatoid factor in rheumatoid synovial tissue and in cells of synovial fluid. (*Top left*) Rheumatoid factor in perivascular lymphoid aggregate. (*Top right*) IgM immunoglobulin in cells of synovial fluid. (*Bottom left*) IgM immunoglobulin in synovial fluid cells. (*Bottom right*) $\beta_1c(C'_3)$ component of complement in synovial fluid cells. (From preparations of Dr. John McCormick.)

suspensions were tested with immunofluorescent reagents. The simultaneous presence of IgG immunoglobulin and of the β_1C component of complement was demonstrated in the cytoplasm of most of the A(M) (phagocytic) cells of the synovia in 15 of 17 samples from both sero-positive and sero-negative patients. In the sero-positive cases, discrete cytoplasmic inclusions were found composed of IgG immunoglobulin and the β_1C component, or of IgG with rheumatoid factor.

Although the formation of immune complexes in rheumatoid synovial tissue and their presence in synovial fluid seems certain, it is not clear that the lesions of rheumatoid arthritis are analogous with those of experimental immune complex disease (Germuth and Pollack, 1967). It is however thought that complexes formed in these sites are rapidly phagocytosed. The evidence relating to the phagocytosis of immune complexes by synovial polymorphs is discussed on p. 102. The data of Kinsella, Baum and Ziff (1969), among others, confirms that a similar process is commonplace within synovial cells. The phagocytosis of complexes, themselves chemotactic to polymorphs through the activation of components $C'3$, $C'4$ and $C'5$ of complement, can itself be a potent factor in exaggerating tissue injury. Thus, particularly in dyslytic states in which phago-cytes are engorged with material engulfed by endocytosis (p. 111), acid lysosomal hydrolases are released and activated. Williamson and Ling (1965) found that when IgG/IgM complexes such as those formed by the interaction of rheumatoid factor and aggregated IgG, are ingested by leucocytes, lysosomal enzymes are liberated into the surrounding medium. The phagocytosis of immune complexes therefore appears to offer one attractive explanation for the high lysosomal enzyme activity recognised in rheumatoid synovial fluid and one explanation for the abnormally high lysosomal enzyme activity now known to be characteristic of the synovial cells at the margin of the articular cartilage (p. 117). Much is now known of the relationship between rheumatoid factor activity and the binding of complement (Messner *et al.*, 1969)—for example, a dissociable factor can induce complement fixation by rheumatoid red blood cells *in vitro* (Gilliland and Turner, 1969)—and rheumatoid factor may interact indirectly with components of complement (Messner *et al.*, 1969) just as it attaches to the Fc portion of IgG antibody, the opsonic site, inhibiting bacterial phagocytosis. The available evidence favours the view that a common con-sequence of this binding process is phagocytosis leading to lysosomal enzyme activation.

Disordered immunoglobulin synthesis (Fig. 9.3)

Occasional patients with rheumatoid arthritis have increased levels of free light chains in the serum, due to increased γ-globulin synthesis. The association of rheumatoid arthritis and myelomatosis is however rare and probably coincidental (p. 155). Patients with hypogamma-globulinaemia may develop rheumatoid arthritis or other systemic disorders of the connective tissue system, evidence which supports the view that the synovitis is influenced by cell-mediated immunological mechanisms rather than by circulating antibodies (Rotstein and Good, 1962).* In a unique report, Zawadzki, Benedek, Ein and Easton (1969) described a male negro patient of 42 who developed rheumatoid arthritis and, at the age of 51, heavy chain disease. No evidence of a malignant tumour of the lymphoid tissues was recognised. The authors suggested that the published evidence, which they survey, supports the view that heavy chain disease may be an intermediate evolutionary form between plasma cell myeloma and malignant lymphoma. The association between longstanding rheumatoid arthritis and the heavy chain disease they think may not be purely coincidental.

Cellular immunity and rheumatoid synovitis (Figs. 9.2, 9.4)

The established synovial lesions in rheumatoid arthritis have always brought to mind the histological changes recognised during a delayed hypersensitivity response such as that typified by the skin reaction, in a sensitive patient, to the intradermal reaction of tuberculoprotein. How-ever, it has proved to be very much less easy to obtain adequate evidence for the existence of a cell-mediated immunological tissue-damaging mechanism in rheumatoid arthritis than to estab-lish the local secretion of immunoglobulins and the phagocytosis of immune complexes (Stroescu and Mihailescu, 1970). Even now, there is no certainty that those features of cell-mediated immunity in rheumatoid arthritis that have been shown to be present are anything more than incidental phenomena in the course of a longstanding inflammatory disease, phenomena which may in fact be provoked, as may the persistent inflammation itself (p. 203), by sensitisation to the mediators of the inflammatory reaction (Philips, Kaklamanis and Glynn, 1966; Willoughby

* But see A. R. Rich's penetrating criticism of the paper by Janeway *et al.* (1956) on the occurrence of 'collagen diseases' in children with hypogammaglobulinaemia.

and Ryan, 1970). Nevertheless, the frequency of rheumatoid arthritis in agammaglobulinaemia (Good and Rotstein, 1960; Rotstein and Good, 1962) has always appeared to be important circumstantial evidence for the involvement of cellular immunological reactivity.

During the past 2 years, considerable progress has been made in analysing the delayed hypersensitivity reaction now known to be mediated by sensitised lymphocytes, by the use of a leucocyte migration inhibition test (M.I.T.). Considerable information, incidentally, has become available concerning the physiology of leucocytes in such circumstances (Bodel *et al.*, 1966). In this procedure white cells, harvested from the peripheral blood, are encouraged to migrate outwards into a culture medium from the end of a capillary tube (Bendixen and Søborg, 1969). In the presence of antigen to which the patient has developed allergy, leucocyte migration is inhibited; an inhibition 'index' can be calculated by planimetric measurement of the zone of spreading. By adopting a microtechnique, sufficient white cells can be obtained from 10 to 15 ml. of blood to permit tests to be conducted with very small amounts of any antigen that it is wished to examine (Federlin, Maini, Russell and Dumonde, 1971).

The M.I.T. has been applied to the white cells of patients with rheumatoid arthritis in attempts to demonstrate a state of delayed hypersensitivity to antigens such as those of the corynebacteria recognised within rheumatoid synovial cells (Maini, Stewart and Dumonde, 1970; Rothenberger and Thiele, 1970). So far, no evidence is available that rheumatoid lymphocytes are more sensitive to these organisms than to other, control corynebacteria; however, a comparable study of leucocyte behaviour in response to the sonicated cell membranes of mycoplasmataceae isolated from cases of rheumatoid arthritis has revealed significant migration inhibition in 67% of tests in 43 patients (Williams, Brostoff and Roitt, 1970), suggesting that the chronicity of the disease, at least, is due to an hypersensitivity response to this organism.

A further method for detecting cell mediated immunity that has been applied to the cells of rheumatoid arthritis patients is the lymphocyte transformation test. Lymphocytes in a resting state can be transformed nonspecifically to blast cells by exposure to agents such as phytohaemaglutinin. The transformed cells have large nuclei rich in DNA and abundant cytoplasmic RNA, actively synthesising protein. An identical but specific transformation can be brought about by exposing lymphocytes to an antigen to which they have previously been specifically sensitised. In this way, allergic responsiveness to suspected antigens can be sought. The test has been made quantitative by incorporating ^{3}H-thymidine in the culture medium during the period following the introduction of antigen. The number of labelled cells or the proportion of isotope incorporated can be measured by liquid scintillation counting. The application of such tests for the detection of lymphocyte transformation by suspected antigens or lymphokine factors in rheumatoid arthritis is in its infancy (Maini *et al.*, 1969). The results obtained by Lycette and Pearmain (1965) were incomplete. However, Astorga and Williams (1969) investigated the lymphocytes from 22 patients with rheumatoid arthritis and found that 14 showed evidence of antigenic stimulation, indicated by transformation, when cells from patients with unrelated diseases were added to the rheumatoid cells in culture. Sixteen of 22 patients reacted in the same way when rheumatoid cells were cultured with normal cells, but when rheumatoid cells were added to cultures of normal cells 19 of 22 displayed transformation. Astorga and Williams concluded that there was evidence that some rheumatoid patients' lymphocytes provoked mutual lymphocytic stimulation when studied with cells from other patients. Presumably, this supports the hypothesis that a feature of rheumatoid arthritis, and perhaps one cause of synovial tissue injury, is cell-mediated immunity to an, as yet, unidentified antigen.

By contrast, there is considerable support for the view that cellular immunity in rheumatoid arthritis is impaired; the impairment may be a result of nonspecific debility (Jennings, 1971).

Rheumatoid factor and tissue injury

The serum proteins in rheumatoid arthritis commonly show a number of alterations (p. 108). An increase in the globulin fractions is frequent and among the abnormal globulins are found an IgM iso-antibody; C-reactive protein; and antinuclear factors. Cecil and his colleagues in the early 1930's had isolated streptococcal strains from rheumatoid tissues. They showed that anti-streptococcal antibodies could be detected in the sera of many active cases, an association that implied an aetiological affinity with rheumatic fever in which experimental evidence for the role of an immunological mechanism had been obtained by Klinge (1929, 1930a, b, c, 1933, 1934) and others. However, the circulating antibacterial antibodies in rheumatoid arthritis were found to be equally active in agglutinating staphylococci; the nonspecificity of the streptococcal agglutination test in this disease was consequently acknowledged.

During investigations of these serological phenomena Waaler (1940) found that rheumatoid sera would agglutinate not only bacteria but also sensitised red blood cells, a phenomena redis-covered independently by Rose and his colleagues (1948) and quickly established as the basis of a nonspecific diagnostic test for rheumatoid arthritis. The circulating 'rheumatoid factor'(Vaughan, 1969) responsible for this agglutination of antibody-coated sheep or rabbit red cells was found to be a gamma globulin of molecular weight approximately 900,000 and with a sedimentation constant of 19S in the analytical ultracentrifuge. Subsequently, immunoelectrophoresis estab-lished that the globulin 'factor' was an IgM immunoglobulin with a nonspecific affinity for IgG antibody globulin that had been uncoiled by procedures such as heating, or for IgG antibody altered by combination with specific antigen. The macroglobulin could be shown to combine *in vitro* with altered IgG immunoglobulin and tended to exist *in vivo* as a larger IgG/IgM complex having a sedimentation constant of approximately 22S. The site at which rheumatoid factor is believed to combine with the IgG antigen is located within the Fc fraction of the IgG immunoglobulin molecule (Walton, 1968b).

The IgM immunoglobulin of rheumatoid factor, it is now clear, is an antibody against auto-logous, uncoiled IgG. It has a strong, nonspecific affinity for connective tissue (Svartz, 1969, 1970). Rheumatoid factor is present in the synovial fluid and reaches this situation from the blood (Hannestad and Mellbye, 1967). Rheumatoid factor is also synthesised locally. In the sense that the factor is an autologous antibody, it is an autoantibody; to this extent the serological distur-bances characteristic of rheumatoid arthritis can be said to indicate that this is an autoallergic disease. However, comparable IgM rheumatoid factor-like substances and antiglobulins of the IgG and IgA groups are formed in other chronic diseases and it is by no means clear whether rheumatoid factor, found inconstantly in rheumatoid arthritis but usually in those patients with severe disease, is fundamentally related to the pathogenesis of the disorder or whether it is an incidental consequence of it.

Kellgren and Ball (1959) suggested that the presence of rheumatoid factor, detectable in a proportion of the population that does not have rheumatoid arthritis, may indicate an inherited abnormality of protein metabolism predisposing to the disease (Burch, 1968). On the other hand, rheumatoid factor *activity* (that is, anti-IgG iso-antibody activity, as distinct from defined IgM rheumatoid factor) develops not only with time in older persons but also occasionally, in related conditions such as systemic lupus erythematosus and in a number of apparently *unrelated* diseases such as subacute bacterial endocarditis, leprosy, syphilis, chronic liver disease, sarcoidosis and visceral larval migrans (Messner, Laxdal, Quie and Williams, 1968). In these circumstances the formation of anti-IgG rheumatoid factor *activity* may represent no more than a response to high IgG levels in sustained infection and is unlikely to be related to the precise nature of the infective agent. This view is supported by the observation that activity has also been shown in noninfective conditions such as the postrenal transplant state (Waller *et al.*, 1965).

The significance of rheumatoid factor formation for the pathogenesis of rheumatoid arthritis remains debatable. The problem is discussed more fully on p. 195. Hollingsworth (1968) comments that the only systemic complication caused directly by a high rheumatoid factor titre is the hyperviscosity syndrome (Abruzzo *et al.*, 1970).

Rheumatoid factor apparently exists *in vivo* as an antigen/antibody complex. It is seldom present early in rheumatoid arthritis (Kaplan, 1963) but is found more frequently with time. Rheumatoid arthritis with subcutaneous nodule formation usually displays the presence of rheumatoid factor (sero-positivity). An association has also been shown between other lesions encountered in rheumatoid arthritis such as digital arterial obstruction and diffuse interstitial pulmonary fibrosis. In general, the presence of rheumatoid factor correlates with continuous, active disease judged by the number of joints involved, X-ray progression and loss of functional capacity (Cats and Hazevoet, 1970) but the role of the factor in mediating tissue damage is disputed. It may be, of course, that technical difficulties such as insensitive measurements have led to the neglect of the possible formation of other classes (IgG, IgA) of antiglobulins in rheumatoid arthritis, as Roitt has suggested, and that the time of formation, specificity and titre of these immunoglobulins might correlate better with tissue damage than is evident when only the IgM immunoglobulins are considered.

Some evidence relating to the role of the antiglobulins in causing tissue damage has been obtained from the demonstration that aggregated γ-globulins exposed to rheumatoid factor in synovial fluid form complexes that are readily phagocytosed *in vitro* by white blood cells (Vaughan, Jacox and Clark, 1969). The evidence is considered more fully on p. 102. Complicated experiments, conducted on patients with rheumatoid arthritis have shown that when altered IgG γ-globulin from one rheumatoid patient is injected locally into a non-inflamed joint of another patient with this disease, local inflammation is produced provided that (1) the recipient has circulating rheumatoid factor and that (2) recipient and donor have in common at least 2 inherited Gm factors (Hollander *et al.*, 1966). If the recipient is sero-negative, if more than two Gm factors do not match or if normal, instead of altered IgG γ-globulin, matched for at least two inherited Gm factors, is injected, then no inflammatory reaction is caused.

By contrast with those studies that have shown that rheumatoid factor is localised in joint tissues in rheumatoid arthritis and which suggest that the factor may be responsible for joint damage, there is some conflicting evidence that the factor may have protective properties. Thus, it has been found that rheumatoid factor under some circumstances inhibits complement fixation. The binding of complement is a process normally necessary for injuries, such as those of the Arthus phenomenon, caused by antigen/antibody interactions in tissues and probably due to activation of $C'5$, 6 and 7. The corollary, that complement prevents the adsorption of rheumatoid factor by altered human γ-globulin, has also been demonstrated. In other experiments it has been recognised that after the intraperitoneal injection of aggregated human γ-globulin, rheumatoid factor may inhibit the lowering of serum complement, diminishing the immunological effect of the injection. However, when aggregates of human γ-globulin are given intravenously, complement depression is not modified by the factor. These studies have led to the view that rheumatoid factor may have a protective effect extravascularly in sites such as the synovial space and that in these situations the factor may assist phagocytosis, perhaps by limiting the damaging action of antibody/antigen interaction.

A tendency for sero-positive patients to fare unfavourably (Duthie *et al.*, 1967) and a correlation between the presence of rheumatoid factor and of subcutaneous nodules is often accepted as circumstantial evidence supporting the idea that the factor may be harmful. The presence of the rheumatoid factor macroglobulin and of the third and fourth components of complement can be shown in or near rheumatoid synovial cells by immunofluorescent techniques (p. 97). It is *very* difficult to be certain of the function of these immunological agents in this situation. It has always appeared possible, nevertheless, that the macroglobulin, which is remarkably nonspecific in its capacity to react with denatured IgG, may play a part in the early tissue injuries of rheumatoid arthritis.

McCormick *et al.* (1969) have produced important circumstantial evidence that rheumatoid serum can act synergistically to injure tissues by demonstrating that nephrotoxic nephritis is exacerbated when rheumatoid factor is given simultaneously with nephrotoxic globulin. However, other *in vitro* investigations suggest that the factor impairs complement fixation, preventing injury to complement-sensitive mitochondrial systems (Davis and Bollet, 1964; Gough and Davis, 1966). It may therefore possess a protective action in immunological tissue injuries such as rheumatoid vasculitis that may be produced by antigen/antibody complexes. Against this view, again, is evidence that the localisation of complement in rheumatoid synovia corresponds to the situation of IgG γ-globulin but not to that of rheumatoid factor (Rofman *et al.*, 1967).

Among the few injurious effects that can be attributed to the presence of high titres of circulating rheumatoid factor, is the development of the hyperviscosity syndrome (Meltzer *et al.*, 1966; Hollingsworth, 1968; Jasin, LoSpalluto and Ziff, 1970). Hypergammaglobulinaemia with abundant rheumatoid factor causes raised plasma viscosity, a bleeding diathesis and, occasionally, vasculitis. The pathogenesis of this rare syndrome is attributable to the union of rheumatoid factor with intermediate immune complexes to form large molecular conglomerates.

Rheumatoid arthritis (RA) cells ('ragocytes')

In nearly all the unstained preparations of rheumatoid synovial fluid searched for crystal inclusions, Hollander and his colleagues found 0·5–1·5 μm granules within the numerous white blood cells (Hollander, McCarty, Astorga and Castro-Murillo, 1965). Ninety-five per cent of the rheumatoid fluids tested contained leucocytes within which were inclusions, the proportion of cells having such inclusions varying, in individual fluids, from 3 to 97%. The majority of the inclusion positive cells were polymorphs that retained their mobility and were distinct from degenerate cells. The included granules did not contain RNA but the positive cells, which resembled 'glitter' cells (granular motility cells) were sometimes difficult to distinguish from the inclusion cells of septic or gouty joints.

Leucocytes from rheumatoid synovial fluid in which these 'rheumatoid arthritis' (RA) cells had been indentified, yielded rheumatoid factor, identified by a latex fixation test, after washing and sonication. These observations brought to mind the demonstration by Parker and Schmid (1962) that precipitates of heat-aggregated gammaglobulin and rheumatoid factor underwent phagocytosis *in vitro*, a phenomenon which could not be caused when albumin was substituted for serum or when either serum or rheumatoid factor were absent. Parker and Schmid interpreted their observations to show the similar treatment accorded to immune complexes and to rheumatoid factor–gammaglobulin aggregates by phagocytes. Their observations, they thought, supported the suggestion that rheumatoid factor macroglobulin was an anti-7S (IgG)-gammaglobulin antibody.

Hollander *et al.* (1965) had, therefore, fortuitously confirmed that rheumatoid immune complexes produced intracellular aggregates sufficiently large to be recognisable by light microscopy.

Extending this work, Rawson, Abelson and Hollander (1965) examined 55 synovial fluids and detected 7S/19S globulin particulate material in 75% (29 cases) of rheumatoid arthritis and in 88% of synovial fluids from the variants (p. 168) of rheumatoid arthritis that they tested. Osteo-arthrotic, septic and pseudo-gout synovial fluids were negative but 2 gouty fluids of 5 were positive. These figures were, broadly speaking, confirmed by Delbarre, Kahan, Amor and Krassinine (1964) working independently. These authors introduced the term 'ragocyte' rather than RA cell and showed that the inclusion-positive phagocyte was recognisable in only 1 of 15 control synovial fluids, but that they were almost always present in fluids from sero-positive rheumatoid arthritics and from cases of Felty's syndrome. In Reiter's syndrome, psoriatic arthropathy and gout the fluids were found not to contain ragocytes.

It appeared at first that the presence of RA cells in a synovial fluid might be of diagnostic significance (Astorga and Bollet, 1964). However, this early view is now in doubt since ragocytes have been identified in a number of other conditions and in sero-negative as well as in sero-positive rheumatoid arthritis. Thus, Fallet, Boussina and Fellman (1968), examining 67 rheuma-toid and 73 other synovial fluids, identified RA cells in 94% of sero-positive cases but in 85% of sero-negative. Similar cells were found less often in other conditions. Fallet et al. preferred the term 'ragocyte' to 'RA cell', a view that would appear to support the strong criticism by Bluhm and Zawadzki (1969) of the application to these cells of any kind of terminology implying speci-ficity. Fallet et al. believe that not all the inclusions observed in rheumatoid synovial leucocytes are, in fact, immune complexes.

Whatever the specificity of the original 'ragocyte', the phenomenon led Restifo, Lussier, Rawson, Rockey and Hollander (1965) to elegant studies in which the pathogenetic significance of their intracellular synovial leucocyte complexes was examined, experiments that have been extended by other workers with inconclusive results. Aggregated or non-aggregated autologous gammaglobulin was injected into the clinically uninvolved knees of a series of sero-positive rheumatoid patients. If the synovial fluid contained rheumatoid factor, then immune complexes, it was postulated, should have formed. The complexes, in turn, would be phagocytosed and phagocytosis would provoke the activation and liberation of leucocytic lysosomal enzymes. These enzymes, it was believed, (p. 113) might be the cause of the synovial inflammation in rheumatoid arthritis. The limited clinical evidence that emerged from these experiments supported this view. Five of 6 cases given autologous rheumatoid gammaglobulin developed acute inflammation. Purified rheumatoid gammaglobulin caused no reaction in osteoarthrotic knees nor was inflam-mation caused by homologous rheumatoid 7S gammaglobulin injected into an uninvolved knee. However, 'purified' (and consequently 'uncoiled') non-rheumatoid gammaglobulin injected into uninvolved rheumatoid knees was inflammatory in 5 of 6 cases.

The evidence, which clearly implied the role of an inherited antigenic determinant in the production of tissue-damaging immune complexes in rheumatoid arthritis, has remained con-troversial. The view that immune complexes can cause tissue injury by activating lysosomal hydrolases (p. 113) has however been substantially extended (Astorga and Bollet, 1965). Thus, cell abnormalities are detectable in the aqueous humour of patients with rheumatoid arthritis and iridocyclitis (Wirostko and Johnson, 1970). This observation suggests that cytotoxic immunological mechanisms may cause injury in sites other than the synovium and subcutaneous tissue. Astorga and Bollet (1965) found that homogenates of ragocytes gave positive tests for rheumatoid arthritis, 15 of whom were sero- and synovial fluid-negative (14 of 71 control cases gave positive tests). On the other hand, a 'rheumatoid rosette' test devised by Bach, Delrieu and Delbarre (1970) gave comparable results for seropositive and seronegative cases. The demonstration that rheumatoid factor (Fraction II globulin precipitates) activates lysosomal enzymes in vitro appears to support the concept that similar enzymes are activated and can cause rheumatoid synovitis *in vivo* (Astorga and Bollet, 1965).

The inclusions of RA cells have been studied by immunofluorescence microscopy (Krassinine, 1966) and by electron microscopy (Zucker–Franklin, 1966) (p. 52) but the electron microscopic studies have failed to distinguish the inclusions of RA cells from the numerous other grey-globular bodies and the phagosomes present in rheumatoid synovial leucocytes. Evidence that the leucocyte gammaglobulin inclusion body phenomenon was not specific for rheumatoid arthritis led Vaughan, Barnett, Sobel and Jacox (1968) and Vaughan (1969) to an extensive survey to determine the nature of the inclusions both in rheumatoid arthritis and in other conditions. Complement (C'3) was detectable within synovial leucocytes in 50% of cases examined, both in rheumatoid and non-rheumatoid cells. In those cases of rheumatoid arthritis in which the serum latex test for rheumatoid factor was positive, intracellular IgM immunoglobulin was more frequent than in sero-negative cases. Furthermore, all joint fluids having low complement activity displayed the presence of gammaglobulin inclusions in synovial fluid leucocytes. This observation accorded with the suggestion that the characteristically low relative levels of synovial fluid complement in rheumatoid arthritis were attributable to the continual local consumption or adsorption of complement during the union of rheumatoid factor with specific IgG antigen (Winchester *et al.*, 1969; Zvaifler, 1969). The formation of complexes could, in this way, be held to account both for the development of the granular 'RA' inclusion bodies and, initially, for leucocyte migration, an aggregation promoted by the known chemotactic properties of C'3 and C'4.

The role of rheumatoid factor in promoting the phagocytosis of material from synovial fluids was further explored by Hurd, LoSpalluto and Ziff (1970). Normal polymorphs phagocytosed IgG, IgM and β_1C (C'3)-containing inclusions from the synovial fluid of seropositive cases but not from cases where the fluid did not contain rheumatoid factor. The addition of rheumatoid factor to these negative fluids promoted the formation of complexes that could be phagocytosed so that it seemed reasonable to assume that altered IgG molecules were present in effusions devoid of autologous rheumatoid factor.

Antinuclear factors

The possibility that other autoantibodies in addition to rheumatoid factor contribute to the cellular phenomena in rheumatoid joints has also been examined. Thus, antinuclear factors (ANF) with an affinity for granulocyte nuclei have been identified both in rheumatoid synovial fluids and in sera (Barnett, Bienenstock and Bloch, 1966; Faber and Elling, 1966; McSween *et al.*, 1968; Elling, Graudal and Faber, 1968) but whether these factors influence synovial leucocyte structure is improbable. Positive tests are very common in Felty's syndrome. It is more likely that ANF are formed as a result of leucocyte injury following lysosomal activation. The frequency with which ANF are demonstrable has varied considerably. Faber and Elling (1966) based their conclusions on a survey of 30 sera reacting specifically with polymorphs, including sera from 14 cases of rheumatoid arthritis. Barnett *et al.* (1966) found ANF activity in 9 of 21 rheumatoid synovial fluids. McSween *et al.* (1968) stated that 28% of 161 rheumatoid arthritis sera contained ANF activity, 22% of synovial fluids. In 75% the ANF activity was in the IgM fraction, in 22% in the IgG and in 3% in both. In 3 patients, activity was demonstrable in the synovial fluid only and in one of these activity was detected in only 1 of 2 joints tested. This important evidence, they believe, suggests that ANF may be formed locally. Condemni *et al.* (1965) reported 35% of ANF-positive sera in 68 patients. Elling, Graudal and Faber (1968), perhaps using tests of greater sensitivity, recognised ANF activity in 64% of rheumatoid sera and in 62% of rheumatoid synovial fluids. There was significantly less reaction with nuclei other than those of polymorphs and the organ specificity of ANF activity detected in systemic lupus erythematosus was not recognised in rheumatoid sera. Granulocyte specificity of the ANF activity was shown to be correlated with low synovial fluid polymorph- but not with synovial fluid mononuclear-counts.

CHAPTER 10

Chemical Pathology

A substantial number of chemical abnormalities have been demonstrated in rheumatoid arthritis. It remains quite uncertain whether any or all of these disturbances are related to the pathogenesis of the disease or whether they are secondary consequences of a type found in other comparable crippling, chronic disorders. Because of the improbability of finding patients for biochemical investigation at the onset of the rheumatoid arthritis it is always important to bear in mind that longterm therapy with anti-inflammatory or analgesic drugs may have influenced the metabolic pathways being investigated. This makes it very difficult to explain these abnormalities with any degree of certainty on the basis of what is known of the molecular pathology of the disease.

West (1970) has recently surveyed the whole field of disordered biochemistry in rheumatoid arthritis. The short account that follows owes much to his careful analysis and, for convenience, follows a similar classification of chemical compounds.

Fibrous proteins. Hydroxyproline is an important part of the collagen macromolecule. In disorders such as rheumatoid arthritis in which the musculoskeletal structure of the body is disturbed, it has long been suspected that the turnover of collagen and the metabolism and excretion of breakdown products such as the numerous known hydroxyproline-containing peptides and polypeptides, might be abnormal. There is limited, conflicting evidence for this view: it would accord with the classical suggestion that rheumatoid arthritis and related diseases might be system disorders of collagen. Although prolyl-hydroxyproline and the end-products of collagen metabolism are excreted in the urine normally in rheumatoid arthritis (Bienenstock and Kilbrick, 1969) earlier evidence of an abnormal pattern of urinary peptides had been presented (Kilbrick, Hashiro and Safier, 1962). The synovial fluid hydroxyproline concentration is raised (Igari, Tsuchizawa, Obara and Ono, 1968). Levels of plasma free- and peptide-hydroxyproline are unchanged but protein hydroxyproline is raised as it is in other comparable skeletal diseases (LeRoy and Sjoerdsma, 1965).

Very little is known of the biochemistry of the reticular fibres, of basement membrane material, or of elastin and elastic material in rheumatoid arthritis. The light microscopic distinction between reticular and collagen fibrils on the basis of silver impregnation techniques is puzzling for the electron microscopist and biochemist: chemically, reticular material may be a form of collagen and perhaps a precursor comparable with tropocollagen. West (1970) dismisses elastin as a connective tissue element of little importance in rheumatoid arthritis. This may not be wholly correct: arterial and pulmonary disease are commonplace rheumatoid disturbances. Elasto-genesis is likely to be a significant factor in vascular and lung repair, elastic breakdown an important contributor to their pathogenesis. If this is accepted, then disorders such as copper deficiency, the experimental influence of amine oxidase inhibitors such as the aminoproprionitriles and the methods now being used for the analyses of these conditions are seen to be relevant to the study of some of the tissue abnormalities of rheumatoid arthritis (Kadar and Gardner, 1970; Kadar, Bush and Gardner, 1971; Kadar, Gardner and Bush, 1971*a, b*).

Connective tissue matrix. The literature has been reviewed (Muir, 1971). There is limited evidence in rheumatoid arthritis of a generalised defect in the biosynthesis of intercellular, non-fibrous material (West, 1970). Physiological support for this view has been obtained from tests of skin permeability and charge density (Bywaters, Holborow and Keech, 1951; Herp *et al.*, 1966; Laskin *et al.*, 1961). That rheumatoid arthritis is a systemic disorder of intercellular material has long been suggested (Klemperer, 1955). The pathological lesions encountered in rheumatoid arthritis are, however, mainly of a focal character. The significance of the generalised disturbance of skin physiology is that it offers an explanation for one way in which joint trauma, local vascular change or immunological insult not capable of disturbing normal connective tissue, could nevertheless cause regional connective tissue injury in a rheumatoid person.

The excretion of hexosamine, one indication of glycosaminoglycan turnover, was found at an early date to be raised both in rheumatoid arthritis and in other comparable diseases (Boas, Bollet and Bunim, 1955). A raised excretion of non-dialysable polysaccharide fragments including chondroitin-4 and chondroitin-6 sulphates was subsequently recognised (Thompson and Castor, 1966). The inconstant urinary excretion of total glycosaminoglycan reported by DiFerrante (1967) in rheumatoid arthritis has been found in other diseases. However, Bitter (1969) confirmed by the 9-aminoacridine precipitation method of Muir, that there was a greatly increased urinary excretion of glycosaminoglycans in severe rheumatoid arthritis.

With regard to the plasma as well as the urine, West (1970) concludes that group assays for glycosaminoglycans have nothing to contribute to the chemical pathology of rheumatoid arthritis. In the synovial fluid of rheumatoid arthritis, however, Balazs, Watson, Duff and Roseman (1967) found that hyaluronate molecules were smaller than normal, that hyaluronate concentration was lower, sialic acid and hexosamine concentration higher. These changes, particularly decreased polymerisation, are believed to be one consequence of the higher rate of synthesis that results from synovitis. An abnormal hyaluronate protein has also been detected in rheumatoid synovial fluid but this protein is also present in gouty synovitis (Hamerman and Sandison, 1963).

Unlike the hyaluronate of normal synovial fluid which can be depolymerised *in vitro* by low concentrations of ascorbic acid, the hyaluronate in rheumatoid arthritis does not respond in this way (Abrams and Sandson, 1964), perhaps due to the presence of abnormally high concentrations of α_2-globulins such as caeruloplasmin (p. 158).

Micro-determinations of proteoglycans have, until very recently, been subject to considerable technical limitations. Methods for the separation of proteoglycans in aliquots as small as 15 mg of fresh cartilage are, however, now becoming available using techniques such as those of McDevitt and Muir (unpublished observations) based on acrylamide gel agarose electrophoresis. Methods for tissue assay are also being developed on the basis of the electron microprobe analysis of 10–50 μm freeze-dried sections. Divalent cations such as calcium are enabled to bind to the anionic proteoglycans and a subsequent analysis made of calcium content (Maroudas, 1970). The changes in glycosaminoglycan synthesis identified by the study of rheumatoid synovial cells in culture have been reviewed previously (p. 39).

Enzymes (p. 35). In an early, short report Hamerman, Stephens and Barland (1961) and, in a longer account, Woessner (1965) surveyed the activities of the numerous enzymes that have now been demonstrated in synovial tissue. In addition to abnormally high activities of lysosomal hydrolases such as acid phosphatase, naphthylamidase and β-glucuronidase, oxidative enzymes of the Emden–Meyerhof pathway have been detected in normal and in rheumatoid synovial tissue by qualitative histochemical assessment and by biochemical determination. The altered enzyme activities of cultured rheumatoid cells, like the changes in proteoglycan synthesis referred to earlier, persist through many generations of cells. Knowledge of the characteristics of the synovial cell enzymes has been extended by the use of quantitative histochemical techniques in which the activity of the enzymes of the synovial cells, as opposed to the subsynovial connective tissues, can be assayed indirectly by the integrating microdensitometric measurement of insoluble reaction products (Chayen et al., 1969). This method, which has confirmed the high manifest activity of lysosomal enzymes such as acid phosphatase in synovial lining cells, has also revealed excessive lysosomal permeability in rheumatoid arthritis. Precise morphological distinction, particularly important in assessing the roles of the surface and subsurface tissues in rheumatoid arthritis, has shown that the catheptic activities of the synovial membrane are not uniformly distributed between the surface and the deeper cells.

There is no reason yet to suppose that any of the altered enzyme activities recognised in the synovial tissue cells stand in direct relationship to the cause of the disease (p. 37). Even less likely is a direct role of the enzymes of the synovial fluid and synovial tissue leucocytes. The phagocytic rheumatoid arthritis cells and their inclusions and the nature of rheumatoid synovial fluid are discussed on other pages (p. 102 and p. 84). The metabolic activities of these cells are altered. Dimitrov, Stjernholm and Weir (1969) have obtained evidence that ^{14}C-labelled propionic acid is used less actively than normal by rheumatoid leucocytes especially when a patient has leucopenia. Contrary to the findings in normal or abnormal controls, Dimitrov et al. (1969) identified ^{14}C-β-alanine in rheumatoid leucocytes of patients with leucopenia. The capacity to phagocytose immune complexes and the possibility that this process may activate lysosomal enzymes some of which can degrade nearby connective tissue matrix, is reviewed on p. 103.

The significance of the changed activities of plasma enzymes in rheumatoid arthritis is not known (West, 1970). Low plasma fibrinolytic activity (Fearnley and Chakrabarti, 1964) is common. This low activity runs in parallel with the low synovial fluid activity and the high synovial fluid fibrin content that are believed to contribute to the chronic character of rheumatoid arthritis. The low plasma fibrinolytic activity correlates with disease activity (Fearnley and Chakrabarti, 1964; Andersen and Winther, 1969). As West (1970) points out, the activity of proline hydroxylase, an enzyme whose activity might be expected to be of particular interest in rheumatoid arthritis because of the suspected increase in collagen turnover, is apparently normal. The demonstration of increased aldolase activity, however, may reflect widespread muscle disease (Wegelius, Pasternack and Kuhlback, 1969) (p. 162).

Characteristic differences have been recognised in the esterase and peroxidase/iso-enzymes present in the synovial tissue of rheumatoid arthritis by comparison with normal. The significance of these differences is quite uncertain. A comparison has been made on the basis of the number of bands detected by acrylamide gel electrophoresis and of migration velocities: there was higher activity and more bands in the rheumatoid tissue (7 esterase, 9 peroxidase) as opposed to control (5 and 8 respectively) tissue.

There is abundant evidence to support the view that *protein* metabolism in rheumatoid arthritis is abnormal (Lövgren, 1945); not all the data, however, is related to the stage, activity and duration of the disease and many abnormalities may, it is suspected, be incidental secondary consequences. Plasma albumin levels are lowered (Wilkinson et al., 1965), plasma globulin levels raised. The significance of the impaired enzyme-binding capacity shown by Potter, Duthie and Alexander (1961) is not known. The glycoprotein trypsin inhibitors detected in the urine in many systemic disorders including pregnancy are recognised in patients with rheumatoid arthritis in whose serum and synovial fluid they are also present. Raised levels of plasma fibrinogen and of gamma-globulin are found, and gamma-globulin turnover is increased (Claman and Merrill, 1966). Metabolic studies with ^{131}I-fibrinogen prepared from autologous plasma (Takeda, 1967) indicate that both intravascular and interstitial fibrinogen levels are raised and that the transcapillary transfer rate, and catabolic and synthetic rates for fibrinogen are also greatly increased. The primary disturbance, proportional to the severity of the disease, is apparently increased fibrinogen synthesis. Increased albumin destruction but normal synthesis have also been shown; by contrast, the high serum IgG levels accompany very high synthetic and high catabolic rates (Andersen and Jensen, 1965).

Amino acids. Many variables may influence tissue, plasma, extracellular and urinary amino acid levels and, at best, demonstrable changes in the levels of amino acids or their precursors and derivatives can only shed limited light on the tissue disturbances in rheumatoid arthritis.

The demonstration that patients with this disease display abnormal tryptophane metabolism (McMillan, 1960), an abnormality which could be corrected by giving pyridoxine (Bett, 1962a, b, 1966; Flinn et al., 1964) led to a suggestion (Flinn et al., 1964), subsequently confirmed (McKusick et al., 1964), that there was a relative functional deficiency of vitamin B_6. Spiera (1963) demonstrated that a tryptophane metabolite, 3-hydroxyanthranilic acid, was excreted in excess. Alternatively, abnormal tryptophane metabolism could be the explanation of increased tryptophane pyrrolase activity or of a shunting of tryptophane along the pathway to kynurenine (Spiera and Vallarino, 1969). To support the evidence that vitamin B_6 was functionally deficient, Rylance (1969) examined the urinary levels of taurine and of sulphate as guides to the efficiency of conversion of cysteine to taurine, another pathway probably dependent on vitamin B_6 activity. However, he demonstrated hypertaurinuria in rheumatoid arthritis rather than decreased excretion and suggested that this abnormality, as in the hypertaurinuria found in conditions such as advanced carcinomatosis and muscular dystrophy, might be a result of cellular damage by the 'rheumatoid process'; he could not, of course, exclude primary over-production of taurine.

Similar, but less intense interest has centred on the essential amino acid histidine. In rheumatoid arthritis, the plasma concentration of histidine, itself the precursor of the inflammatory mediator histamine, is abnormally low (Borden et al., 1950; Nettelbladt and Sandell, 1963; Gerber and Gerber, 1967; Gerber, Sakamoto, Carmody and Perry, 1969). West (1970) implies that these observations, made under differing circumstances with different techniques, should be confirmed before their significance is considered. In particular, values obtained for patients with other analogous chronic diseases are required and the sensitivity of the technical methods for the measurement of minor variations in the metabolism of amino acids should be confirmed. As West (1970) reminds us, plasma tyrosine levels in rheumatoid arthritis have been said to be raised, lowered or normal. Since the catecholamines, with an important presumptive role in the vascular phenomena of rheumatoid arthritis, are derived from tyrosine, the possibility of abnormal tyrosine or catecholamine metabolism in this disease is still an interesting question: correspondingly variable results have been described in measurements made for arginine, glutamine and glutamic acid, and taurine.

Keele (1969), reviewing the possible contribution of the kinins to the symptomatology of rheumatoid arthritis, refers to the normal salivary kallikrein activity and the low urinary kinin activity. The significance of the kinin system for the pathogenesis of rheumatoid arthritis is not yet understood although an important contribution by kinins derived from the plasma to the increased vascular permeability and local inflammatory phenomena of rheumatoid arthritis is suspected.

Trace elements. The changes that have been detected in iron (p. 157), copper (p. 158) and manganese (p. 76) concentrations in the blood, tissues and urine are described on other pages. A recent study by Cockel and his colleagues (1971) (Table 10.1) suggests that blood levels of calcium and sodium may also be marginally decreased. Potassium concentrations, however, probably do not differ from normal in the absence of complicating renal and gastrointestinal disorder.

Corticosteroid metabolism in rheumatoid arthritis is no longer the focus for the intense biochemical activity which prevailed in the decade from 1950 to 1960. At that time there was a distinct possibility that an abnormality in steroid metabolism could be associated with rheumatoid

TABLE 10.1. *Mean values (± 2SD) obtained in 100 rheumatoid patients and 100 matched controls, together with statistical analysis using Student's 't' test.*

Test	Rheumatoid patients		Matched controls		P at 5% level
Calcium (mg/100 ml.)	9·32	(± 1·62)	9·75	(± 0·8)	< 0·001
Albumin (g/100 ml.)	3·53	(± 1·08)	4·35	(± 0·68)	< 0·001
Alkaline phosphatase (KA units/100 ml.)	13·5	(± 17·2)	8·74	(± 6·2)	< 0·001
Globulin (g/100 ml.)	3·72	(± 2·06)	2·75	(± 0·72)	< 0·001
Sodium (mEq/l)	140·7	(± 8·4)	142·7	(± 5·2)	< 0·001
Cholesterol (mg/100 ml.)	215·0	(± 90·0)	244·0	(± 82·0)	< 0·001
Iron (µg/100 ml.)	44·8	(± 68·0)	102·0	(± 96·0)	< 0·001
Potassium (mEq/l)	4·29	(± 0·98)	4·4	(± 0·98)	0·05 > P > 0·02
Urea (mg/100 ml.)	39·1	(± 70·4)	31·1	(± 14·3)	0·05 > P > 0·02
Creatinine (mg/100 ml.)	0·96	(± 1·12)	0·96	(± 0·32)	NS
Uric acid (mg/100 ml.)	4·49	(± 4·6)	4·65	(± 2·4)	NS
Glucose (mg/100 ml.)	120·0	(± 90·0)	110·0	(± 74·0)	NS
Bilirubin (mg/100 ml.)	0·45	(± 2·4)	0·54	(± 0·48)	NS
Glutamic-oxaloacetic transaminase (units/ml.)	9·64	(± 23·6)	8·59	(± 13·6)	NS

NS = not significant

(From Cockel, Kendall, Becker and Hawkins, 1971.)

arthritis but this view was not substantiated. Individual investigators have pursued this field of enquiry (Pal, 1967) but, in the United Kingdom, a decreasing use of corticosteroids in treatment has led rather to additional work on the metabolism of alternative therapeutic compounds such as natural and synthetic ACTH, radioimmuno-assays for which are coming into regular use (Glass, 1971).

CHAPTER 11

Role of Lysosomes

Marginal cartilage destruction is an invariable preliminary to the later diarthrodial joint deformities in rheumatoid arthritis. In organ culture, and in experimental arthritis lysosomal enzymes have been shown to be responsible for the degradation of cartilage matrix. Investigations of the nature, origin, structure and functions of lysosomes have, consequently, contributed substantially to present views on the mechanism of cartilage lysis in rheumatoid arthritis (de Duve, 1959, 1963a, b; Weissman, 1967; Barrett, 1969; Dingle, 1969b; Dingle and Fell, 1969).

Significance of lysosomes

Lysosomes. De Duve (1959) was able to show that a number of important mammalian enzymes demonstrated increasing activity if the tissue in which they were present was permitted to auto-lyse, was deprived of a normal supply of oxygen or intermediary metabolites or was physically disrupted (de Duve *et al.*, 1955). The enzymes were all hydrolases with acid pH optima and displayed low activity in fresh tissue: they comprised ribonuclease, deoxyribonuclease, acid phosphatase, cathepsins, glycosidases and sulphatases. The disruptive procedures successfully used to reveal latent enzyme activity included osmotic lysis, alternate freezing and thawing, and ultrasonic vibration.

When preparations of tissue made by these disruptive methods were examined, it was found that enzyme activities were not distributed uniformly. Indeed, when a series of fractions was obtained by subjecting the preparations to sucrose density gradient centrifugation, it became clear that the greater part of the hydrolytic enzyme activity was present in a single fraction in which was much finely particulate material. The examination of this fraction by electron microscopy revealed large numbers of small, electron dense bodies, presumably of cellular origin; the particles came to be called lytic bodies or *lysosomes* because of the enzyme activities with which they were associated. The fraction contained few mitochondria or other known organelles (Novikoff, Beaufay and de Duve, 1956).

Subsequent investigation revealed that lysosomes are present, in widely varying numbers, in the majority of mammalian cells including those of the synovia and cartilage. Lysosomes are thought to have a double unit membrane characteristic of intracellular structures such as the mitochondria, but by a single membraneous lamina. It was deduced that lysosomes could be the normal sites of a number of important enzymes, latent because of their retention behind a membrane which is impermeable to small molecules including substrates and coenzymes. In disease, or as a consequence of physical or chemical disruption *in vitro*, the permeability of the retaining membrane was thought to increase, permitting a local change in pH and the interaction of enzyme with substrate and cofactors.

In *health*, functions subsequently attributed to lysosomal enzymes included, for example, the intracellular digestion of material engulfed by endocytosis and retained within a phagocytic vacuole or phagosome prior to metabolic processing; the imperceptible enzymatic digestion of

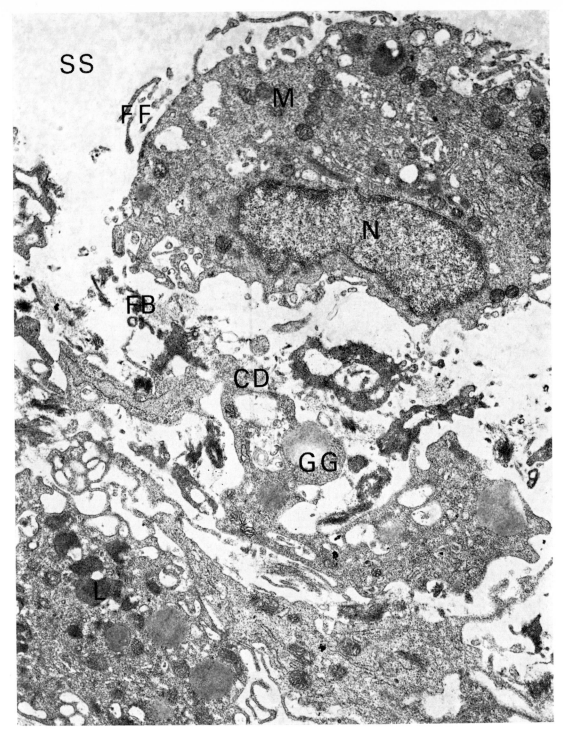

Fig. 11.1 Synovial surface. Cell debris and transected portions of cytoplasmic processes from adjacent cells inter-mingle to give the variegated appearances commonly seen in rheumatoid arthritis. There is no certainty that the grey-globular bodies identified by electron microscopy are identical with the immune complexes thought to be one cause of the inclusions seen in rheumatoid arthritis cells but this view has been suggested. Part of the cross-striated material lying free on the cell surface is fibrin, part other plasma proteins. With the majority of preparative techniques that are still in use, glycosaminoglycans and other non-fibrillar materials that lie upon and normally cover the synovial surface, and which comprise much of the intercellular matrix, are lost during fixation and dehydration and cannot be seen at subsequent microscopy. Ruthenium red (Fig. 5.1) can be used to preserve these matrix structures. They can also be shown in cryostat section or demonstrated indirectly by the electron microprobe scanning of sections stained with the copper-containing dye Alcian blue. (From a micrograph of Dr. A. J. Palfrey.)   (× 12,000)

tissue during metamorphosis; the insiduous replacement of zones of provisional cartilage mineralisation during vertebrate endochondral ossification; and the digestion of normal cell constituents as a response in starvation.

In *disease*, interest has tended to focus on the properties of cells such as those of the liver and the neutrophil polymorph in which lysosomes are abundant and easily identified (Weissman, 1967; Lack, 1969; Page Thomas, 1969). Chemotactic migration of polymorphs towards sites of injury, a common event in bacterial infection and in complement-mediated tissue damage, was shown to be followed by the local liberation of lysosomal proteases and other hydrolases. These enzymes appeared also to be responsible for the intercellular digestion of tissue derivatives that occurs in zones of infarction and in ischaemic atrophy.

Lysosomes in rheumatoid arthritis

Origin of investigations. The development of knowledge of the relationship of lysosomal function to cartilage lysis in rheumatoid arthritis has been admirably summarised by Barland, Novokoff and Hamerman (1964a, *b*), Weissman (1967), Lack (1969), Page Thomas (1967, 1969), and by Chayen and Bitensky (1971). Other enzyme activities and different distributions of isoenzymes, in addition to lysosomal enzymes, are, of course, also of interest (Eberl and Altmann, 1970).

The principles by which lysosomal hydrolases digest and degrade heterologous and autologous materials in rheumatoid synovitis appear to be identical with those that determine the role of these enzymes in other circumstances. Thus, *foreign* material, such as bacterial protein, is ingested by endocytosis and tends to lie within vacuoles (phagosomes) into which lysosomal enzymes pass, and are activated, when the vacuolar and lysosomal membranes unite to form a phagolysosome. Because of the origin of the material to be digested this structure has been termed a *heterolysosome*. *Autologous* cellular and intercellular (autophagic) vacuoles that unite with nearby lysosomes form *autolysosomes*. Simultaneous digestion of autologous and of heterologous material may of course take place within a single phagocyte. The products of lysosomal digestion remain within phago-lysosomes or autolysosomes until extrusion takes place by the process of exocytosis.

Investigations of lysosomal activity in rheumatoid arthritis can be traced to the observations of Thomas (1956) who demonstrated the lysis and collapse of rabbit ear cartilage following an in-travenous injection of the proteolytic enzyme papain. Enzymes such as papain, it was shown, destroy cartilage matrix by degrading the protein-polysaccharides, causing a histological loss of metachromatic material (Spicer and Bryant, 1958). Dingle (1961) and Lucy, Dingle and Fell (1961) had described an analogous breakdown of cartilage rudiments in organ culture under the influence of vitamin A added to the culture medium. Their work derived from the demonstration by Fell and Mellanby (1952) that there was a loss of cartilage metachromasia when cartilage was maintained under these conditions. Because of these observations, it was natural to assume that identical degradative mechanisms might be responsible for cartilage matrix loss both as a result of vitamin A excess and because of the activity of injected papain. This suggestion was supported by the results of Fell and Thomas (1960) who found that vitamin A fed to rabbits degraded cartilage matrix proteoglycans. Advances in the understanding of lysosomal functions made it appear probable that matrix degradation in each of these studies resulted from the release and activation of lysosomal hydrolases, a release caused by the disturbance of chondrocyte lysosomal membranes (Weissman, 1965; Fell, 1969).

Synovial fluid lysosomal enzymes

The synovial fluid in rheumatoid arthritis displays high acid hydrolase activity (Jacox and Feldmahn, 1955; Smith and Hamerman, 1962; Lehman, Kream and Brogna, 1964; Caygill and Pit-keathly, 1966; Page Thomas, 1969). The enzymes are those known to be situated characteristically within lysosomes. Since rheumatoid synovial fluid also contains excessive numbers of polymorphs, and since polymorph granules are lysosomes, it appeared logical to attribute the synovial enzyme activity to the liberation and activation of polymorph granule acid lysosomal hydrolases. This hypothesis was an attractive explanation for evidence showing that acid hydrolases extracted from polymorph granules can cause a marked reduction in the vicosity of solutions of cartilage protein-polysaccharides, a change presumably due to enzymatic degradation of these macro-molecules. These alterations in cartilage macromolecules can, moreover, be induced by homo-genates of polymorphs that have been prepared by methods that conserve and activate lysosomal enzymes.

It was found, however, that raised enzyme activities in rheumatoid synovial fluid were not confined to lysosomal hydrolases. Lactate dehydrogenase activity, a cytoplasmic enzyme, was significantly increased and it appeared probable that the presence of this raised activity was a result of polymorph cell disintegration rather than of activation and release following the phago-cytosis of material such as exogenous infective agents (p. 188), immune complexes (p. 102) or the products of inflammation (Riddle, Bluhm and Barnhart, 1965) (p. 18). Against this view, was the additional evidence that the alkaline phosphatase characteristic of human polymorphs was not present in increased amounts in rheumatoid synovial fluid. This suggested that disintegration of other cells in continuity with the synovial fluid, perhaps synovial, subsynovial or chondrocytic, was the source both of the lysosomal hydrolases and of the other enzymes.

Synovial and cartilage lysosomes

One of the most conspicuous features of the histological changes in rheumatoid arthritis, and one that has been known since the earliest pathological studies, is the formation of a marginal pannus of vascular granular tissue that progressively replaces articular cartilage (p. 27). Pannus formation is, of course, not pathognomonic of rheumatoid arthritis, in which it is a characteristic feature, but is encountered in other forms of infective and non-infective inflammatory joint disease. Pannus formation is seen, for example, in human tuberculous arthritis and in experi-mental turpentine arthritis (Fig. 5.6).

The fact that the greater part of the articular surface in rheumatoid arthritis appears, by light microscopy, to remain intact until a late stage and that cartilage loss is confined to the circum-ference, argues against the participation of free, activated synovial fluid lysosomal enzymes in this important phase of the disease. For this reason, for those stated on the previous page, and because of the close approximation of the inflamed synovial tissue to the articular cartilage margin, the conclusion seems inescapable that cartilage lysis by lysosomal hydrolases can only be the result of the local, circumferential activity of enzymes normally held latent within peri-pheral chondrocytes themselves, within nearby synovial or subsynovial cells, or within the inflammatory cells which aggregate in rheumatoid synovial tissue. Recent observations on the differential susceptibility of cartilage surfaces and deeper cartilage to enzymatic degradation, suggests, however, that understanding of pannus formation is incomplete (Reynolds, 1970).

On the basis of Dingle's (1969a) work it appears quite possible that rheumatoid cartilage lysis, as in the case of the lysis of cartilage maintained in organ culture, can be caused by the local, pericellular action of chondrocyte hydrolases. Lysosomal membranes fuse with the chondrocyte plasma membrane; acid hydrolases are released and activated; and the locally digested matrix is phagocytosed, the phagosome fusing with further intracellular lysosomes prior to continued intracellular digestion. But to postulate this mechanism in rheumatoid arthritis begs the question as to why matrix degradation should be confined to marginal articular cartilage. One explanation would be (p. 136) that this is the tissue first affected by the vascular phenomena of rheumatoid synovitis; another, that this zone is first injured by the factor provoking the synovitis. In either event, it is now quite generally assumed that the marginal cartilage 'erosions' of rheumatoid arthritis are caused by synovial or subsynovial cells or by the inflammatory cells infiltrating the synovia. Local release and extracellular activation of lysosomal hydrolases is postulated.

The first clear proposition that this might be so appears to have been that of Dingle (1962) whose work had been concerned both with the metabolism of synovia and with the effects of vitamin A on cartilage rudiments in culture (Fell and Dingle, 1963). Weissman (1964) accepted the same principle and found evidence that the release of acid lysosomal hydrolases could be antagonised by cortisone (Weissman, 1963). Evidence in support of Dingle's hypothesis was obtained by Luscombe (1963) who found increased activity of acid phosphatase and a cathepsin in rheumatoid synovia, and by Hendry and Carr (1963). These authors demonstrated that there was a relationship between clinical disease activity in four groups of diseases (acute and quiescent cases of internal knee derangements, osteoarthrosis and rheumatoid arthritis), and the activity, in synovial tissue homogenates, of β-N-acetyl-glucosaminidase, an enzyme shown by Pugh and Walker (1961) to be active in rat synovia. Although there was a wide scatter of results and no demonstrable correlation with serum rheumatoid factor activity, the importance of these findings was obvious.

Subjective histochemical evidence had meanwhile been gained for the increased activity of lysosomal enzymes such as acid phosphatase in rheumatoid synovial tissue (Hamerman, Stephens and Barland, 1961; Smith and Hamerman, 1962) and Burstone (1962) reported corresponding increases in the activity of another lysosomal enzyme, leucine aminopeptidase,* in rheumatoid subcutaneous nodules (p. 122). Lysosomes obtained from rheumatoid cells were found to be more fragile than normal (Barland, Novikoff and Hamerman, 1964a). High leucine aminopeptidase activity in the synovia of rheumatoid arthritis was confirmed by the qualitative observations of Vainio (1966, 1970) whose investigations led him to support the concept that this enzyme may be responsible for the digestion of phagocytosed rheumatoid factor (p. 100).

Further investigations of enzymes such as acid phosphatase and lysozyme activated by sonication of the cells from rheumatoid synovial fluid, suggested that the supernatant obtained after centrifuging the preparations, displayed enzyme inhibitory properties. Comparable inhibition for lactate dehydrogenase was shown by the synovial fluids from rheumatoid arthritis and from gout. The significance of these apparently non-specific inhibitory characteristics is not yet understood but it is clear that the presence or absence of 'inhibitors' in sites such as articular cartilage margins could be an explanation for the limited, marginal and zonal cartilage lysis by rheumatoid pannus.

Cytological studies of lysosomes

The subjective evidence that lysosomal hydrolases displayed increased activity in rheumatoid arthritis, based on studies made with an acid phosphatase as a 'marker' for lysosomal activity led to a series of cytological investigations. Many reports of the electron microscopic appearances of the synovial and inflammatory cells in rheumatoid arthritis were published—they are reviewed on p. 44—but few studies reported of the chondrocytes of nearby articular cartilage. The experiments of Coimbra and Lopes-Vaz (1967) exemplify those that concentrated on the survey of lysosomes and their derivatives. These authors (1967) surveyed the neutrophil polymorphs of the

---

* Better termed a naphthylamidase and no longer universally accepted as lysosomal (Barrett and Poole, 1970; Weissman, 1970).

synovial fluid from 3 patients with rheumatoid arthritis and showed that at least 4 types of cyto-plasmic bodies were present: (a) dense; (b) digestive endocytotic vacuoles; (c) residual (auto-phagic) vacuoles; and (d) multivesicular and lipid. The localisation of acid phosphatase activity to the dense bodies (lysosomes) was demonstrated by electron histochemistry. In further work the same authors (Lopes-Vaz and Coimbra, 1967) found that the larger bodies present in the synovial fluid white blood cells from rheumatoid arthritis and from ankylosing spondylitis were of two kinds. The first, secondary lysosomes, were acid phosphatase-positive, as was to be expected from earlier light-microscope histochemistry. The second were believed to be the antigen/antibody complexes that Zucker–Franklin (1966) (p. 52) found it difficult to identify with certainty. Later, Petrescu *et al.* (1970), like Zucker–Franklin (1966) recognised 'grey-globular' leucocyte inclusions in the cells of rheumatoid synovial fluid but could obtain no proof that these structures corresponded to the immune complexes of fluorescence light microscopists.

The morphological surveys of synovial cells made by electron microscopy (p. 44) have been reviewed by Ghadially and Roy (1969), and by Davies and Palfrey (1971). They agree that the A(M) cells of rheumatoid synovia contain increased numbers of dense bodies that are probably lysosomes, that there are numerous vacuoles, and that the Golgi complexes are often prominent.

It can be concluded that there is light and microscopic evidence for the presence in rheumatoid synovial cells of increased numbers of organelles with the appearance of lysosomes. The purely morphological demonstration of the site of acid phosphatase activity is not, of course, an indica-tion of the extent of this activity *in vivo*. There is, indeed, some reason to suspect that the tech-niques that have been used in the past for electron histochemistry may inactivate substantial proportions of the latent enzyme activity. The electron microscopic evidence should not therefore be taken as more than an indication that lysosomal activity in rheumatoid arthritis is increased. Even the presence of increased numbers of dense bodies thought to be lysosomes cannot neces-sarily be termed significant; the factors responsible for determining numbers of synovial cell lysosomes remain quite unknown.

Microchemistry of lysosomes

To overcome the difficulties inherent in studying tissue sections qualitatively and to permit a measurement of synovial cell lysosomal enzyme activity, as opposed to a subjective estimate on the visual survey of coloured reaction products, new techniques have been devised. The synovial cells form a narrow lamina, normally 1–4 cells deep but as much as 1–10 cells thick in rheumatoid arthritis. Homogenates made from aliquots of whole synovial tissue for biochemical measurement of enzyme activities invariably contain all the additional, subsynovial and possibly irrelevant, components of the subjacent connective tissue—blood vessels, lymphatics, nerves, fibroblasts, mast cells and collagen—together with the inflammatory cell infiltrate which had proved trouble-some in earlier experiments when the metabolism of synovial tisssue was being measured (Dingle and Page Thomas, 1956) (p. 41).

An entirely different quantitative technical approach for the study of synovial lysosomal enzyme activities was therefore adopted by Chayen, Bitensky, Butcher and Poulter (1969). These authors made use of cryostat sections of rheumatoid synovia rather than homogenates of synovial tissue. They reacted synovial sections for selected lysosomal enzymes and measured the reaction products formed in relation to single synovial lining cells, by scanning and integrating micro-densitometry. They showed, in control experiments, that indirect measurements of enzyme activity obtained in this way replicated those made with analogous samples analysed by spectro-photometric techniques after homogenisation. It was possible to use a recording microdensito-meter for the same purpose (Altman, 1971).

The advantages of microdensitometric measurement of deposits such as formazan crystals and diazo dyes at sites of enzyme activity are to enable assays of reaction products related only to synovial surface cells. Readings can be taken over single cells and compared to a baseline, such as the Feulgen-positive DNA, measured from sections of the same tissue. The disadvantage of this technique is that the analysis can only be an indirect guide to enzyme activity. This disadvantage can, perhaps, be overcome by microanalytical techniques such as those modified from Lowry et al. (1954) and used by Laing and Gardner (1964), Gardner and Laing (1965), Wyke and Gardner (1970) and Gardner and Wyke (1970), for measuring enzyme activities in non-homogeneous tissues such as arterial walls after rapid-freezing, freeze-drying, and micro-dissection. However, there is very considerable difficulty in separating synovial surface cells from those of the underlying subsynovial connective tissue (there is no intervening basement membrane) and the necessity for micro-weighing imposes slowness of analysis.

Roberts, McLees and Kerby (1967) provided a partial solution to this problem by devising an attractive and precise method of dissecting synovial cells from the remaining subsynovial tissue. By this means, they were able to measure synovial cell metabolism using ^{14}C-labelling and to make a correction for the part which tissue red and white cells might contribute in terms of lactate production and ^{14}C-CO_2 formation. They confirmed the raised metabolic activity of rheumatoid synovial tissue and demonstrated that the Embden–Meyerhof pathway was a major energy pathway. The Pasteur effect (p. 41) was again noted in normal synovium but, when glucose was being metabolised, the tricarboxylic acid cycle was not significant as an energy source. Pentose shunt pathway activity was found, suggesting the possible importance of lipid and of steroid metabolism in synovial tissue. The addition of proteins, including γ-globulin and rheumatoid factor euglobulin to the preparations under study, altered carbohydrate metabolism non-specifically. When comparisons between villous and non-villous synovial tissue were made, in the manner adopted by Page Thomas and Dingle (1956), the former displayed higher rates of lactate production and of $^{14}CO_2$ formation (from glucose-1-^{14}C) than the latter.

Whichever technique is adopted in the study of the rheumatoid lysosomal enzymes, it is evidently essential to distinguish between latent (bound) and manifest activity. The distinction has been achieved by Chayen et al. (1969) and it has been shown that, in rheumatoid arthritis, the lysosomal membrane, normally an effective barrier to the access of the lysosomal acid hydrolases to appropriate substrates, becomes ineffective. Free activity of enzymes such as acid phosphatase is therefore high. In further studies Chayen, Bitensky, Butcher and Cashman (1971) measured naphthylamidase activity in the synovial lining cells of 80 patients, half of whom had rheumatoid arthritis. A distinction was made, anatomically and in terms of the influence of puromycin, between the surface cells and those of the deeper, subsynovial connective tissue. In non-rheumatoid cells the ratio of freely available enzyme activity to total activity was always between 1:2 and 1:1·5. In rheumatoid cells, all enzyme activity was freely available, practically none latent within intact lysosomal membranes. Lysosomal membrane behaviour was, apparently, grossly disordered in rheumatoid arthritis.

In searching for an explanation for the mechanism by which the lysosomal membranes in rheumatoid synovial cells become defective barriers to substrate access, Chayen et al. recognised that rheumatoid synovial tissue in short-term organ (maintenance) culture retains its histological integrity better at pH values more acid than those (ca. 7·8) that they regard as optimum for normal synovial tissue. Determinations of tissue redox potentials then suggested an imbalance by which rheumatoid synovial cells were in an hydrogen-rich state. This observation encouraged the speculation that lysosomal membrane permeability was increased because of redox imbalance, an hypothesis that received some support when it was shown that the addition of hydrogen-acceptors such as 2-methyl-1-4-naphthoquinone to the culture fluid reversed the trend towards poor preservation.

Experimental demonstration of lysosomal activity in synovitis

The observation that a number of therapeutic anti-inflammatory agents effective in alleviating rheumatoid synovitis, exerted an influence on lysosomal membranes, decreasing permeability and reducing free enzyme activity, encouraged the experimental investigation of lysosomes in relation to synovial injury (Figs. 11.2, 11.3).

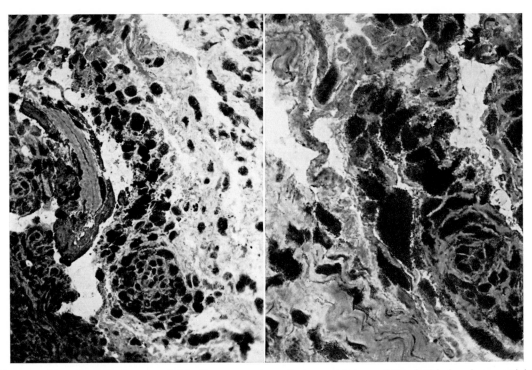

Fig. 11.2 Experimental adjuvant arthritis. Cryostat sections of rat synovial tissue. Sites of acid phosphatase activity (*left*) are indicated by concentrations of black and grey-black granules. They are related to surface synovial cells and to the considerable numbers of histiocytes and polymorphs that surround a synovial artery and lie free within the subsynovial connective tissue. (*Right*) Higher power view of part of similar tissue showing concentration of acid phosphatase (lysosomal) activity in relation to surface synovial cells.   (*Left* × 500; *right* × 1,140)

Among agents used experimentally to cause the direct discharge of lysosomal hydrolases into the cytoplasm were: (1) streptolysin S, which preferentially disrupts lysosomes (Weissman, 1967); (2) leucocytes, antileucocyte-antibody and complement; and (3) photosensitising substances that concentrate in cells (Allison, 1968). Weissman and Thomas (1964) prepared lysosome suspensions from leucocyte granules and demonstrated that it was possible to promote an experimental synovitis in rabbits by an intraarticular injection either with this suspension or with intact leucocyte lysosomes followed, 6 hours later, by the administration of endotoxin. Weissman and Spilberg (1965) later used streptolysin S, said to be non-antigenic, and examined the effects of this lysosomal enzyme activator on rabbit cartilage. Comparable observations have been made in rabbits and goats. Lack (1966) extended this work by repetitive injections into rabbit joints. He showed that a single injection of streptolysin S causes no generalised cartilage lysis. Three injections, however, given at weekly intervals, were found to cause transient inflammation while 4 or more weekly injections led to a chronic rheumatoid-like arthritis with pannus formation and synovial lymphocytosis, accompanied by fibrin deposition on the synovial surfaces. There was little doubt, therefore, that streptolysin S, a known activator of lysosomal hydrolases, could effectively provoke an experimental arthritis. Whether the mode of action of the provocative agent is upon lysosomes or not is still not entirely certain and Taylor (1970) has found that the mitogenic fraction of streptolysin S can itself cause round cell infiltration and cartilage erosion.

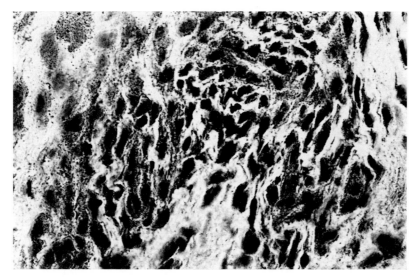

Fig. 11.3 Experimental adjuvant arthritis. Cryostat section of synovial tissue showing sites of naphthylamidase activity. The black and grey-black granules illustrate concentrations of reaction product produced in response to the activity of this proteolytic enzyme.   (× 1,260)

Effects of lysosomal activation

Lysosomal enzyme activation may, it is proposed, result from rheumatoid synovitis. Equally, the increased local hydrolytic enzyme activities may cause, provoke or prolong inflammation. One way in which this may be brought about is by the liberation of kinins or by the activation of Hageman factor. The digestion of cartilage matrix by lysosomal enzymes liberates chondroitin sulphate and this polysaccharide itself activates Hageman factor. The lysosomes of synovial fluid polymorphs are likely to play some part in this sequence and thus to prolong rheumatoid synovitis. That they may also digest other forms of cartilage is suggested by the demonstration of elastinolytic activity in the granules of polymorph leucocytes (Janoff and Scherer, 1968).

Recent evidence has been gained that under experimental conditions, anti-lysosomal protease enzyme antibodies can effectively inhibit cartilage degradation (Weston, Barrettt and Dingle, 1969). Weston and his colleagues tested organ cultures of chick embryo cartilage and demonstrated that the digestion of cartilage by pure cathepsin D, and autolytic digestion, could be inhibited by an IgG fraction from a rabbit anti-chick cathepsin D serum. Cathepsin D activity, found to be localised at selected sites intracellularly by immunofluorescence microscopy (Poole, 1970), is believed to contribute to the autolytic degradation of intercellular connective tissue matrix and may even be the main agent responsible for it. The role of this enzyme and of anti-bodies to it, in rheumatoid arthritis, remains to be determined; different cartilage layers and different zones are likely to display differential susceptibility (Dingle, Barrett and Weston, 1971; Gardner, 1972).

Immunological phenomena in relation to lysosomal activity

The wide variety of immunological phenomena that have been proposed in rheumatoid arthritis are likely to provoke secondary changes in the lysosomal systems of synovial, lymphoreticular and cartilage cells (Coombs and Fell, 1969). The lymph nodes in rheumatoid arthritis are often cytologically abnormal; macrophage lysosomal enzymes play a part in processing soluble and particulate antigens and may be invoked in rheumatoid lymphoid responses. Any exogenous infective agent that can be shown to cause rheumatoid synovitis is likely to induce lysosomal activity. Further, there is little doubt that some of the inclusion bodies of the RA cell (p. 102) are immune complexes; cellular ingestion of these complexes appears to release lysosomal enzymes (Williamson and Ling, 1965; Astorga and Bollet, 1965). There is also the possibility that some of the ingested material in synovial fluid cells may be fibrin that may itself be immunogenic (Ghadially and Roy, 1967).

Weissman (1964) suggested that the lysosomal hydrolases might play a part in causing auto-allergic phenomena in the systemic connective tissue diseases and in particular, in rheumatoid arthritis. The products of extracellular lysosomal digestion, ingested by endocytosis, might be so changed that their antigenic structure could lead to a humoral or cellular immunological response; or, in a more subtle way, synovial cells, failing to respond adequately to excess exogenous material by endocytosis, or reacting in autophagy by permitting the escape of altered autologous material, might cause a fault in the autoallergic suppression mechanism. It would also be possible, in theory, for increased endocytotic activity to lead to increased autophagy, a process that may perhaps provoke the formation of modified antigenic determinants capable of causing auto-allergic reactions.

As matters stand at present, three main explanations have been proposed to account for synovial cell lysosomal enzyme 'triggering' in rheumatoid arthritis: (a) the response to the phagocytosis of one or more exogenous infective agents; (b) the response to the phagocytosis of immune complexes; and (c) the response to the phagocytosis of products of inflammation such as fibrin. Additional agencies may induce chondrocyte lysosomal activity; and the reactions of synovial fluid cells that attracted so much initial interest can now be seen as incidental to the marginal cartilage destruction of rheumatoid synovitis. Further, the role of enzyme inhibitors and activators may be much more important than has so far been suggested. Comparing two lysosomal enzymes (acid phosphatase and lysozyme) with two glycolytic enzymes (lactate and pyruvate dehydrogenases) Kerby and Taylor (1967) found that a synovial supernate partly inhibited lysozyme; rheumatoid synovial fluid also partially inhibited lactate dehydrogenase. It is possible therefore that (at present unknown) inhibitors and activators hold the balance in the regulation of synovial tissue—as well as synovial fluid enzyme activities and that knowledge of these inhibitors and activators may contribute to a better understanding of the phases of synovial inflammatory activity.

In summary, it is very generally agreed with Weissman (1966) that, whatever the initiating cause of rheumatoid arthritis, the role of the lysosomal enzymes may be to act as a '*final common pathway*' for tissue injury. And this seems indeed to be a wholly reasonable explanation for the part that lysosomes play in exacerbating cartilage damage. Lack (1969) accepted this view but stressed the possible importance of alternative mechanisms for the release of cartilage cell lysosomal enzymes such as the action of raised oxygen tension (Sledge and Dingle, 1965), an agent well known for its capacity to induce fibroplasia (Strickfield, 1962). This sequence is the diametric opposite to that proposed by Gardner (1965) to account for cartilage lysis in rheumatoid arthritis. No direct evidence has been obtained to show whether the oxygen partial pressure of the extracellular fluid of cartilage is increased or diminished (p. 31) but synovial fluid partial pressures tend to be extremely low.

CHAPTER 12

Systemic and Extraarticular Lesions

Patients with rheumatoid arthritis often display pathological evidence of visceral disease (Christie, 1954; Sinclair and Cruickshank, 1956; Thomson, 1966; Pearson *et al.*, 1966). The relationship between these lesions, which may not be readily apparent, and the primary disorder, has attracted great interest. Thus, Baggenstoss and Rosenberg (1941, 1943), in early reports, drew attention to cardiac changes in rheumatoid arthritis, and pulmonary disease began to be recognised. That 20% of patients with rheumatoid arthritis develop subcutaneous nodules had long been appreciated (Collins, 1937; Keil, 1938) but the full extent of the visceral lesions that may accompany rheumatoid arthritis has only been grasped during the past 15 years. Many of these lesions are of limited clinical significance. In discussing the systemic changes it should be remembered that the duration of rheumatoid arthritis is long, the variety of therapeutic agents very great. The possibility always exists therefore, that a visceral lesion may have been caused by an incidental disorder during the course of the illness or by the action of a drug (Hart, 1969, 1970). Furthermore, patients with rheumatoid arthritis are particularly prone to secondary infection (Parker, 1965) and to silent bacterial joint disease.

In an important paper which followed an early account (Gruenwald, 1948) of the visceral lesions in rheumatoid arthritis, Bevans *et al.* (1954) introduced the description 'malignant rheumatoid arthritis' for cases with a fulminating clinical course. Their patients displayed pericarditis and pleurisy; necrotic and granulomatous lesions in all stages of healing and evolution were found in the heart, lungs, kidneys, skeletal muscle and synovia. The underlying disorder was apparently a 'fibrinoid necrosis' (p. 18) involving the walls of small blood vessels and resulting in widely disseminated lesions resembling the rheumatoid subcutaneous nodule. Many aspects of these systemic lesions of rheumatoid arthritis have recently been reviewed by Hollingsworth (1968), and by Waaler (1967); the less common manifestations of the disease are outlined by Weiss and Keller (1967).

There is no doubt that Bevans *et al.* (1954) performed a valuable service in drawing attention to this group of cases and in distinguishing the cardiac lesions of rheumatoid arthritis from those of rheumatic fever. However, it is questionable whether the best term for this group of cases was chosen. The adjective 'malignant' is properly reserved for invasive tumours and in the present context it would be preferable to talk of 'accelerated' rheumatoid arthritis just as 'malignant' hypertension is better described as 'accelerated' hypertension.

(a) Subcutaneous nodules

Approximately 20% of cases of rheumatoid arthritis develop subcutaneous granulomata called 'nodules' (Collins, 1937; Keil, 1938; Collins, 1949; Bywaters, Glynn and Zeldis, 1958; Cochrane *et al.*, 1964). The incidence of nodule formation varies in different populations. Nodules may occasionally develop before clinical signs of rheumatoid arthritis appear; their presence, moreover, is correlated with that of rheumatoid factor (p. 100) in the blood. This state of 'sero-positivity' is frequently accompanied by other visceral disorders and particularly by arteritis and lung disease. Rarely (Lowney and Simons, 1963) nodules indistinguishable from those of rheumatoid arthritis develop in patients in whom neither this disease nor rheumatic fever ever become manifest (Akers, 1965). Conversely, occasional patients with pneumoconiosis develop rheumatoid pulmonary granulomata before clinical evidence of rheumatoid arthritis is detectable although tests for rheumatoid factor are usually positive. There is also evidence that nodule formation, even in unusual sites such as the epi- and pericardium, the thoracic aorta or the lungs (p. 139) (Gürich, 1968), can be related to corticosteroid treatment.

Rheumatoid granulomata appear insidiously near body surfaces exposed frequently to pressure or stress; but they are not confined to these zones. The nodules are at first painless and perhaps of greater cosmetic than of clinical interest; they range in size from a few millimetres to several centimetres in diameter. Typical situations in which nodules are encountered include the skin overlying the olecranon process of the ulna, the occiput, the skin adjoining the ischial and femoral tuberosities and areas in relation to the heads of the phalangeal or metacarpal bones.

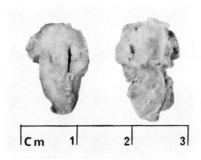

Fig. 12.1 A rheumatoid nodule excised at operation and bisected. The centre is soft and a cleft illustrates where fluid debris has escaped. The remainder of the nodule is moderately firm, grey-yellow, or yellow-white in appearance, and closely associated with nearby connective tissue. The nodule was excised from near an elbow joint. (From Gardner D. L., *Pathology of the Connective Tissue Diseases*, London: Arnold, 1965.)

The young nodule may appear clinically to be an entity but microscopic evidence shows that a single gross lesion can be a conglomeration of individual structures. There is a tendency for rheumatoid nodules to increase slowly in size and it is occasionally possible to demonstrate a direct relationship between enlargement and physical irritation. Thus Glynn (personal communication) tells of a case in which an elderly rheumatoid arthritic developed a nodule in the area of the index finger used to support her pen. She overcame this disability by transferring her pen to the support of her second and third fingers and, when, in turn, these developed nodules, to that of the third and fourth fingers, and so on.

Dissection of a rheumatoid nodule reveals that the compact margin, formed of collagenous connective tissue of moderate to high density and of moderate to low vascularity, is in continuity with adjacent, less dense subcutaneous or peri-articular connective tissue (Fig. 12.1). At first soft and vascular, the nodule margins become dense and sclerotic as the collagen content increases. The firm margins, which may have a yellow or yellow-white colour due, apparently, to a local accumulation of lipochrome pigments, enclose a softer, irregular centre the contents of which are often liquid or semi-fluid.

The older, macroscopic subcutaneous nodule is composed microscopically of a series of irregular necrotic zones of widely varying size and shape, bounded by collagen that welds the whole zone into the single mass seen clinically. The individual microscopic, necrotic zones differ little in detailed structure. However, the clinical evidence shows clearly that discrete subcutaneous nodules may grow steadily in size and may form in succession in several or many body areas. Although of different size, they are not necessarily of different age. When excision is attempted, failure to remove a nodule completely appears to leave a 'locus minoris resistentiae' which, for reasons not yet understood, but perhaps because of a defective blood supply to the necrotic zones, is particularly subject to indolent local infection. This state of affairs, in a patient under treatment with corticosteroids, may be the stimulus for the onset of systemic, antibiotic-resistant staphylococcal or fungal infection.

The unit of which the conglomerate macroscopic granuloma is formed is an irregular, limited zone of tissue necrosis, the margins of which are found, on section, to have a serpiginous form (Figs. 12.1 and 12.2). The boundary is usually a pallisade-like array of elongated cells resembling histiocytes or fibroblasts, arranged with their long axes directed radially towards the centre of the necrotic zone. It is suggested (Sokoloff, 1966) that the radial arrangement of these cells is determined by the disposition of adjacent reticular fibres but the converse seems more probable. These marginal cells contain lipid droplets but do not appear to be capable of taking up neutral red, one index of phagocytic capacity. The radially arranged cells may, nevertheless, be of phagocytic origin since they display abundant acid phosphatase activity, presumably of lysosomal origin. Among the pallisade cell layer, and sometimes within the nearby connective tissue, occasional multinucleated giant cells of 'Touton' type are encountered. The morphological characteristics of these cells are closely reminiscent of those seen in the xanthomata; the ingestion of fat may, indeed, determine their structure. The giant cells are smaller than the mulberry-cells of the virus exanthemata; the reason for their presence is not understood. They are distinct from the synovial giant cells described above (p. 23) although nodule-like zones of necrosis are not rare in rheumatoid synovial tissue.

The necrotic zone of the rheumatoid nodule includes abundant eosinophilic amorphous material. The lesion is sterile and no bacteria or other micro-organisms can be identified in, or at the margins of the necrotic zone by light or by other forms of microscopy. Intact reticular fibres extend into or through the nodule. Nuclear debris abounds in the zone of necrosis, interspersed with structureless material that stains positively for fibrin, faintly for collagen, and positively for neutral fat, phospholipid and cholesterol. There is, indeed, so much fat that a xanthomatous appearance may be simulated (Watt and Baumann, 1967).

It is now known, from studies with the electron microscope (Cochrane et al., 1964; Gieseking, 1969; Gieseking, Baümer and Backman, 1969) that the necrotic central part of a rheumatoid nodule contains a dense network of fibrin, fragments of cells and nuclear debris, and scanty residues of the relatively large fibres of partly digested, mature collagen. The results of electron microscopy provide evidence for the view that the marginal pallisade cells of the nodule are of phagocytic rather than of fibroblastic (secretory) character. The necrotic zone includes glycosaminoglycans, demonstrable with the Alcian blue techniques, and other plasma proteins. Calcium deposits, however, are rare. Proteolytic enzyme activity has been shown (Maldyk and Kalczak, 1968) and enzymes of lysosomal origin have been found to be active (Burstone, 1956).

The necrotic centre of the rheumatoid nodule is interpreted variously as (1) a result of local ischaemia, due to nearby arterial disease (Bannatyne, 1896; Sokoloff, McCluskey and Bunim, 1953; Sokoloff, 1963); as (2) a reaction to chemical toxins or infective agents; or as (3) a focus in connective tissue of the cytotoxic consequences of an antigen/antibody interaction. Careful dissection and serial section, it is claimed, show a constant relationship to a diseased artery. However, the way in which histiocytes are arranged in the serpiginous margins of the nodule,

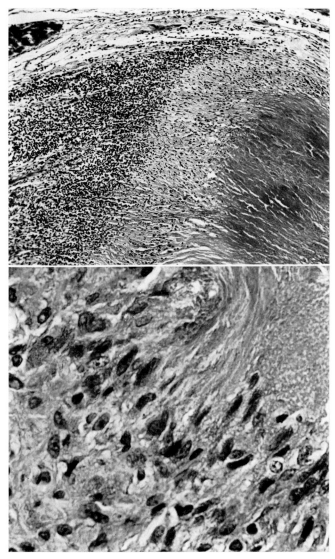

Fig. 12.2 Rheumatoid granulomatous nodules, present in 20% of clinically affected rheumatoid arthritics, have a characteristic but not pathognomonic structure. (*Top*) Zone of necrosis (*right*) in cardiac nodule adjoins vascular granulation tissue that is extensively infiltrated (*left*) by lymphocytes and some plasma cells. (From Gardner D. L., *Pathology of the Connective Tissue Diseases*, London: Arnold, 1965.) (*Bottom*) The margin of a rheumatoid subcutaneous nodule is characteristically composed of fibroblasts and histiocytes arranged in a radial fashion with their axes towards the centre of the necrotic zone of the nodule. At this margin, morphological distinction between fibroblasts and histiocytes is difficult. Occasional lymphocytes but few polymorphs are present. Lymphocytes are more abundant in the adjacent connective tissues. (*Top* ×72; *bottom* ×475)

with the long axes of the cells lying radially, suggests that they are directed towards or repelled from a chemical or microbial agent within the necrotic centre. Coarse, amorphous masses have been seen and are believed, from the evidence of Zucker–Franklin (1968), to be antigen/antibody complexes. This observation suggests that the nodule, like the other lesions of rheumatoid arthritis, may be the result of a direct immunological injury to collagen (Klemperer, Pollack and Baehr, 1942). Although chemical analyses for hydroxyproline do not support this suggestion (Bywaters and Glynn, 1970), the possibility that the local accumulation of antigen/antibody complexes can be responsible for granuloma formation is substantiated by recent experimental work (Spector and Heesom, 1969).

The microscopic structure of the rheumatoid nodule often requires to be distinguished from that of traumatic, fungal, bacterial and viral granulomata, from the smaller nodule of rheumatic fever (Dawson, 1933), from foreign body reactions, from chemical irritation and from the effects of vascular disease.

The nodules are very similar in form and location to certain cases of synovial tuberculosis and to the granulomata of candidiasis (Gardner, Krieg and Chapnick, 1962). There is a less close resemblance to the small nodules of granuloma annulare, to the acute subcutaneous nodule in rheumatic fever and to the lesions of necrobiosis lipoidica. However, the granulomata are larger than the evanescent nodules of rheumatic fever, and tend to be firm, dense and long-lasting. They may simulate epidermoid cysts (Wilson and Sokoloff, 1970). They are bound to adjacent connective tissue from which they can be freed with difficulty. Their structure and natural history recall those of the infectious granulomata such as those of tuberculosis, syphilis or yaws rather than of the smaller, less dense nodule of rheumatic fever or the paediatric lesion, granuloma annulare. Nodule formation is uncommon in juvenile rheumatoid arthritis and this is a reminder of the possible association between nodule formation and the production by the adult patient of the IgM anti-IgG gamma globulin, rheumatoid factor.

Something of the nature of rheumatoid nodules may be learnt by considering the pathogenesis of other, analogous granulomata. The cause of granuloma annulare remains, of course, unknown. The cause of tissue damage in rheumatic fever is apparently an immunological response on the part of cardiac, synovial and subcutaneous tissues to antibodies formed against antigenic determinants shared with Group A, β-haemolytic streptococci. The action of mycobacteria on connective tissue is mainly one of direct chemical injury but allergy is known to play a part in mycobacterial granuloma formation. None of these analogies gives an entirely convincing reason for deducing the pathogenesis of the granuloma of rheumatoid arthritis. The available evidence supports the view that an extrinsic agent causes the focal granulomata but suggests that the precise sites at which the lesions develop is determined by local vascular, mechanical or chemical factors. A so-called 'pseudorheumatoid' subcutaneous nodule must be distinguished (Mesara, Brody and Oberman, 1966).

It is recognised that small granulomata similar to those found in the subcutaneous tissues occur within the synovial tissue of affected joints where their presence is of diagnostic significance. Granulomata have also been encountered in tendon sheaths, in the sclera, in relation to the base of heart valves, in the pharynx, within the dura mater (Maher, 1954; Gardner, unpublished observations), in the subdural or extradural spaces (Linquist and McDonnell, 1970; Friedman, 1970), in the pleural margins of the lungs (Rubin, Gordon and Thelmo, 1967), and in the parenchyma of the lung in coal-workers with many of the known forms of pneumoconiosis (p. 140). Small nodules have been described in the perineural sheath of peripheral nerves (Leichentritt, 1943).

In all these situations, the basic structure of the nodule, with its central necrotic zones, marginal pallisaded histiocytes and surrounding collagen, closely resembles that of the prototype sub-cutaneous nodule. In different organs additional distinctive regional structural features may, however, be encountered. Hollingsworth (1968) records one case in which a rheumatoid granu-loma caused a 'saddle-nose' deformity. Another, most unusual manifestation was the develop-ment in 2 patients of linear subcutaneous bands across the chest wall, extending from the axilla and formed of coalescing granulomata (Dykman, Galens and Good, 1965). Basal cell carcinoma may be simulated (Healey, Wilske and Sagebiel, 1967). A strange granuloma of the head and neck of the femur was attributed to rheumatoid arthritis (Hunder, Ward and Ivins, 1965) and 2 similar cases were reported by Colton and Darby (1970).

Attempts have been made to provoke nodule formation in the skin of patients with rheumatoid arthritis and in animals by the injection of insoluble material such as bentonite or fibrin. The reactions vary markedly according to whether the implant is of autologous or heterologous origin. A particularly vigorous experimental reaction is provoked when foreign fibrin is implanted in a sensitised recipient. Massell, Coen and Jones (1952) injected small amounts of a patient's own blood into the skin overlying the olecranon and knee, producing nodules which resembled the evanescent foci found in rheumatic fever rather than the chronic granulomata of rheumatoid arthritis. Salicylates did not affect these experimental lesions the size and activity of which were related to the activity of the patient's disease. Saline could cause similar nodules; local trauma appeared to be necessary for this response. Trypsin and hyaluronidase were found to have the same local influence and it was clear that the reaction was nonspecific and probably unrelated to rheumatoid arthritis.

Immunofluorescent analyses of rheumatoid subcutaneous nodules have shown that the exu-dation and tissue destruction are likely to be the result of interactions between rheumatoid factor as antibody and IgG immunoglobulin as autoantigen (Nowoslawski and Bryzosko, 1967b). The central necrotic areas contain much IgG in the form of an IgG/IgM complex. IgG im-munoglobulin occurs as granules and as bumpy deposits filling the distended spaces between collagen fibres. The deposits interact both with aggregated human IgG and with heterologous immunoglobulin. They bind labelled rheumatoid factor and guinea-pig complement but do not contain the homologous $\beta_1 C$ component.

Analyses of the blood vessel walls in relation to the margins and centre of the rheumatoid nodule have demonstrated that there has been an uptake of fibrin and an 'incrustation' with IgG immunoglobulin with a specific affinity for rheumatoid factor and an avidity both for guinea-pig complement and for rheumatoid factor. In addition, the immunofluorescent analyses have shown that some blood vessels were occluded by large, bumpy precipitates of globulin and of fibrin or fibrinogen.

(b) Cardiovascular system

(i) Heart

It is important to distinguish the features described in ankylosing spondylitis (rheumatoid spondylitis) (Clark, Kulka and Bauer, 1957) from those of rheumatoid arthritis. Aortic incom-petence, for example, is rare in rheumatoid arthritis in which, however, aortic stenosis has been described (Lassiter and Tassy, 1965).

Patients with rheumatoid arthritis are found at times to have peri-, myo- and endocardial disease (Hollingsworth, 1968). Heart disease is more common in seropositive patients (Bonfiglio et al., 1969). Of the various lesions recognised clinically, pericarditis has attracted most interest. Pathologically, the possible relationship between valvulitis and subvalvular granulomata, and earlier rheumatic carditis remains an important question. The valvular lesions have usefully been reviewed (Roberts *et al.*, 1968). Until quite recently, cardiac lesions found in patients with rheumatoid arthritis were generally attributed to silent rheumatic disease (Baggenstoss and Rosenberg, 1941; Baggenstoss and Rosenberg, 1944; Collins, 1949). Thus in 23 cases of rheumatoid arthritis, Bayles (1943) found 6 with valvular and myocardial damage similar to that encountered in rheumatic fever. Five of the 6 appeared inactive. By contrast, Clark and Bauer (1948) surveyed 45 necropsies on patients with rheumatoid arthritis. The patients had a mean age of 51, a mean duration of the disease of 12 years. Only 2 had a previous history of rheumatic fever but 50% had evidence of some form of heart disease before death. Of these hypertension (50%) and rheumatic heart disease were nevertheless the most frequent. Pericarditis (14%) and valvular disease (16%) were common features of the suspected rheumatic heart disease. Aortic atherosclerosis (p. 131) was found frequently; focal non-rheumatic myocarditis was present in 16%, pericarditis in 44% and valvulitis in 20%. In only two cases were rheumatoid cardiac granulomata identified. In further series ranging in number from 10 to 105 necropsies, cardiac lesions, thought to be rheumatic, were described in proportions ranging from 5 to 66% (Bywaters, 1950; Sokoloff, 1953).

More recently it has come to be accepted that granulomata in rheumatoid heart disease are usually of rheumatoid origin (Christie, 1954; Sokoloff and Bunim, 1957). Rheumatoid pericarditis has also been identified as an entity. Bywaters (1950) was among the earliest to attribute pericarditis and nonspecific myocarditis to the systemic effects of rheumatoid arthritis. Cruickshank (1954) found evidence of coronary arteritis, often of a subacute character, in 15 of 72 necropsies: he regarded 6 as of rheumatic, 9 as of rheumatoid origin.

There is no doubt now, consequently, that all parts of the heart can be affected by rheumatoid disease.

Pericarditis (Gardner, 1969) was recognised frequently by Cruickshank (1958) in a survey of cardiac lesions in 100 fatal cases of rheumatoid arthritis. Those with pericarditis included 2 patients with rheumatoid granulomatous endocarditis (1 healed, 1 fibrotic), 2 with rheumatic endocarditis, 6 with nonspecific endocarditis (4 fibrotic) and 2 with myocarditis unaccompanied by endocarditis (1 fibrotic, 1 subacute with arteritis). As Sokoloff (1964) has pointed out, pericarditis represents one of the most constant findings in necropsy studies of patients with rheumatoid arthritis, approximately 40% of cases showing evidence of this condition. However the majority of cases show pericardial fibrosis, a minority active granulomatous pericarditis (Fig. 12.3).

Until very recently, reports of symptomatic rheumatoid pericardial disease had been infrequent. During the past 9 years, beginning with reports such as those of Wilkinson (1962), it has been recognised that fibrous rheumatoid pericarditis may cause constriction (Sutton, 1967; Harrold, 1968). Kirk and Cosh (1969) confirmed clinically that pericarditis may be a good deal more frequent than had been thought: 10 unsuspected examples were found among 100 rheumatoid arthritics; 45 were symptomless. There was no relationship to the duration of the disease but high titres of rheumatoid factor, anaemia, nodule formation and high erythrocyte sedimentation rates were usual. Resection of the shrunken, fibrous pericardial sac effectively alleviated the signs of obstructed venous return (Lange, Weiss and Ochsner, 1965; Kennedy, Partridge and Matthews, 1966; Batley, Uddin and Kelly, 1969).

Microscopically, the pericardial sac in fibrotic cases is largely composed of dense, collagenous connective tissue. Where active inflammation persists, there is young vascular granulation tissue, focally infiltrated with varying numbers of plasma cells and lymphocytes and occasionally displaying zones of fibrin and a subacute arteritis. The changes recall those seen in the joints in longstanding and relatively inactive rheumatoid synovitis with fibrous ankylosis: they are not specific and can be made the basis of diagnosis only by exclusion. No immunofluorescent investigations have been made.

Granulomatous lesions with a structure fundamentally similar to that of the subcutaneous granuloma (p. 122) were encountered by Cruickshank (1958) in 5 of 100 necropsy cases. Some were microscopic. Sokoloff found granulomata usually of the valve, valve ring, myocardium or

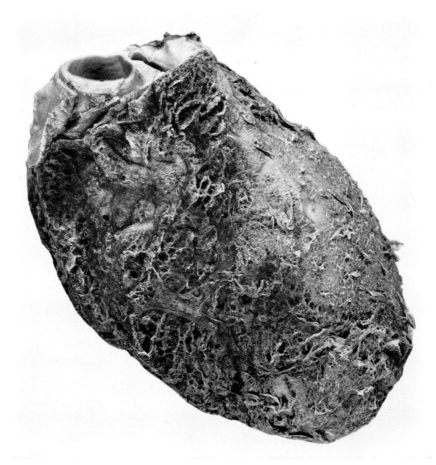

Fig. 12.3 Acute fibrinous pericarditis in rheumatoid arthritis with amyloidosis and uraemia. The appearances are those characteristic of fibrinous pericarditis. In the present case, that of an elderly woman with longstanding rheumatoid arthritis, the pericardial effusion was haemorrhagic. In most instances, evidence of pericarditis takes the form of collagenous connective tissue, partially or wholly obliterating the pericardial sac. Microscopically, subacute pericarditis is an occasional finding.

epicardium, in 2 of 19 patients, figures which compared with 2 of 62 cases (Lebowitz, 1963), 7 of 36 (Goehrs, Baggenstoss and Slocumb, 1960) and 10 of 43 (Levin *et al.*, 1955). Rheumatoid granulomata are often accompanied by subacute coronary arteritis, pericarditis or interstitial myocarditis and the coincidence of these individually nonspecific lesions helps to validate the diagnosis. Cardiac, subcutaneous and pulmonary granulomata (Ziff and Scully, 1967) may coexist but the absence of subcutaneous granulomata does not signify that cardiac nodules in the same patient are not rheumatoid. Where cardiac granulomata are present in the absence of rheumatoid arthritis (Good *et al.*, 1970) it is important to recall that comparable granulomata may be the result of other diseases such as bacterial or fungal infection (Gardner, Krieg and Chapnick, 1962).

Myocardial granulomata in rheumatoid arthritis are usually asymptomatic but may cause bundle branch (Lebowitz, 1963; Carpenter, Golden and Roberts, 1967) or complete (Gowans, 1960; Sobin and Hagstrom, 1962) heart block. In a recent report the detailed necropsy of a single case was described by Harris (1970). Congestive cardiac failure had been associated with bradycardia. A rheumatoid granuloma was found within the left coronary cusp of the aortic valve, covered by a vegetation. Similar granulomata were present in the right coronary cusp. Fibrosis and inflammatory cell infiltrates accompanied these and a nodular granuloma of the base of the anterior cusp of the mitral valve. Other granulomata were identified within the upper part of the muscular interventricular septum and in the interatrial septum. Almost the whole extent of the atrioventricular conducting tissue was infiltrated by inflammatory cells and many zones of necrosis, considered to be of rheumatoid granulomatous origin, were present.

Interstitial myocarditis. Focal interatrial collections of lymphocytes, plasma cells and histiocytes were encountered by Cruickshank (1958) in 11 of 100 cases, 6 with concurrent granulomatous or nonspecific endocarditis. The cell foci were sometimes close to blood vessels but 5 patients displayed independent vascular changes. The left ventricle in the region of the mitral valve was most frequently affected, the right ventricle or all four chambers less often. Sokoloff (1964) emphasised that the myocardial cell infiltrates may be extensive and indistinguishable from Fiedler's myocarditis. They occasionally include numerous eosinophils; these cells may be one consequence of allergy, drug toxicity or viral infection complicating treatment with corticosteroids. There is sometimes focal myocardial fibrosis (Schwartz, 1967).

The coexistence of myocarditis with pericarditis, arteritis and granulomata allows a firm diagnosis of rheumatoid heart disease to be attempted. Cardiac amyloidosis must be excluded.

Arteritis involving divisions of the coronary arteries may be of a low-grade, subacute variety (p. 135) or a necrotising lesion (p. 131). Karten (1969b) recognised diffuse vasculitis in 6 of 102 rheumatoid patients in 4 years: 2 also had myocardial infarcts. Coronary arteritis was demonstrated in one of these cases and was suspected in the other. An additional survey of 95 other cases, 7 of which had myocardial infarcts, failed to reveal further cases of coronary arteritis. Rheumatoid coronary artery involvement, found in 20 of Cruickshank's (1958) 100 cases, is usually accompanied by arteritis in other viscera. Sokoloff (1964) could not distinguish a significantly raised incidence of arteritis in patients previously treated with corticosteroids. Active arteritis may coexist with other inactive, healed cardiac lesions.

In diagnostic terms, the site, nature and clinical features allow rheumatoid cardiac disease to be distinguished from rheumatic. Rheumatoid granulomata resembling the subcutaneous nodule are not easily mistaken although features of acute mycotic cardiac lesions recall those seen at an early stage in rheumatoid arthritis (Gardner *et al.*, 1962). Aschoff bodies are not seen in cases with focal myocardial lymphocytic infiltration ('myocarditis'). Arteritis is of a subacute variety; and the dense, fibrotic pericardium shows no histological features of tuberculosis or of rheumatic fever. When calcific aortic stenosis coexists with rheumatoid arthritis, it is generally not possible to be certain whether one of the several suspected causes of this disease, such as brucellosis, has been operative. But aortic valvular insufficiency with regurgitation, and accompanied by nonsyphilitic thickening of the vasa vasorum is most unusual in rheumatoid arthritis in spite of its evident association with ankylosing spondylitis (Clark *et al.*, 1957).

(ii) *Blood vessels* (Sokoloff, 1963; Kulka, 1966)

Both the muscular arteries and arterioles are frequently sites for vascular disease in rheumatoid arthritis, particularly in the more severe forms of the disorder and when rheumatoid factor is detectable in the serum. Abdominal apoplexy is also recognised (Webb and Payne, 1970). Arterial disease can now be diagnosed with some certainty by rectal biopsy (Schneider and Dobbins, 1968) a technique already widely adopted in rheumatoid arthritis for the recognition of amyloidosis (p. 166). So far as I am aware, rheumatoid factor has not been demonstrated in or in relation to the arterial or arteriolar lesions in spite of its presence in the synovia and regional lymphoid tissue of the same patients (Douglas, 1965; Paronetto, 1969). The aorta is often atherosclerotic in older patients with rheumatoid arthritis but, notwithstanding suggestive changes in the level of serum α-globulins, the incidence of atherosclerosis is no less than in control, non-rheumatoid populations (unpublished personal observations).

The microvasculature has been studied in some detail (Kulka, 1966). Using the freeze-fixation technique developed by Kulka, Goldie (1969) obtained evidence which suggested that the inflammatory tissue damage in rheumatoid synovia comes from a gradual stagnation of the circulation through venular and capillary plexuses, with a temporary persistence of flow in preferential arteriolar-venular channels. Comparable *in vivo* observations have been made by Bakowska and Gardner (1971) in the vessels of animals with allergic arthritis. There have not yet been any reports in rheumatoid arteritis of the virus-like inclusions seen in the capillary endothelial cells of muscle in polymyositis, in the small vessels in scleroderma and systemic lupus erythematosus (Norton, 1969), and, more recently, in dermatomyositis (Norton, Velayos and Robinson, 1970) (p. 193). In these diseases, in which many vascular changes analogous with those of rheumatoid arthritis have been discovered, the inclusions may represent virus ribonucleo-protein. They recall the structures reported in capillary cells infected by poliomyelitis virus.

Necrotising arteritis (Fig. 12.4)

It has been clear since 1949 (Graef, Hickey and Altman, 1949; Christie, 1950) that an inflammatory arteritis may complicate or be associated with rheumatoid arthritis (Fig. 12.4). Sokoloff, Wilens and Bunim (1951) drew attention to an arteritis of skeletal muscle and Ball (1954) described a necrotising arteritis indistinguishable from that of classical polyarteritis nodosa. This observation was confirmed by Radnai (1953, 1969). Radnai investigated 30 patients and recognised arteritis in 14, 9 of which he classified as acute or subacute. Cruickshank (1954) however, in a necropsy study based mainly on cardiac and skeletal muscle, synovial and nerve tissue, emphasised that in the majority of cases of rheumatoid arthritis the lesions were of a subacute variety (p. 135) and could be differentiated from those of polyarteritis nodosa, rheumatic fever, systemic lupus erythematosus, temporal arteritis, dermatomyositis and scleroderma. A full review of the literature was provided by Alexander (1967) in relation to his physiological studies of the skin circulation in rheumatoid arthritis.

The manifestations of necrotising arteritis complicating rheumatoid arthritis may be as protean as are those of polyarteritis nodosa. Thus, examples of rheumatoid mesenteric infarction were recorded by Bienenstock, Minick and Rogoff (1967) and of polyneuropathy by Topp and Hart (1967). The latter demonstrated that the prognosis in necrotising rheumatoid arteritis, as in polyarteritis nodosa, is by no means uniformly bad. However, cases of rheumatoid arthritis in which arteritis develops are usually sero-positive and of a severe variety.

Arteritis may cause visceral lesions resembling those of polyarteritis nodosa clinically. Alternatively, the arterial disease may be recognised by chance at necropsy in clinically inactive cases. In one instance of arteritis observed personally (case 36) focal cerebral, testicular and adrenal infarction caused by necrotising arteriolitis were found at necropsy in an elderly man whose synovitis was clinically inert. It is not yet certain whether active arteritis is caused by the same agent(s) that provokes active rheumatoid synovitis. A primary virus arteritis similar to that detected in equine viral arteritis, could accompany and be part of early rheumatoid synovitis. The later course of rheumatoid synovitis, maintained by autoallergic mechanisms, may, equally,

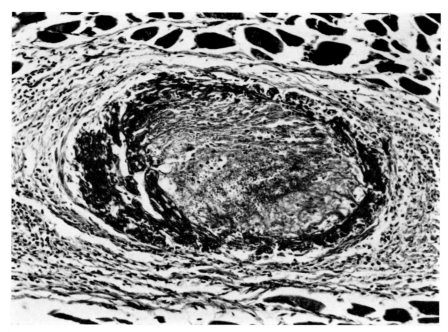

Fig. 12.4   Necrotising arteritis in rheumatoid arthritis. A skeletal muscle, medium-size artery, the wall of which is necrotic. Deeply eosinophilic (black) material occupies much of the wall of the vessel the lumen of which is occluded by a loose fibrin and platelet thrombus. Surrounding the necrotic vessel are moderate numbers of lymphocytes, plasma cells and some polymorphs. The appearances closely resemble those of polyarteritis nodosa. (From Gardner D.L., *Pathology of the Connective Tissue Diseases*, London: Arnold, 1965.)   (× 170)

be responsible for an autoallergic arteritis. In 1957 a report by Kemper, Baggenstoss and Slocumb suggested that necrotising arteritis in rheumatoid arthritis could be precipitated by the therapeutic use of corticosteroids. Because necrotising arteritis can occur in rheumatoid arthritics in the absence of this form of treatment, it remains uncertain whether this suggestion can be substantiated. Evidence that might prove this result of corticosteroid treatment is not easy to obtain since the current trend in the United Kingdom is either to avoid corticosteroids or to use very small doses.

Intimal proliferation (Figs. 12.5, 12.6)

In investigations that have been mainly clinical, it has been established that peripheral vascular insufficiency in rheumatoid arthritis is often associated with inadequate filling of the digital arteries by injected contrast media (Bywaters, 1957; Scott *et al.*, 1961). The frequency of this digital vascular disease has been investigated by Cats and Pit (1969). These authors found digital lesions in 10% of males from a group of 146 cases of whom 49% had rheumatoid nodules, 79%

rheumatoid factor and 45% antinuclear factor. The corresponding figures for the female cases were 30%, 24%, 74% and 28% respectively. A comparable study was made by Skrifvars, Laine and Wegelius (1969); radiological changes were identified in the blood vessels of 15·4% of 370 patients with rheumatoid arthritis and of 3·4% of 438 control cases.

The underlying vascular changes are those of intimal proliferation or endarterial fibrosis ('endarteritis') and they are not readily distinguished from those encountered after prolonged exposure to cold or vibration. The digital arteries (Fig. 12.6), and less often those of the synovia and viscera, come to be partly or almost wholly obstructed by a proliferation of intimal connective

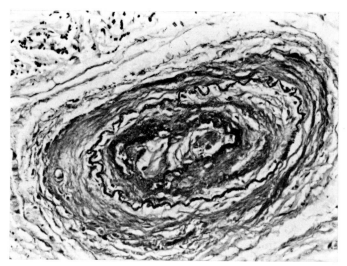

Fig. 12.5 Small artery in rheumatoid arthritis showing occupation of lumen by abundant new intimal connective tissue, a process of endarterial fibrosis. The connective tissue is thought to comprise prolific proteoglycan matrix within which are elongated cells, some of smooth muscle type. Note little new elastic formation. *Elastic—van Gieson.* (×160)

tissue and smooth muscle cells and by the new synthesis of intimal proteoglycans. The change, according to its location, accompanies, causes or is caused by diminished blood flow to the tissues to which the diseased arteries run. The physiological disturbances that result include Raynaud's phenomenon, pulmonary hypertension and visceral ischaemia. The arterial disease recalls that observed at the base of peptic ulcers: and, as in this disorder, the term endarterial fibrosis has succeeded 'endarteritis obliterans' as a more rational description of the condition since it is by no means certain whether arterial obstruction leads to or results from the nearby inflammatory reaction.

Thrombosis may cause an inconvenient localised digital gangrene and, occurring in viscera and in channels as important as the vertebral arteries (Webb, Hickman and Brew, 1968), may lead to death. There is at least a generic similarity between the obliterative arterial disease of rheumatoid arthritis and the intimal connective tissue multiplication recognised in the skin and viscera in progressive systemic sclerosis, although the quantity of new connective tissue matrix detected in the latter disorder, as in the renal arteries in some cases of accelerated hypertension, is greater than in the more cellular and less fibrous lesions of rheumatoid arthritis. The similarity between these occlusive arterial lesions is sufficient to suggest that in this respect, as in the common sharing of interstitial cystic pulmonary fibrosis, rheumatoid arthritis and systemic sclerosis lie at different points on a common spectrum of disorder. Digital arterial obstruction in rheumatoid arthritis is almost always associated with the persistence of sero-positivity (Bywaters and Scott, 1963) but the cause of the intimal reaction is more likely to be the local aggregation of antigen/antibody complexes than the local cytotoxic action of autologous antiglobulin (Douglas, 1965).

The skin lesions caused by vascular insufficiency in rheumatoid arthritis include small areas of infarction, and overt gangrene (Bywaters, 1957). These changes, with their corresponding zones of ulceration or discolouration, cannot be assumed to be caused only by intimal proliferation

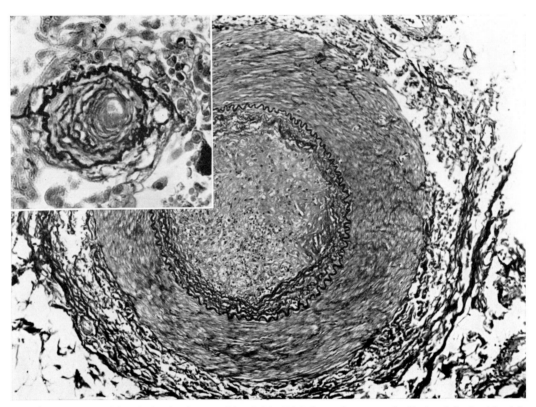

Fig. 12.6   Digital arterial occlusion in rheumatoid arthritis. Digital vessels commonly display defective blood flow. In the vessel demonstrated in this Figure there is reduplication of the internal elastic lamina. Recent thrombus has occupied the vessel and has undergone organisation. Small capillary channels can be recognised: the thrombus contains small numbers of inflammatory cells. (*Inset*) Pulmonary arteriole to show elastic reduplication and intimal proliferation in rheumatoid pulmonary vascular disease. (From Gardner D. L., *Pathology of the Connective Tissue Diseases*, London: Arnold, 1965.)   (× 160; *inset* × 375)

since it has now been demonstrated that they may also result from acute or subacute arteritis (O'Quinn, Kennedy and Baker, 1965).

In rare instances (Gardner *et al.*, 1957) the digital arterial occlusion of the sero-positive rheumatoid arthritic may be accompanied by comparable changes in the lungs (Fig. 12.10), leading to a form of pulmonary hypertension. Nothing is known of the pathogenesis of the obliterative pulmonary vascular lesions that are readily distinguished from the occasional case of necrotising pulmonary arteritis seen in rheumatoid arthritis, from the upper respiratory infarcts of Wegener's granulomatosis and from the pulmonary vascular changes in systemic sclerosis (Collins, Darke and Dodge, 1958) and systemic lupus erythematosus (Cruickshank, 1966).

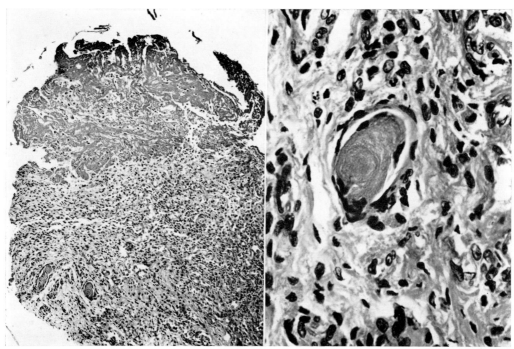

Fig. 12.7 Rheumatoid synovitis in thrombotic thrombocytopenic microangiopathy. (*Left*) Surface of rheumatoid synovial villus with numerous polymorphs and lymphocytes infiltrating tissues. (From Gardner D. L., *Pathology of the Connective Tissue Diseases*, London: Arnold, 1965.) (*Top*) Abundant fibrin containing small numbers of inflammatory cells. Note (*bottom left*) two venules containing microthrombi. (*Right*) Part of previous figure seen at higher magnification, to show microthrombus, covered by endothelial cells, lying within a synovial venule. Surrounding the vessel are moderate numbers of histiocytes and occasional polymorphs. (*Left* ×90; *right* ×360)

Thrombotic microangiopathy (Fig. 12.7)

Two cases of rheumatoid arthritis have been described in which the microangiopathic haemolytic anaemia syndrome (Editorial, 1969) with thrombotic microangiopathy (Moschowitz's syndrome) has been associated with the therapeutic use of phenylbutazone (Dunea, Muehrcke, Nakamoto and Schwartz, 1966; Thomson and Gardner, 1969) (Fig. 12.7). The pathogenesis of this rare syndrome in rheumatoid arthritis remains speculative but it is interesting to note that the venules of the inflamed rheumatoid synovia may come to contain fibrin and platelet thrombi just as do those of the viscera (Thomson and Gardner, 1969).

Subacute arteritis

One variety of arterial disease commonly encountered in necropsy specimens in rheumatoid arthritis is a low-grade, subacute arteritis. Cruickshank (1954) made a microscopic survey of a large series of blocks of cardiac and skeletal muscle, and of nerve. The lesion comprises a moderate intra- and periarterial infiltration by lymphocytes and histiocytes but with few plasma cells. There is usually little evidence that this arterial disease has caused clinical signs or symptoms but an association with the nerve lesions in laryngeal rheumatoid arthritis suggests that these focal arterial disturbances may not always be innocuous (Wolman, Darke and Young, 1965). They are not easy to distinguish from the occasional arterial lesions in rheumatoid arthritis that result from systemic, secondary bacterial or fungal infection (Gardner et al., 1962).

Venulitis

The role of the small vessels in the pathogenesis of rheumatoid arthritis has been closely studied by Kulka (1966). Current evidence favours the view that venules, rather than capillaries, mediate the local phenomena of inflammation (Curran, 1967). Kulka has drawn attention to the frequency of venular and capillary dilatation in synovial, nodular and visceral lesions in rheumatoid arthritis and has devised a *schema* for the pathogenesis of the disease based on both *in vivo* and *in vitro* studies. He believes that the small vessel changes are an end-result of focal capillary–venular dilatation and increased permeability. The venulitis ranges in intensity from fibrin infiltration, endothelial necrosis and thrombosis, through a cellular inflammatory infiltrate, to intimal proliferation and endothelial hyperplasia.

Pathological physiology (Alexander, 1967)

Pathological investigations of the vasculature in rheumatoid arthritis have complemented those on microcirculatory physiology, electron microscopy and immunology. It has been appreciated for many years that the skin circulation in this disease might be abnormal and 'capillaritis' is known to occur (Dequeker and Rosberg, 1967). Studies such as those of Potter and Duthie (1961) have defined capillary resistance to negative pressure and have shown that there is a negative correlation between capillary resistance and environmental temperature in rheumatoid arthritis. The capillary resistance measured in these tests was, it was concluded, a 'measure of some property of the connective tissue ensheathing small cutaneous vessels and particularly the collecting venules' (Zweifach, 1955). The relationship between these temperature-dependent alterations to physical stress and the sequence of changes in the venules that Kulka (1966) believes play an important role in the inflammatory lesions of rheumatoid arthritis, is uncertain. However, it appears possible that a primary alteration in the physical characteristics of the vascular or perivascular connective tissue could simultaneously contribute to the increased susceptibility to negative pressure and to increased vascular permeability in the inflammatory reaction.

Brånemark et al. (1969) surveyed the pathological physiology of the blood vessels in rheumatoid arthritis and made light and electron microscopic investigations of the synovial vasculitis. Plasmatic vasculosis (Lendrum, 1969) is occasionally encountered (unpublished personal observations). The work of Brånemark et al. (1969) was an extension of *in vivo* observations made on conjunctival and synovial tissue in which these authors had concluded that the disposition of the vascular lesions was haphazard (Brånemark et al., 1963). Brånemark et al. (1969) confirmed the presence of venulitis but found the arterioles to be normal. They deduced from their electron microscopic studies that the pathological features described by other authors (Hirohata and Kobayashi, 1964; Paul, 1967) were either not different from those detected in normal, control material or were due to artefact. Brånemark et al. (1969) admitted that sampling for electron microscopy introduced problems of interpretation. Their work is difficult to understand and their failure to confirm by electron microscopy the lesions which they and others had found by light microscopy can perhaps be explained by the fact that they did not use thick (0.5–$1.0\,\mu$m), Epon- or araldite-embedded sections for survey purposes.

(c) **Respiratory system** (Table 12.1 and Fig. 12.8)

Contrary to the earlier views of Aronoff, Bywaters and Fearnley (1955), Gibberd (1965) and Short, Bauer and Reynolds (1957), respiratory disease is very common in rheumatoid arthritis

TABLE 12.1. *Frequency of lung and bronchial disease at death, determined for 142 patients with rheumatoid arthritis dying in hospital*

Pleural fibrosis	56	(41%)
Bronchopneumonia	54	(40%)
Emphysema	31	(23%)
Pulmonary embolism	14	(10%)
Tuberculosis	13	(10%)
Pulmonary hypertension	9	(7%)
Pulmonary infarction	8	
Acute pleuritis	8	
Pulmonary primary tumours	7	
Abscess	6	
Bronchiectasis	6	
Atelectasis	5	
Interstitial fibrosis	4	

(Scadding, 1969). Sievers, Aho, Hurri and Perltala (1964) showed a significantly raised incidence of radiological abnormalities when sero-positive rheumatoid patients were compared with sero-negative controls, an observation suggesting the possibility that rheumatoid factor was related to the genesis of lung disease in rheumatoid arthritis. Cruickshank (1959a) recorded 8 instances of interstitial pneumonia from among approximately 100 necropsy cases, an incidence perhaps exaggerated by bias in selection, but Patterson, Harville and Pierce (1965) also believed the lungs in rheumatoid arthritis to be 'exceptionally reactive'. Pulmonary vascular changes, characteristically parietal hyalinosis, are frequent (Roujeau and Amouroux, 1968) and pleural fibrosis, one index of previous pulmonary inflammation, is recognisable in almost half of all patients dying with rheumatoid arthritis.

Four main groups of pathological change (Christie, 1954) can therefore be described. They frequently coincide:

1. Pleuritis, with or without effusion;
2. Pulmonary granulomata, pleural or intrapulmonary in location, and very occasionally coexisting with pneumoconiosis (Caplan's syndrome);
3. Pulmonary necrotising arteritis; and pulmonary intimal proliferation;
4. Bronchiectasis; interstitial pneumonitis with bronchiolitis and cystic change.

The four groups are reviewed by Spencer (1968). Earlier publications report less complete findings (Spencer, 1955).

In spite of clinical usage, there is very little justification for the term 'rheumatoid lung' which, except in the case of pulmonary granulomata, describes clinical association rather than pathological entity. None of the changes listed above is individually characteristic and all may be encountered in other inflammatory disease, particularly those of the systemic connective tissues.

Pleural effusion (Dodson and Hollingsworth, 1966) is a particularly frequent clinical sign (Editorial, 1968) and has been variously reported as being present in 2·3–22·2% of patients (Walker and Wright, 1967, 1968). 'R.A.' cells (p. 102) have been encountered in the fluid

(Carmichael and Golding, 1967; Nosanchuk and Naylor, 1968). The question of the cytodiagnosis of rheumatoid pleurae effusions has recently been examined in detail by Boddington *et al.* (1971). 19 pleural effusions were studied. In 7 cases there were degenerating polymorphs, amorphous extracellular material and epitheliod cells, many of which were multinucleated. In 5 further cases, only the first 2 phenomena were noted. The amorphous material reacted with

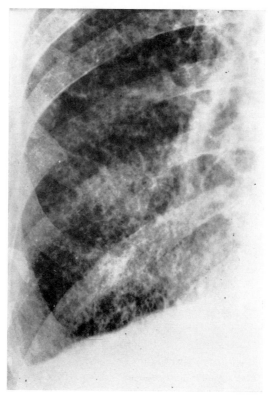

Fig. 12.8 The lung in rheumatoid arthritis illustrating the honeycomb-like, reticular pattern characteristic of longstanding lower lobe disease. The appearances correspond to those shown microscopically in Figure 12.13. They closely resemble those encountered in systemic sclerosis. (From Gardner D. L., *Pathology of the Connective Tissue Diseases*, London: Arnold, 1965.)

anti-IgM antisera and positive precipitin tests both for IgM and IgG were obtained. The conclusions seemed clear that with care, and by appropriate techniques, rheumatoid effusions could be differentiated from others. Necropsy studies, in which examination can be more complete, reveal an even higher incidence of pleural disease. Talbott and Calkins (1964) reported that more than half of their series of 37 cases (51·6%) had pleural disease compared with 38·9% of a similar number of control cases. Evidently pleural fibrosis is common among older people whether or not they have rheumatoid arthritis. Very occasionally, evidence of pleuritis can be found before arthritis is detected. In my own series, 56 of 142 necropsy cases showed more or less evidence of pleural fibrosis. A substantial proportion of patients with rheumatoid arthritis develop lung infections during life (Walker, 1967)—at least 40% show signs of bronchopneumonia at necropsy—and the pleuritis (Schools and Mikkelsen, 1962) must, in most cases, be regarded as a remote secondary consequence of the underlying rheumatoid disease. Impaired mobility and diminished resistance to infection predispose to viral, bacterial and fungal invasion. Decortication has occasionally proved necessary (Brunk, Drash and Swineford, 1966).

Pleural granulomata closely similar to those found in the subcutaneous tissues and, less commonly, in the other viscera (p. 122) are a much more serious proposition (Bennett, Zeller and Bauer, 1940; Raven, Parkes Weber and Price, 1948; Heller, Kellow and Chomet, 1956; Price and Skelton, 1956; Schools and Davey, 1960; Rubin, Gordon and Thelmo, 1967; Champion, Robertson and Robinson, 1968). They may be extra- or intrapulmonary in position and may be related to the parietal or to the interlobular pleural surfaces. Although guidance with the histological diagnosis of material obtained from such cases can be obtained by the finding of a low pleural fluid glucose level, the interpretation of biopsy material can be perplexing (Carr and

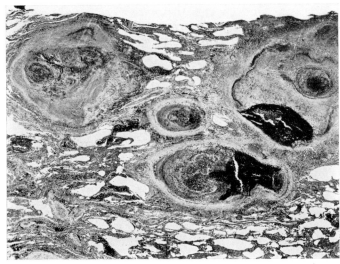

Fig. 12.9 Pulmonary rheumatoid nodule formation (Caplan's nodule). A series of adjacent and merging rheumatoid nodules, deeply laden with carbon pigment, in the emphysematous and fibrotic lung of a coalminer with pneumoconiosis. The confluent nodules that have zones of necrotic material, assume a characteristic gross appearance radiologically. (From Gardner D. L., *Textbook of the Rheumatic Diseases*, ed. Copeman W. S. C., 1968, pp. 87–152.)
(×7)

Mayne, 1962; Mattingley, 1964; Poppius and Tani, 1964). The minute portion of tissue obtained by aspiration needle may contain vascular connective (granulation) tissue infiltrated with mononuclear cells, including considerable numbers of plasma cells. Subacute or necrotising arteritis may be recognised. The presence of granules resembling those of mast cells has been shown by electron microscopy (Bischoff, Harrison, Bucci and Nelson, 1969). But the cellular and vascular changes are nonspecific in themselves; they can only be of confirmatory value when clinical and serological criteria for the diagnosis of rheumatoid arthritis are established, or by the exclusion of neoplastic or other disease (Carr and Mayne, 1962; Ward, 1961).

According to Walker and Wright (1968), 43 patients with *intrapulmonary granulomata* had been reported. Others, naturally, have been seen but not described (Case 139). The majority of patients with pulmonary nodules also have subcutaneous granulomata. The number quoted by Walker and Wright (1968) is almost certainly an underestimate and an additional, typical case is described by Hollingsworth (1968).

The granulomata may persist unchanged for years. They occur, as do rheumatoid granulomata generally, in sero-positive patients with severe arthritis and tend to be peripheral in location, an opinion usually based more on radiological assessment than on pathological dissection. Where confluent nodules are encountered in the outer part of the lung, peripheral carcinomata, meta-stases, tuberculous foci, and infarcts may be simulated. A proportion of the reported cases has been detected by pleural biopsy (Walker and Wright, 1968) or at necropsy (Ellman and Ball, 1948; Gruenwald, 1948; Horler and Thomson, 1959; Schools and Davey, 1960; Hindle and Yates, 1965). The nodules may coexist, misleadingly, with more serious lung lesions such as bronchial carcinoma, and may become overtly infected. Liquefaction, cavitation (Portner and Gracie, 1966; Stengel, Watson and Darling, 1966) and rupture are described. Pyopneumothorax or pneumothorax (Portner and Gracie, 1966) may be consequences.

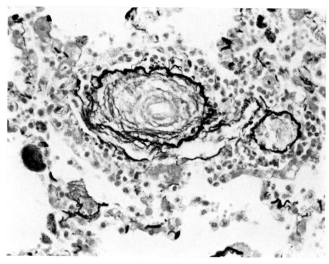

Fig. 12.10 Compare with Figure 12.6 (*inset*). A further field to show arteriolar occlusion in rheumatoid pulmonary hypertension. There is reduplication of the normally single elastic lamina and new connective tissue formation that occupies the intima and occludes the blood vessel. Small numbers of nearby inflammatory cells can be seen.

(× 310)

Intrapulmonary rheumatoid granulomata vary in size but are seldom more than 2 cm in diameter. By itself, the size of a nodule is insufficient to cause secondary phenomena such as atelectasis; however, nodules may become confluent and involvement of the pleura may lead to rheumatoid pleuritis. Hypertrophic pulmonary osteoarthropathy (p. 74), as in other forms of lung disease in rheumatoid arthritis, is most exceptional.

The title *Caplan's syndrome* is applicable to the coexistence of rheumatoid intrapulmonary granulomata with coal-worker's pneumoconiosis (Niedobitek, 1969). The radiological appearances are characteristic (Caplan, 1953) and have been fully discussed (Caplan, Payne and Withey, 1962) (Fig. 12.9). Coal worker's pulmonary rheumatoid nodules may be identified before synovitis is detected clinically, suggesting that the rheumatoid process predisposes to this particular form of lung response. Rheumatoid factor is present in the plasma but has not yet been found, to my knowledge, in or in relation to the granulomata. Histologically, there is always a central zone of necrosis (Gough, Rivers and Seal, 1955; Gough, 1959) and the structural features closely re-semble those of the subcutaneous nodule, with, in addition, more or less abundant marginal impregnation with coal dust.

Since Caplan's original account, similar pulmonary nodules have been found in asbestos workers (Richards and Barrett, 1958; Tellesson, 1961), gold miners (Chatgidakis and Theron, 1961), chalk miners (Lamvik, 1963) and other industrial workers (Campbell, 1958; Caplan, Cowen

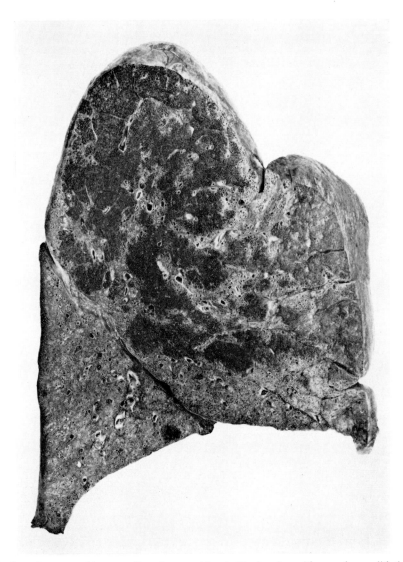

Fig. 12.11 The lung in a case of longstanding rheumatoid arthritis showing widespread consolidation, fibrosis and cyst formation in the lower lobe and lower part of the upper lobe. The greater part of the upper lobe retains a grey-black appearance where zones of congestion and haemosiderin pigmentation are confluent. In this case, Case 148, the diagnosis of systemic lupus erythematosus at age 55, had been succeeded by some years of corticosteroid treatment. Later, peripheral vascular insufficiency was accompanied by pulmonary hypertension, cor pulmonale and congestive cardiac failure. (From Gardner D. L., *Textbook of Rheumatic Diseases*, ed. Copeman W. S. C., 1968, pp. 87–152.)

and Gough, 1958; Posner, 1960) but less is known of the microscopic structure of these granulomata than of those found in the coal miner.

Pulmonary vascular disease in rheumatoid arthritis, by contrast with the changes in polyarteritis nodosa and in Wegener's granulomatosis, has attracted little clinical interest. A necrotising arteritis may occur (Ellman and Ball, 1948; Gardner, 1966) giving rise to zonal infarcts which must be distinguished from pulmonary granulomata. Intimal arteriolar and arterial proliferation with new elastic and smooth muscle formation may develop, apparently in isolation and may cause otherwise unexplained pulmonary hypertension (Gardner *et al.*, 1957). Focal arteritis results from, and is incidental to, interstitial pulmonary fibrosis (Price and Skelton, 1956). When lung disease is sufficiently severe to cause cystic or honeycomb-like changes (Fig. 12.13), many small arteries in the affected lobules show pronounced intimal proliferation, possibly as a consequence of segmental thrombosis.

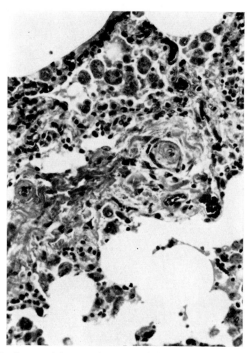

Fig. 12.12 Pulmonary arteriole (*upper right centre*) occupied by excess new intimal connective tissue material. Numerous pulmonary, haemosiderin-laden macrophages are present, part of the process of congestive cardiac failure; other inflammatory cells, mainly lymphocytes and occasional polymorphs, lie within the pulmonary interstitium.

(× 195)

Diffuse *interstitial pulmonary fibrosis* (Heppleston, 1951; Lee and Brain, 1962; Walker and Wright, 1969) was recognised clinically in 1·6% of 516 patients with rheumatoid arthritis (Walker and Wright, 1968). These authors discovered an additional 115 cases reported in the literature: approximately 2/3 were men. Many cases not examined in hospital must remain undetected. A probable sequence of events for the development of the lung changes was outlined by Cruickshank (1959*a*). This author emphasised first, that a causal relationship between rheumatoid disease and pulmonary lesions was likely, and second, that none of the lesions found in his 8 necropsy cases was specific. A nonspecific reversible, interstitial pneumonia appeared to be the earliest change; persistent inflammation, however, led to increasing fibrosis, followed by bronchiolectasis and, ultimately, honeycomb lung (Figs. 12.8, 12.13) (Heppelston, 1956; Dixon and

Ball, 1957). This sequence conforms closely with what is known of interstitial fibrosis due to lipid pneumonia, sarcoidosis, the Hamman–Rich syndrome and other conditions (Anderson and Foraker, 1960) (Figs. 12.10–12.13). In its fully developed stage, pulmonary arterial intimal proliferation is frequent, arteritis occasional.

The contribution made by vascular disease to the interstitial pneumonitis described above is uncertain and the suggestion that bronchial arterial injury is causal (Ellman and Cudkowicz, 1954) remains unsubstantiated. Distinction from the cystic lung of systemic sclerosis may not be simple in advanced cases but a consideration of the serological and haematological features may enable an opinion to be given. Early interstitial pulmonary fibrosis, in the absence of rheumatoid synovitis, may be associated with the presence of rheumatoid serum factor and, later with the synthesis of antinuclear antibodies (Turner–Warwick and Doniach, 1965). The significance of the inclusions resembling those of mast cells described in the parenchyma of the lung (Bischoff *et al.*, 1969) is not known. Whether the lung lesions are provoked by an antigen/antibody reaction due to protein precipitation or secondary bacterial infection remains uncertain (Hollingsworth, 1968). An association with bronchial carcinoma is reported (Roegel, Weitzenblum, Lenz, Stoebner and Oudet, 1969) but would appear, by contrast with the associations known in dermatomyositis, to be coincidental.

(d) Urinary system

Few patients with rheumatoid arthritis show clinical evidence of impaired renal function. When selected series are investigated more closely, proportions varying from 7 to 72% have, however, been found to have renal disease (Pirani and Manaligod, 1966) and *post mortem* evidence of renal disorder is comparatively frequent. Biopsy studies support this view (Brun *et al.*, 1963). Since 13–17% of hospital patients dying with rheumatoid arthritis have amyloidosis, almost always affecting the kidney (Heptinstall and Joekes, 1960), this process must be considered in reviewing any renal disturbances that may be encountered. This consideration is also relevant in Still's disease in which however amyloidosis is uncommon.

TABLE 12.2. *Organ weights in rheumatoid arthritis and in control cases matched for age and sex (necropsy records)*

	Mean weight (g.)	
	Spleen	Liver
Rheumatoid arthritis	224	1,490
Control cases	120	1,435
Difference	104	55
SE	± 26·1	± 86

Whether there are renal changes specific for rheumatoid arthritis is extremely doubtful—in my view the absence of glomerular disease is one of the most reliable histological means for distinguishing atypical cases of rheumatoid arthritis with a positive LE cell test from classical systemic lupus erythematosus—and there is no justification whatsoever for the use of the term 'rheumatoid kidney'. The significance of glomerulitis is disputed.

As is so commonly the case with the other viscera in rheumatoid arthritis, very much more is recorded of the clinical aspects of the kidney than of the pathological. Histologically, two main disorders have attracted recent interest: glomerulitis; and the vascular and tubular consequences

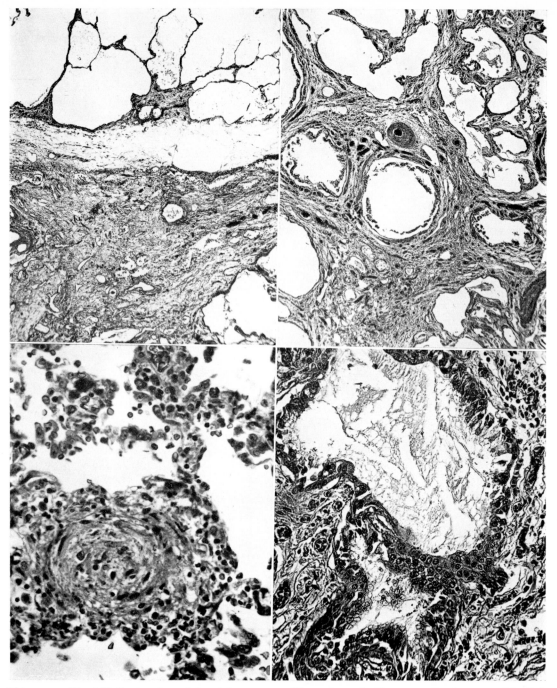

Fig. 12.13 (*Top left*) Section through interlobar septum of lung shown in Fig. 12.12. Emphysema, with slight interstitial fibrosis, of upper lobe (*top*). Lower lobe (*bottom*) extensively occupied by fibrous tissue: few residual alveolar spaces dilated, with lining of low cuboidal epithelium. (*Top right*) Enlarged alveolar spaces, with destruction of intra-aveolar septa, dilated bronchioles with cuboidal epithelial lining and pulmonary arterial branch (*centre*) partly occluded by intimal hyperplasia. (*Bottom left*) Pulmonary arteriole to show greatly thickened wall containing much new fibromuscular and elastic tissue, and increased cellularity of adjacent alveolar septa. (*Bottom right*) In the most severely affected parts of the cystic-appearing lung, the residual air spaces are lined by hyperplastic cuboidal alveolar or low columnar bronchiolar epithelium. The appearances recall those seen in healing lung injuries and in systemic sclerosis. (From Gardner D. L., *Textbook of the Rheumatic Diseases*, ed. Copeman W. S. C., 1968, pp. 87–152.)

(*Top left* ×24; *right* ×24; *bottom left* ×195; *right* ×195)

of phenacetin toxicity. Because of the age distribution of rheumatoid arthritis, hypertensive arteriolar sclerosis is frequent but valid evidence of active or of chronic pyelonephritis has, in my own series of necropsy cases, been less common than anticipated. (But compare Lawson and MacLean's series, below, in which the various forms of pyelonephritis were extremely common.) The microbiological evidence suggests, however, that urinary tract infection in rheumatoid arthritis (5·9%) is no more frequent than among a control population (11·8%) (Mowat, Hothersall and Gould, 1970).

'Glomerulitis' (Baggenstoss and Rosenberg, 1943; Fingerman and Andrus, 1943; Pirani and Bennett, 1951; Sinclair and Cruikshank, 1956), with a slight increase of both endothelial and of mesangial cells, has been described in up to 2/3 of a small series of cases. Doubt has been cast on the frequency and significance of this lesion (Allander, Bucht, Lövgren and Wehle, 1963; Pollak, Pirani, Stech and Kark, 1962), which is followed neither by focal nor by panglomerular fibrosis. However, Pirani and Manaligod (1966) point out that by the exotic technique of glomerular cell counting in renal biopsy specimens (Sørenson, 1967), increased glomerular cellularity can be identified (Brun, Olsen, Raaschou and Sørensen, 1965) and can be assumed to provide evidence of glomerulitis. So far, there is no evidence that the deposits of immunoglobulin, of complement and of fibrinogen that have been recognised in relation to glomerular and tubular basement membranes in ankylosing spondylitis (Linder and Pasternack, 1970) are present in active, untreated rheumatoid disease.

Mahallaway and Sabour (1959) have drawn attention to an increased frequency of arterial disease in the kidneys of rheumatoid arthritis, a finding supported by Pasternack, Wegelius and Mäkisara (1967) who reported arterio- and arteriolosclerosis in 9 of the 20 kidney biopsies which they contrasted with 10 control cases. These authors reached the conclusion, with which I cannot agree, that 'the presence of so-called local glomerulitis and interstitial tissue changes in young patients with the recent onset of rheumatoid arthritis and no heavy analgesic abuse makes the existence of rheumatoid kidney disease at least probable'.

The kidney in rheumatoid arthritis is also susceptible to a necrotising arteritis that closely simulates polyarteritis nodosa (p. 131) (Schmid, Cooper, Ziff and McEwen, 1961).

The extent to which phenacetin is used in the treatment of rheumatoid arthritis varies widely according to the preference of individual physicians and it is my impression from the comparison of the records of cases coming from two large hospitals that the renal complications of phenacetin treatment vary correspondingly. Thus, Lawson and Maclean (1966) analysed the clinical and pathological records of 44 women and of 17 men dying with rheumatoid arthritis, with particular reference to the influence of drug treatment on the incidence of renal disease. Seventy-two per cent of the cases showed evidence of significant renal disease and 21% had renal papillary necrosis. Although detailed interpretation was limited by small numbers, the frequency of renal papillary necrosis in women (27·3%—12 cases) was appreciably higher than in men (5·9%—1 case). By contrast the frequency of amyloid disease without papillary necrosis (ca. 11%), of acute pyelonephritis without amyloidosis or renal papillary necrosis (ca. 5%) and of uncomplicated chronic pyelonephritis (ca. 20%) did not differ between the two sexes. Renal artery disease, however, was found to be 3 times more common in males dying with rheumatoid arthritis than in females so that the overall incidence of renal disease in the two sexes was very similar (males 64·8%, females 74·9%).

The possibility that renal papillary necrosis, a condition normally associated with pyelonephritis in diabetes mellitus, was caused in rheumatoid arthritis by drug treatment was raised by Clausen and Pedersen (1961) in a survey of patients dying with rheumatoid arthritis. Many had pyelonephritis. Subsequent investigations showed that phenacetin was the agent most likely to be implicated and that the chronic or sclerotic form of renal papillary necrosis (Schourup, 1957) was most often encountered (Sanerkin and Weaver, 1964).

Lawson and Maclean's findings confirmed these observations and demonstrated that non-obstructive pyelonephritis was significantly more common in patients receiving phenacetin (24/37) than in those not so treated (5/24). At the same time they showed a comparable difference in the frequency of renal papillary necrosis in the two groups (11/37 and 2/24 respectively). Whether patients also received salicylates did not appear to influence the incidence of these disorders.

Experimental evidence has suggested that corticosteroid treatment accelerates amyloid deposition. There is considerable concern regarding the influence of these drugs in human disease. The observations of Gardner (1962) (Table 12.3) who studied 54 patients dying with rheumatoid

TABLE 12.3.   *Incidence of amyloidosis in patients treated before and after the introduction of corticosteroids*

	Treated with Corticosteroids	Not given Corticosteroids
54 cases rheumatoid arthritis dying 1935–1950 Amyloidosis	0	5 (9·3%)
54 cases rheumatoid arthritis dying 1954–1960 Amyloidosis	1 (5 further cases given corticosteroids did not have amyloidosis).	7 (14·8%)

(From Gardner, D. L., 1962, *Ann. rheum. Dis.*, **21**, 298–299.)

arthritis between 1935 and 1950, and 54 dying between 1950 and 1960, provided some evidence to support an increase in the incidence of amyloidosis in rheumatoid arthritis but showed that the increase was not confined to cases treated with corticosteroids. However, Lawson and Maclean demonstrated that 8 of their 29 patients receiving corticosteroids had renal amyloidosis compared with only 2 of 32 patients not treated in this way. The two series, based on different hospitals in the same region, differ markedly in the proportion of patients given steroid treatment.

No evidence for the influence of myocrisin or of phenylbutazone on the incidence of renal disease has been obtained (Lawson and Maclean, 1966) but the literature contains cases in which an adverse effect of gold on renal structure (Pollak *et al.*, 1962) and the production of membranous glomerulonephritis as a result of gold hypersensitivity (Steples, Toome, Kirby and Kag, 1962) have been recorded. Microangiopathy affecting renal vessels and associated with phenylbutazone therapy has been described (Thomson and Gardner, 1969).

(e) **Alimentary system**

Almost all parts of the alimentary system may be found at times to be abnormal if a sufficiently large number of cases of rheumatoid arthritis is reviewed. However, a small group of disorders is characteristic if not pathognomonic. The oral and salivary gland changes in the Sjögren syndrome, the gastric atrophy of megaloblastic anaemia, the hepatic lymphocytic infiltrates, the lingual and rectal amyloid deposits and the mesenteric arterial lesions indicate the diversity of rheumatoid changes that may be encountered. They are occasionally found together.

The pathological characteristics of the Sjögren syndrome are described on p. 168. But salivary gland changes are not confined to the sicca syndrome. Ericson (1968), for example, comparing 92 rheumatoid arthritics with 92 normal persons, found histological abnormalities, including salivary duct ectasia, duct strictures, salivary calculi and glandular atrophy, more frequently in the former group. There is now strong reason to suspect that the lymphoid cells infiltrating the salivary glands are immunologically competent and reactive and that there is an association between the salivary disorder and the hepatic lymphoreticular change which is also commonly found in this disease. Thus, Talal, Asofsky and Lightbody (1970) made an important analysis of the capacity of salivary gland lymphocytes in the Sjögren syndrome to synthesise immunoglobulins, measured by radioimmuno-electrophoresis. The lymphocytes were collected by lip biopsy. These authors reviewed both controls and 20 cases of the Sjögren syndrome. The lymphocytes taken from the latter produced greater amounts of IgG, IgM and IgA immunoglobulins, the extent of IgM and IgG synthesis correlating with the degree of lymphocytic infiltration of the gland tissue but not with the concentration of plasma immunoglobulin. Their evidence supported a suggested extra-salivary source for the lymphoid cells and showed greater immunoglobulin synthetic activity by the cells of rheumatoid patients with the 'sicca' syndrome than in those with uncomplicated rheumatoid arthritis.

Peptic ulcer may offer clinical difficulties when salicylates are prescribed (Atwater et al., 1965). Even in the absence of clinical signs, and in the presence of normal levels of gastric acid secretion, biopsy may reveal inflammatory changes, atrophy, mucosal thickening, and capillary proliferation. In the report by Fenyohazi et al., (1970) inflammation was detected in 38% of 35 rheumatoid patients, atrophy in 61%, mucosal thickening in 43% and capillary proliferation in 72%. In control cases the corresponding last three figures were 28·5%, 17% and 28·5%.

The suggestion that liver function tests become abnormal in rheumatoid arthritis has been examined but no evidence of altered bile pigment metabolism, excretory or detoxicating activity or enzyme activity has been found (Roy et al., 1955). Impaired bromsulphthalein clearance has, however, been shown, particularly where amyloidosis is present (Castenfors, Hultman and Lovgren, 1964). Although disturbed serum amino acid levels are described, the general pattern of urinary excretion of amino acids is not changed (Roy et al., 1955; Trnvská and Sitaj, 1960) (p. 109). Nevertheless, the plasma albumin/globulin ratio is reduced (Wilkinson et al., 1965) and thymol turbidity tests are positive. Liver carbohydrate metabolism is slightly impaired. Increased urinary copper ligand activity has been found (Gerber, 1966), possibly associated with the use of salicylates, but not attributable to the increased excretion of histidine and 3-methylhistidine. Decreased serum histidine concentrations have been described (Trnvská and Sitaj, 1960; Nettlebladt and Sandell, 1963).

Evidence of structural liver changes in this disease, with the exception of amyloid, is nevertheless scanty (Movitt and Davis, 1953; Lefkovits and Farrow, 1955). In my experience, sparse portal tract infiltrates with lymphocytes and occasional plasma cells may be encountered, but fibrosis is rare. In Felty's syndrome the situation is different. Blendis et al. (1970) studied 12 cases, 6 of whom were anaemic. Of these, 5 had a normal red cell mass although in 1 the red cell mass was increased. In the 6 anaemic patients, the anaemia was due to an increase in plasma volume, unlike the anaemia of uncomplicated rheumatoid arthritis (p. 156). In 2 patients the anaemia was accompanied both by haemolysis and by a sequestration of red blood cells within the spleen. Eight of the 12 cases had normal latex fixation tests. Histological study of 8 cases revealed a lymphocytic sinusoidal infiltration in 5, sometimes of portal distribution, with portal fibrosis. In only 1 case was there macronodular fibrosis but in 3 apparent nodule formation was seen without true cirrhosis.

There is now a strong suspicion that the 'sicca syndrome' and liver disease occur together more often than can be due to chance. Liver dysfunction is frequent in patients with the 'sicca complex' (Whaley, 1970); conversely, the 'sicca syndrome' may accompany liver disease (Golding, Brown, Mason and Taylor, 1970). The latter authors showed that signs of Sjögren's syndrome were frequent in 63 patients with liver disease. In active chronic hepatitis 42% of patients had evidence of the 'sicca syndrome' and 1 case had rheumatoid arthritis. In primary biliary cirrhosis, 72% had signs of the 'sicca syndrome' but in cryptogenic cirrhosis, only 38%. A single case in each of the first two groups had rheumatoid arthritis. Liver disease has also been encountered in psoriasis (Berge et al., 1970).

The intestinal mucosa has not been examined systematically by stereomicroscopy and no changes comparable to those found in systemic sclerosis have been reported. In my own series, blocks of small and large intestine were surveyed in paraffin section but no consistent abnormality characteristic of rheumatoid arthritis was recognised. The intestine occasionally perforates as a result of infarction caused by mesenteric arteritis (Parker and Thomas, 1959) but there has been a tendency to attribute this phenomenon to corticosteroid treatment rather than to the underlying disease.

(f) **Lymphoreticular system** (Figs. 12.14–12.16)

Since the time of Felty (1924) there has been a suspicion that the lymphoreticular organs in rheumatoid arthritis are grossly and microscopically abnormal (Michelazzi, 1937; Motulsky, Weinberg, Saphir and Rosenberg, 1952; Marshall, 1956). The literature on the immunological phenomena of rheumatoid arthritis is very large; those parts relevant to the tissue changes are reviewed in Chapter 8 which should be read in conjunction with the present section. From what is known experimentally of the responses to antigenic stimulation, the evidence is compatible with the view that the reticuloendothelial system, the central lymphoid organs, including the thymus, and the peripheral lymphoid follicular tissue of the spleen, nodes, tonsils and gut, may all at times be involved, simultaneously or in sequence, in the antigen-determined reactions causing or related to the origin of rheumatoid arthritis (Glynn and Holborow, 1965; Glynn, 1968; Gardner, 1968a).

Pathological studies of the lymphoreticular tissues in rheumatoid arthritis have been limited until recently by technical considerations which have not curtailed experimental studies. The use of paraffin-embedded, fixed material, although suitable for autoradiography after ^{3}H-thymidine labelling and for classical histological investigations, has many serious disadvantages and can shed limited light on pathological physiology. Imprints and smears, histochemical and immunofluorescent analyses of fresh tissue, cell culture, methods for identifying transformation in response to antigenic stimuli and electron microscopy are now being widely used in the study of the immunological phenomena of rheumatoid arthritis (Maini, Stewart and Dumonde, 1970). Investigations have also been handicapped because patients are seldom encountered at the time of onset of the disease, permitting serial immunological studies to be made, and because lymphoreticular tissues tend to atrophy with age. The effects of rheumatoid arthritis must therefore be distinguished from those of age, of longstanding disease and from the incidental effects of treatment. Even if material from early untreated cases of the disease were readily available for study, the nature of the local lymphoid response would allow of no easy interpretation. In making an analysis of the demonstrable cytological changes, it is essential to remember therefore that much of the evidence relating lymphoid tissue responses to antigenic stimulation comes from the study of animal tissues. The human analyses, for the most part, whether cytological, physiological or in tissue culture, have been based on material taken from adults with established disease. Comparison

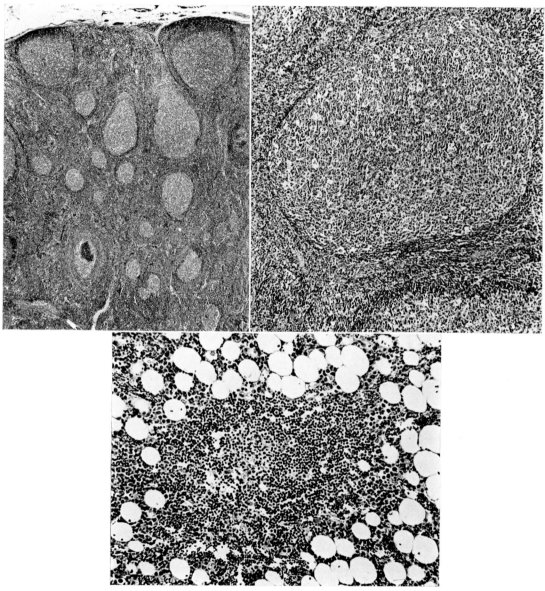

Fig. 12.14 (*Top left*) Lymph node in rheumatoid arthritis. Numerous large germinal centres are present. Their size and extent may suggest the diagnosis of follicular lymphoma. However (*top right*) the germinal centres contain only moderate numbers of lymphoblasts and the cells are not of neoplastic character. Surrounding the germinal centre are layers of plasma cells and, externally, lymphocytes. (*Bottom*) Lymphoid follicles are found in excess in the bone marrow in established rheumatoid arthritis. Germinal centre formation, however, is rare.

(*Top left* ×22; *right* ×85; *bottom* ×125)

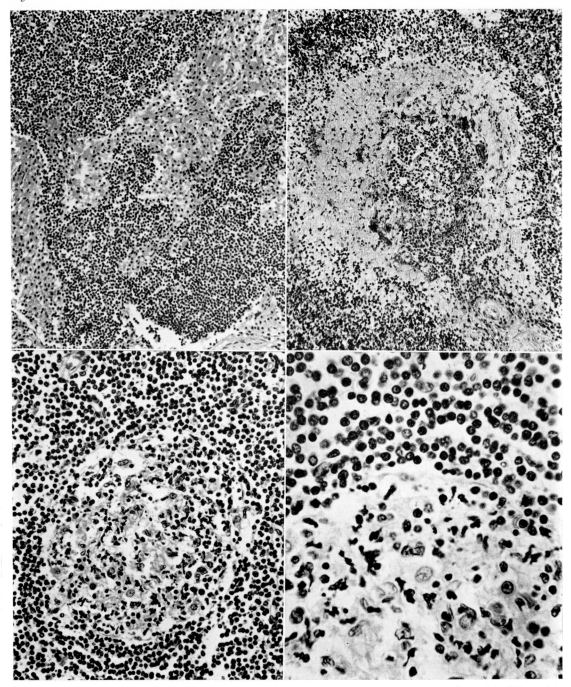

Fig. 12.15 Lymphoid tissue. (*Top left*) Sinus cell hyperplasia in a fatal case of rheumatoid arthritis. (*Top right*) Lymph node amyloid formation. A wide zone of amyloid is recognised outside an apparently compressed follicle. (*Bottom left*) Germinal centre from axillary lymph node in fatal case of rheumatoid arthritis. Many precursor cells are present with open vesiculate nuclei. There is abundant nuclear debris and a surrounding broad rim of small lymphocytes, reticular cells and plasma cells. (*Bottom right*) Higher power view of field shown in previous figure illustrating individual cell types. (From Gardner D. L., 1968, in *Rheumatic Diseases*, ed. Duthie J. J. R., and Alexander W. R. M., Edinburgh: University Press, pp. 105–121.)   (*Top left* ×140; *right* ×130; *bottom left* ×250; *right* ×500)

with lymphoid material from young animals with experimental disease of short duration and of an acute character, is particularly difficult.

It is possible to consider the lymphoreticular tissues in rheumatoid arthritis in 3 categories: (1) those with reticuloendothelial activity; (2) central, thymic lymphoid tissue and the thymic-dependent lymphocytic activities that are controlled centrally and determine cell-mediated immunity; and (3) peripheral, gut-associated lymphoid tissue and the lymphocytic activities, including those of the bone marrow, responsible for the synthesis of circulating antibody.

(1) There is good evidence that the reticuloendothelial system is frequently abnormal in rheumatoid arthritis. Whether this disorder is an early feature of the disease is less certain. The principal organs of the RE system—the spleen, liver, lymph nodes and bone marrow—are often abnormal histologically and there is sufficient evidence of altered phagocytic activity to allow this to be regarded as a constant feature of established rheumatoid arthritis.

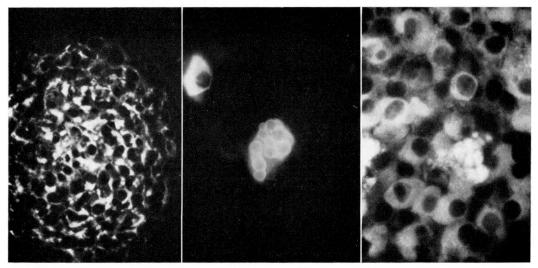

Fig. 12.16 Immunufluorescent localisation of rheumatoid factor IgM in lymph nodes. (*Left*) Rheumatoid factor in germinal centre of lymph node. (*Centre*) Rheumatoid factor shown by same technique in plasma cell containing numerous elementary Russell bodies. (*Right*) IgG immunoglobulin in medullary plasma cells. (From preparations of Dr. John McCormick.)

The spleen is usually enlarged in fatal hospital cases and may be rather more than twice the normal weight at death (Gardner and Roy, 1961) (Table 12.2). The first description of this enlargement was that of Chauffard and Ramond (1896). The clearance from the blood stream of particulate material, high molecular weight dyes (Roy, Alexander and Duthie, 1955) and oil/glycerine emulsions (Mills, Salky and Diluzio, 1964) is enhanced and more iron is retained within reticuloendothelial phagocytes (Gardner and Roy, 1961) including type A(M) synovial cells (Muirden, 1966) and lymph node macrophages (Muirden, 1970a) than normal. Thus, Gardner (1957) discovered more histologically stainable iron in axillary lymph nodes in rheumatoid arthritic patients who had been treated with iron than in the nodes of patients to whom iron had not been given therapeutically. Muirden (1970a) confirmed these results and described haemosiderin-containing macrophages in 9 of 11 cases, demonstrating by electron microscopy that the reticulum cells in 2 cases contained abundant ferritin (Figs. 12.17, 12.18); he measured the iron content of the excised lymph nodes, as Gardner and Roy (1961) had done previously, and confirmed a significant difference in the concentration of chemically measurable iron in the nodes of iron-treated and non-treated patients.

(2) The central, thymic lymphoid tissue is not morphologically changed and there is no evidence of any characteristic thymic disorder in this disease (Gardner, 1968a). In spite of this, thymectomy has been attempted, without success, in acute cases of the disease not responding to any other form of treatment (Milne *et al.*, 1967). The synovial changes seen in rheumatoid arthritis (p. 19) recall those of a cell-mediated, delayed hypersensitivity reaction but investigations of cell-mediated immunity are still in their infancy.

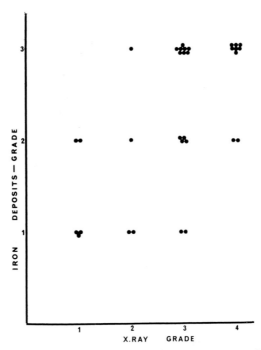

Fig. 12.17   The relationship between the histological grade of recognisable iron deposit in rheumatoid synovial tissue and the X-ray grade of disease activity is shown. More iron appears to be present in cases of greater clinical activity. (From Muirden K. D., 1970, *Aust. Ann. Med.*, **19**, 97–104.)

(3) In the case of the lymphoid (plasma) cells responsible for circulating antibody synthesis (gut-dependent immunocytes), the site(s) of sensitisation probably determines the main foci of subsequent antibody secretion. Popliteal and inguinal lymph nodes, for example, form antibody actively when the ipsilateral foot is experimentally injected with antigen; after intraperitoneal injection, the thoracic nodes are the sites for antibody synthesis. In each case, the soluble or particulate antigen is probably ingested, digested and altered by reticulo-endothelial cells, an activity mediated by lysosomal hydrolases. From the phagocyte, a unit containing RNA, perhaps with an attached fragment of antigen, is thought to be transferred directly to the regional lympho-reticular antibody-synthesising immunocytes, cells which assume the morphological appearance of plasmacytes or divide to give daughter cells with these appearances. Although Burnet's (1969) theories are criticised (Mitchison, 1967), an alternative role of processed antigen locally may be

to permit the proliferation and synthetic activity of a clone of cells containing the inherited information required for appropriate antibody synthesis rather than to instruct antibody protein synthesis directly.

In rheumatoid arthritis it would seem relevant to seek for histological evidence both of *primary* and of *secondary* lymphoreticular responses to antigen in regional lymph nodes draining joints with signs of early inflammation. It could be supposed, for example, that an exogenous infective agent existing within cells might give rise to immunological reactions demonstrable in regional lymph nodes when its biological activities began to cause cell injury and inflammatory disease.

In the case of an early *primary* reaction, mitotic activity in precursor blast cells might be anticipated. Medullary immunocytes would remain scanty and would not be demonstrable in

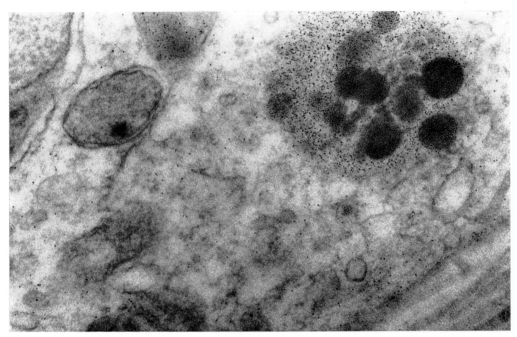

Fig. 12.18 Accumulation of ferritin, seen as minute electron opacities, in relation to lysosomal bodies in synovial cell in rheumatoid arthritis. Electron micrograph kindly supplied by Dr. K. D. Muirden. (Muirden, K. D., 1966, *Ann. rheum. Dis.*, **25**, 387–401.) (× 116,000)

germinal centres. The entire cellular response could be difficult to detect after more than 2 weeks. In the *secondary* response, many more cells throughout the medullary cords and at the borders of primary follicles would be expected to show antibody formation. The immunocytes would resemble plasma cells and would have abundant pyroninophilic cytoplasm due to the presence of the extensive endoplasmic reticulum associated with the polyribosomes known to be responsible for encoding the primary amino acid sequences of antibody peptides.

One important histological question therefore must be to determine to what extent the lymphoreticular changes in untreated, uncomplicated, early rheumatoid arthritis resemble those known, from experimental observation, to be associated with immunoglobulin synthesis. Fluorescein-conjugated anti-IgG and anti-IgM sera can be used to show that protein of antibody type is localised to these nodes: it is a long and difficult task to prove whether this response is caused by an agent disturbing regional synovial tissue, whether the response is caused by an unrelated, incidental antigen or whether the reaction is part of the disease process in rheumatoid arthritis but not causal.

The lymphoid follicles of the peripheral lymph nodes in rheumatoid arthritis are often large (Nosanchuk and Schnitzer, 1969). Secondary, germinal centre formation is frequent (32%) and, occasionally, the germinal centres are huge. Amyloid may be present. In my cases examined at necropsy, excess plasma cells were found in 49% and sinus cell hyperplasia (Fig. 12.15) in 70% of cases (Gardner, 1968a) (Table 12.4). The latter reaction is common when coincident infection is prominent. Structureless, eosinophilic material is often seen among the cells of the germinal centre and this area is surrounded by a zone of small lymphocytes, plasmablasts and plasma cells.

TABLE 12.4. *Cellular characteristics of lymph nodes in 51 fatal cases of rheumatoid arthritis*

	Prominent germinal centres	Plasmacytosis	Sinus cell hyperplasia
Lymph nodes (47)	15 (32%)	23 (49%)	33 (70%)
Spleen (51)	9 (18%)	18 (35%)	20 (40%)

Of the 18 spleens displaying plasmacytosis, 8 contained amyloid; amyloid, however, was identified in only 5 of the 23 lymph nodes with plasma cell excess.

Cytological assessments were made on a 5-point scale:

0 Nil	3 Marked
1 Slight	4 Severe
2 Moderate	

and only those cases with moderate, marked or severe reactions are included in this table.

(From Gardner, D. L., 1968a: in *Rheumatic Diseases, Pfizer Medical Monograph No. 3*. Edited by Duthie, J. J. R. and Alexander, W. R. M., University Press, Edinburgh, by permission of the publishers.)

When the cases were analysed in which moderate to severe plasmacytosis were associated with prominent germinal centres or sinus cell hyperplasia no factor was discovered that linked the clinical presentation or behaviour of the cases with the cytology of the lymph nodes (Table 12.5).

TABLE 12.5. *Clinical characteristics of cases of rheumatoid arthritis found to have moderate, marked or severe lymph node plasmacytosis (as recorded in Table 12.4) and in which this change was found in association with (a) prominent germinal centres or (b) sinus cell hyperplasia*

(a) 1. Female, aged 80; active RA; no amyloidosis; death due to hypertensive encephalopathy and bronchopneumonia; no corticosteroids.
   2. Female, aged 58; chronic pyelonephritis with renal papillary necrosis; amyloidosis; no corticosteroids.
   3. Male, aged 48; polyarteritis and myocardial infarction; prepyloric erosions; treated with corticosteroids.
(b) 4. Female, aged 68; chronic pyelonephritis; systemic and pulmonary hypertension; no amyloidosis; no treatment with corticosteroids.
   5. Male, aged 58; essential hypertension with lung oedema; no amyloidosis; no corticosteroids.
   6. Male, aged 56; pyaemia; septic on rheumatoid arthritis; hypoplastic bone marrow; no amyloidosis; no corticosteroids.

(From Gardner, D. L., 1968: in *Rheumatic Diseases*, Pfizer Medical Monograph No. 3. Editors: Duthie, J. J. R. and Alexander, W. R. M., Edinburgh: University Press. By permission of the publishers.)

Further investigations of this type in early cases of the disease and using more refined cytological techniques, would be of value.

Subjective, clinical surveys of lymphadenopathy in rheumatoid arthritis have also been made but few biopsy studies (Motulsky *et al.*, 1952). Thus Robertson *et al.* (1968) compared the axillary, epitrochlear and inguinal lymph nodes in 100 cases of rheumatoid arthritis with those in 100 normal control cases. In the absence of measurements of lymphoreticular function, the results are not easy to interpret. These authors found that lymph node enlargement was usually related anatomically to the lymph drainage from inflamed joints and that enlargement was apparently more common in males than females. In a few cases, enlargement, assessed subjectively, was generalised. As a rule, lymph node enlargement, clinically, was more severe in cases of rheumatoid arthritis with positive tests for rheumatoid factor, in those with active disease and in those with erythrocyte sedimentation rates of over 70 mm/hr.

The important problem of distinguishing histologically between the lymphoreticular change in rheumatoid arthritis and those in the other non-neoplastic disorders of the lymphoid tissues and in the lymphomas has been very fully discussed by Butler (1969). This author lists the lymphoid change of rheumatoid arthritis as a reactive process which simulates lymphoma and is of 'known aetiology' a view with which it is not possible to agree. However, Butler's analysis of the rheumatoid lymph node is of value and his classification of the rheumatoid changes as a form of nodular lymphoma might find general acceptance. He believes that generalised enlargement of lymph nodes in rheumatoid arthritis affects 50–70% of cases and, with Motulsky *et al.* (1952), that lymphadenopathy may precede the clinical appearance of the arthritis. He emphasises the frequency of plasmacytosis but stresses that this feature is not distinguishable from the similar finding in lymph nodes draining zones of chronic inflammation.

Occasional instances are recorded in which the lymph nodes of rheumatoid arthritis have been mistakenly thought to show the microscopic changes of giant follicular lymphoma: but the cause of this 'reticulosis' remains obscure. Furthermore, reactive sinus cell hyperplasia of a kind found in rheumatoid arthritis is encountered in numerous skin and connective tissue inflammatory reactions and is in no sense specific. At the present time the evidence regarding the cause of the cellular changes in the lymph nodes is therefore not sufficiently precise to allow any deductions to be made regarding the aetiology of rheumatoid arthritis. However, this position may very well alter when more refined techniques are used to analyse fresh biopsy material.

The lymphoreticular changes in rheumatoid arthritis, therefore, may mimic those of giant follicular lymphoma and there is other limited evidence that lymphoreticular disorders and rheumatoid arthritis are associated more often than can be due to chance. Fudenberg (1966) states that immunological deficiency, autoallergic disease and lymphoid neoplasms in rheumatoid arthritis occur together in individuals and in families with significant frequency. Moreover, there is some evidence to show that immunological deficiency predisposes to malignant tumours of the lymphoreticular organs. Goldenberg, Paraskevas and Israels (1969) reviewed 112 cases of plasma cell and lymphoid neoplasms and identified 4 cases of rheumatoid arthritis, 2 with multiple myeloma, 1 with Waldenström's macroglobulinaemia and 1 with reticulum cell sarcoma. Sixteen cases of rheumatoid arthritis and 2 with secondary joint diseases were similarly studied by Zawadzki and Benedek (1969). Each had a coexistent paraproteinaemia, antedating the arthritis by 1–44 years. The possibility was raised that a prolonged antigenic stimulus, part of the paraproteinaemia, could be a pathogenic factor in evoking rheumatoid arthritis, a hypothesis which, of course, is not easily confirmed or refuted. Eight of Zawadzki's cases had lanthanic dysimmunoglobulinaemia, 6 multiple myeloma, 1 Waldenströms macroglobulinaemia and 1 'heavy chain' disease. An additional case, in which plasmacytoma and rheumatoid arthritis coexisted, was outlined by Wegelius, Skifvars and Andersson (1970); in this instance, however, rheumatoid arthritis developed *before* the plasmacytoma, a sequence which is difficult to reconcile with the views advanced by Zawadzki and Benedek (1969).

(h) Haemopoietic system

Few signs of rheumatoid arthritis are more characteristic than anaemia. The degree of anaemia is a precise indication of the severity and activity of the disease (Tanner *et al.*, 1970) and the blood haemoglobin concentration is a better guide to the state of the patient than variables, such as the erythrocyte sedimentation rate, that are dependent on plasma protein changes.

For these reasons, the blood and blood-forming organs have been very fully studied in patients with rheumatoid arthritis. A particularly comprehensive series of reports has come from the Rheumatism Research Unit, Edinburgh, where Duthie and his colleagues have systematically investigated the subject during the past 20 years (Mowat, 1971). The anaemia of rheumatoid arthritis has been reviewed by Pitcher (1966) and by Mowat (1971). The cytology of the bone marrow in rheumatoid arthritis was exhaustively reviewed by Richmond, Gardner, Roy and Duthie (1956) and by Burkhardt (1971). The state of the lymphoreticular organs in relation to anaemia has been reported by Gardner and Roy (1961), by Gardner (1968a) and by Muirden (1969, 1970a) and the possible immunological significance of the marrow changes considered by Szasz *et al.* (1968).

The anemia of rheumatoid arthritis is of a normocytic, hypochromic nature and is more severe in females than in males. The red cells, of normal diameter and volume, contain less haemoglobin iron than normal and the serum iron levels are characteristically low. An improvement in the anaemia can be brought about by large doses of saccharated iron oxide but this effect is exerted on the red cell count, not on the hypochromia (Richmond, Roy, Gardner, Alexander and Duthie, 1958). Iron, however, is present in abundance in the organs of the reticuloendothelial system. The spleen, which can be shown at necropsy to be enlarged, shows an iron concentration per unit

TABLE 12.6.   *The peripheral blood in rheumatoid arthritis*

Sex	No. of cases	Peripheral blood values (mean and standard deviation)					
		Hb (g/100 ml.)	Red cell count (millions/cu. mm.)	Mean corpuscular volume (cu. μ)	Mean corpuscular Hb concentration (g%)	Erythrocyte sedimentation rate (mm/hr)	Plasma iron (μg/100 ml.)
Males	26	12·4 ± 1·2 (84%)	4·94 ± 0·37	84·6 ± 2·4	29·1 ± 3·9	39 ± 8	92 ± 11 (23 cases)
Females	38	10·9 ± 0·9 (73%)	4·94 ± 0·56	82·4 ± 3·6	28·7 ± 4·9	52 ± 7	80 ± 29 (35 cases)

(From Richmond, J. *et al.*, 1956, *Ann. rheum. Dis.* **15**, 221.)

wet weight which is at least normal, suggesting that the iron stores are abnormally high (Gardner and Roy, 1961) (Table 12.2). Whether iron is absorbed normally from the intestine is still debated although there is evidence that absorption is unimpaired (Boddy and Will, 1969). The iron-binding capacity of the serum is normal or slightly diminished, a finding which distinguishes the hypochromic anaemia of rheumatoid arthritis from true iron deficiency anaemia in which the iron-binding capacity is usually raised. The low plasma levels can be reversed by corticotrophin treatment (Mowat, Hothersall and Aitchison, 1969). Although insiduous blood loss caused by administration of salicylates or vitamin B_{12} or folate deficiency (Gough *et al.*, 1964; Deller *et al.*, 1966; Omer and Mowat, 1968, 1969) have been shown to be associated with occasional instances of anaemia in rheumatoid arthritis, some of megaloblastic type (Partridge and Duthie, 1963*a*) there is normally no such explanation for the disturbance of haemoglobin synthesis. Nor can the anaemia be adequately explained on the basis of decreased red cell survival, measured by immunological or by isotopic labelling techniques (Richmond, Alexander, Potter and Duthie, 1961). Rheumatoid red blood cells, tested by the mouse macrophage technique of Stuart, Davidson and Cuming (1967) are not more susceptible to adhesion and phagocytosis than are normal red cells of the same blood group (Farkas and Gardner, unpublished observations). There is evidence that an increase in plasma volume may contribute to occasional cases but this, again, is an inconstant finding.

The most important observation in rheumatoid anaemia, appears therefore to be the paradoxical iron deficiency of the red blood cells in the face of an amount of iron in the storage organs of the reticuloendothelial system which is at least normal. This evidence implies a defect in the utilisation of 'available' iron; evidence for a diminished release of iron under comparable experimental circumstances has been obtained (Owen and Lawson, 1966). Yet exogenous iron in the form of transferrin-bound ^{59}Fe can apparently be assimilated and used normally for haemoglobin synthesis and direct evidence of increased storage is difficult to obtain (Lawson, Owen and Mowat, 1967). The nature of the 'block' in iron incorporation in rheumatoid arthritis remains unexplained but it seems quite likely that the substantial iron reservoirs of the reticuloendothelial organs are less readily accessible than had been supposed.

An additional factor contributing to iron sequestration in rheumatoid arthritis has been proposed by Muirden (1969, 1970*c*). In a survey of synovial tissue by light and by electron microscopy (p. 52) Muirden demonstrated that rheumatoid synovia contain abundant iron, a demonstration confirmed by chemical analysis (Muirden and Senator, 1968; Senator and Muirden, 1968; Mowat and Hothersall, 1968). Levels as high as those identified in villonodular synovitis and haemochromatosis were encountered (Senator and Muirden, 1968) but the synovial iron content did not correlate with the serum or synovial fluid iron.

Subsequently, Muirden (1970*c*) showed that the extent of the iron deposits found in 28 cases of rheumatoid arthritis bore a highly significant relationship to the presence of anaemia in spite of the fact that some cases with abundant synovial iron were not anaemic (Figs. 12.17, 12.18). Muirden was also able to show a relationship between the duration of the disease, the extent of radiological joint change and the state of the synovial iron deposits. Somewhat similar observations were made on the content of iron in the axillary lymph nodes of patients not given therapeutic iron, observations conforming with those of Gardner (1957) who had also distinguished between the iron content of the lymphoreticular tissues in patients with rheumatoid arthritis treated with iron and in patients not so treated.

There seems little doubt, therefore, that the synovial tissues accumulate substantial amounts of iron, particularly in patients with the most severe forms of rheumatoid arthritis. In the same way, the available evidence suggests that the organs of the reticuloendothelial system, particularly the spleen and lymph nodes, retain paradoxically large amounts of non-haemoglobin iron in the face of a persistent hypochromic anaemia. Whether the retention of synovial iron contributes significantly to, or provokes the anaemia, as Muirden (1970*c*) implies, is another matter and one to which no easy answer is available. The *quantity* of iron retained in the synovia in this way *could* lead to an hypochromic anaemia if the body had no other accessible iron source. But it may equally be true that, just as the bizarre anaemia of rheumatoid arthritis is incidental to but characteristic of the disease, so the synovial iron accumulation is incidental to the anaemia. Minor degrees of trauma to rheumatoid synovial tissue are common and synovial haemosiderin aggregates are the result. If these aggregates are held to cause or maintain the anaemia, then any similar local trauma or haemorrhage in which haemosiderin iron is retained should have the same result. This hypothesis could be tested in rheumatoid patients in whom local bleeding during fracture repair or following local haematomata causes a prolonged local retention of iron-containing pigments. Is there evidence that during fracture repair the anaemia of a rheumatoid arthritic becomes persistently worse?

The bone marrow in active rheumatoid arthritis contains substantially increased proportions of plasma cells and this plasmacytosis correlates with plasma globulin levels (Fig. 9.1). It is not yet known whether there is any similar correlation with levels of IgG immunoglobulin which bone marrow plasma cells are thought to synthesise in excess during the early active disease. A slight but probably significant increase in normal red cell precursors has been recognised in one survey of the bone marrow cytology in rheumatoid arthritis (Richmond et al., 1956) but megaloblasts are rare. The white cell series, except in cases of Felty's syndrome in which leucopenia is severe, is normal but cases with iatrogenic marrow disease (p. 177) are not infrequent and should be carefully distinguished as, indeed, should those with arrested platelet release or megakaryocyte hypoplasia in thrombocytopenia.

This is a convenient point at which to draw attention to relevant observations on the role of copper in rheumatoid arthritis. The plasma and synovial fluid caeruloplasmin concentrations are raised (Müller, Kluthke and Muller, 1963; Niedermeier, 1965) and the daily turnover of ^{131}I-labelled caeruloplasmin in rheumatoid arthritis significantly accelerated (Koskelo et al., 1966; Koskelo et al., 1967). Niedermeier (1967), further showed that rheumatoid synovial fluid hyaluronate is more resistant to depolymerisation by ascorbic acid than control fluid, possibly due to the raised caeruloplasmin levels.

Penicillamine, an effective agent chelating metal ions, including copper, has been shown to be of some benefit to a small group of patients with rheumatoid lung disease (Lorber, 1966) (p. 137). The rationale of this study, which has not been confirmed, was that the decreased serum protein sulphydryl content of rheumatoid patients could contribute to the presence and binding properties of rheumatoid factor macroglobulins (Lorber et al., 1964). Thiol compounds such as d-penicillamine are known to dissociate polymeric proteins by cleaving disulphide bonds and it seemed reasonable to test this hypothesis by giving the chelating agent to patients with positive serum tests for rheumatoid factor and rheumatoid lung disease (p. 137). The results of this stimulating therapeutic essay, which were equivocal, are open to at least two radically distinct interpretations in view of what is known of copper-binding protein in rheumatoid arthritis (Sternlieb et al., 1969).

(j) Endocrine system

Compared to the flood of papers which accompanied the introduction of cortisone as a therapeutic agent for rheumatoid arthritis (1949) and the clinical and physiological studies of endocrine function which followed, there have been few reports on endocrine pathology in rheumatoid arthritis during the past 10 years with the exception of those dealing with the thyroid gland (Fig. 12.19) and Hashimoto's disease (p. 170). Thus, in 34 unselected cases of Hashimoto's thyroiditis Buchanan et al. (1961) recognised a prevalence of rheumatoid arthritis significantly greater than in a control hospital series. Thyroid auto-antibodies likewise were shown in a higher proportion of an unselected group of rheumatoid arthritics than normal. Six cases were identified in which thyroiditis and rheumatoid arthritis coexisted: both entities, it was thought, could be due to the action of autoallergic mechanisms (Buchanan, 1965).

The deficiency of pituitary basophil cells with aggregates of Schiff-positive granules at the opposite poles of the nuclei (Pearse, 1953) has not been confirmed by more recent histochemical, immunofluorescent or isotope techniques. Indeed, I know of no satisfactory pathological evidence

TABLE 12.7. *Cytological details of bone marrow in rheumatoid arthritis*

Subject	Date	Authors	No. of cases	Principal findings
Iron content	1953	Smith	3	Stainable iron present in two cases and absent in one.
	1954	Pratt and Johnson	5	Iron content greater than normal in four cases.
Cytology	1938	Mester	33	Plasmacytosis.
	1938	Kaether	26	Toxic granulation of neutrophil polymorphs.
	1937	Michelazzi	1	Increase in reticulum cells and plasma cells.
	1940	Fleischhacker and Lachnit	55	Slight increase in plasma cells.
	1945	Merlo and Tortori–Donati	7	'Histiolymphocytosis'.
	1946	Luchesi, Luchesi and Da Silva	32	Plasmacytosis.
	1948	Marmont	21	Plasmacytosis. Eosinophilia. 'Active reticuloendothelial systems'.
	1948	Nilsson	12	Disturbance of erythroid maturation.
	1949	Leitner	2	Plasmacytosis. Eosinophilia. Shift to left of myeloid series.
	1951	Hayhoe and Smith	10	Plasmacytosis in nine cases, associated with hyperglobulinaemia in six where plasma proteins were estimated.
	1951	Jasinski and Staehelin	20	Eosinophilia.
	1951	Finch, Crockett, Ross and Bayles	—	Moderate depression of erythroid series.
	1952	Morelli and Arciello	15	Plasmacytosis in thirteen cases.
	1952	Edgcumbe and Husain	13	Normal plasma cells and eosinophils.
	1953	Jeffrey	16	Plasmacytosis in only three cases. Low proportion of mature normoblasts in seven.
	1953	Klein and Block	8	Described plasmacytosis.
	1954	Houli and Monteiro Marinho	20	Plasmacytosis in only five cases. Eosinophilia in seven.
	1955	Ebaugh, Peterson, Rodnan and Bunim	21	Slight plasmacytosis.

(From Richmond, J. *et al.*, 1956, *Ann. rheum. Dis.* **15**, 217.)

to implicate any part of the endocrine system in the pathogenesis of the disease. The views widely held during the 1950s on this matter must therefore be regarded as unsubstantiated. At that time, a disturbance of the pituitary/adrenal axis was widely canvassed and the structure and function of both glands closely examined. Apart from occasional reports such as that of Elias *et al.* (1966) who describe an adrenal dystrophic change with swelling and lipid depletion, there is no adequate evidence to differentiate a disorder of this organ from those caused by treatment (Fig. 12.20).

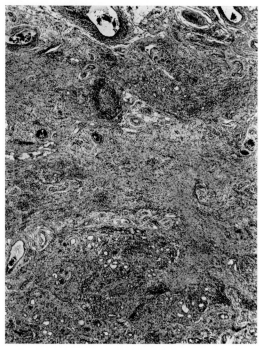

Fig. 12.19   Thyroid gland. Widespread fibrosis and abundant lymphocytic infiltration characteristic of thyroiditis. Lymphoid follicles (*top centre*) occasionally show germinal centre formation. Although thryoiditis has been associated with rheumatoid arthritis on the basis of serological studies, thyroiditis is a commonplace feature in elderly persons and its association with rheumatoid arthritis is less significant than has been supposed. (From Gardner D. L., *Pathology of the Connective Tissue Diseases*, London: Arnold, 1965.)   (×22)

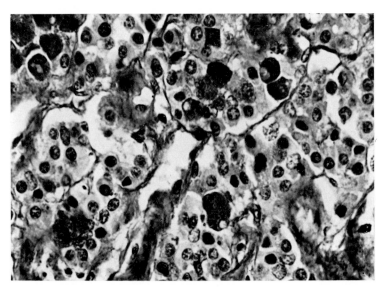

Fig. 12.20   Anterior pituitary in rheumatoid arthritis. A sinusoid runs obliquely (*lower centre*) through the tissue. Its wall is occupied by dark grey-appearing material which displays the staining characteristics of amyloid. (From Gardner D. L., *Pathology of the Connective Tissue Diseases*, London: Arnold, 1965.)   (×540)

TABLE 12.8. *Relationship between duration of disease and plasma cell count in bone marrow in 60 cases of rheumatoid arthritis*

Duration of disease (years)	0–1·9	2–9·9	10 and over
Mean plasma cell count (%)	2·6	1·7	1·3
Standard error of mean	0·344	0·172	0·193
Number of cases	12	26	22

(From Richmond, J. *et al.*, 1956, *Ann. rheum. Dis.* **15**, 223.)

(k) Nervous system

(i) Central nervous system

The dearth of pathological knowledge of the nervous system in rheumatoid arthritis is reflected in the fact that in one recent text the brain receives no mention (Scott, 1969) and in another (Hollingsworth, 1968) the brain rates 7 short lines of text and 2 references.

By contrast, there is widespread appreciation of the influence of basilar and cervical disease on spinal cord function and structure (p. 133) (although, again, the literature is largely clinical) and substantial descriptions deal with peripheral neuropathy either caused by pressure or in association with peripheral vascular disease (p. 132).

In unpublished personal observations, a survey of 5 blocks of tissue taken respectively from the cerebral cortex, cerebellum, basal ganglia, pons and medulla oblongata in 35 cases of rheumatoid arthritis revealed no abnormality which could be said to be characteristic of the disease. In a further case, dural nodules of the type described by Maher (1954) were present but were symptomless. In addition, Hollingsworth mentions a case of rheumatoid arthritis in which extensive granulomata involved the upper cervical and brain stem areas, recalling the granulomata occasionally encountered in the pharynx.

The brain, cord and peripheral nerves are from time-to-time involved incidentally in disturbances which occur in the course of treated or untreated rheumatoid arthritis and which may terminate fatally. Thus, necrotising arteritis occurring spontaneously or in the course of corticosteroid therapy may result in multiple, possible subclinical, micro-infarcts (Case 36). Vertebral artery thrombosis has been described (Webb, Hickman and Brew, 1968) and subaxial dislocation of the cervical spine is a well-recognised cause of death in rheumatoid arthritis following even minor trauma in association with the very common osteoporosis. Hemiplegia in rheumatoid arthritis (Bland and Eddy, 1968; Bland and Winston, 1968) exerts a protective influence on the joints of the immobilised side, presumably due to the enforced rest, an effect which can be mimicked by enforced total immobilisation within plaster (Partridge and Duthie, 1963*b*). Paralytic poliomyelitis and disuse following trauma are occasionally observed to have the same effect (p. 75). It is paradoxical that immobilisation, which prevents or diminishes synovitis, apparently accelerates cartilage degradation.

Nodules, presumed to be of rheumatoid nature, have been encountered in the choroid of the eye and have accounted for retinal detachment, reversible under corticosteroid and cyclophosphamide therapy (Hurd, Snyder and Ziff, 1970). Bilateral lesions are usual and there is a premonitory scleromalacia perforans. Scleral lesions are recognised (Rademakers *et al.*, 1969). Scleritis is a recognised feature of rheumatoid arthritis but episcleritis is rare. In a survey of 142 rheumatoid arthritics and 142 controls, Jayson and Jones (1971) identified 9 examples of scleritis in the former group, none in the latter. The scleral inflammation was usually bilateral and cases with this response tended to have subcutaneous nodules, pericarditis or pleuritis, and arteritis. Choroidal nodules accompany systemic nodule formation in other sites, and, occasionally coexist with arteritis.

I know of no histological evidence dealing with the autonomic nervous system in rheumatoid arthritis with the exception of Sokoloff's (1966) comments. Bennett and Scott (1965), however, showed that the clinical sensory neuropathy found in rheumatoid arthritis is of a post-ganglionic type, corresponding in distribution to the demonstrable sensory loss.

(ii) *Peripheral nerves*

Focal lesions of the peripheral nerves, in association with subacute arteritis and with skeletal muscular lymphorrhages, were among the early systemic lesions to be described in rheumatoid arthritis (Cruickshank, 1952b). There is, however, no pathological evidence to associate these localised and nonspecific peripheral nervous lesions with the clinical onset of sensory neuropathy.

Chamberlain and Bruckner (1970) studied 32 cases of rheumatoid arthritis and neuropathy and discovered that the cases fell into 2 groups. Excluding compression neuropathy such as that which is characteristic of the carpal-tunnel syndrome, it was demonstrated that the peripheral neuropathy of rheumatoid arthritis was not related to the duration of arthritis, the evidence of local joint disease, the nature of the treatment given and the presence or absence of demonstrable antineural antibodies. The 2 groups comprised, first, those with 'benign' rheumatoid arthritis, only moderately sero-positive, commonly without nodules or evidence of erosion, and with a sex ratio as for classical rheumatoid disease. A patchy glove-and-stocking anaesthesia with hypo-algesia involving the feet and, occasionally the hands, was rarely accompanied by minimal evidence of motor weakness. In the second group, a high titre of rheumatoid factor was charac-teristic, erosions were common, morbidity and mortality were higher and motor weakness was often profound. Sensory changes were not conspicuous but there was evidence of severe denervation.

The majority of examples of rheumatoid neuropathy can be explained either by pressure caused by plaster casts or granulation tissue occupying zones such as the carpal tunnel, or by ischaemia. Where arterial disease is the cause, demyelination and axonal degeneration may be identified. The significance of the focal lymphocytic endoneural and perineural aggregates of myelinated nerves is uncertain and similar changes have not been encountered in autonomic ganglia (Sokoloff, 1966). The volume of information available for analysis is, however, limited and there is little doubt that, if the opportunity presented, careful dissection would reveal more evidence of neuronal change.

(l) **Skeletal muscle** (Fig. 12.21)

The variety of neuromuscular changes encountered in rheumatoid arthritis is greater than had been appreciated (Gospodinoff, Gospodinoff and Fiore, 1965a, b; Haslock, Wright and Harriman, 1970). Motor point muscle biopsy by the latter authors in 34 cases permitted the delineation by clinical and histological criteria, of 4 main groups of cases.

In the first, evidence of connective tissue disease was recognised in muscle; in the second, there was nutritional muscular cachexia; in the third peripheral neuropathy (demyelinating or due to polyarteritis); and in the fourth, steroid-induced myopathy. The varieties of muscle disease were found to coexist in a number of patients. The possibility that muscle disease might be reflected in changed cholinesterase activity was considered by Milstoc (1970) who found the rheumatoid red cell enzyme activity to be higher than normal, the whole blood level to be slightly raised but the plasma level to be reduced. It was not clear whether the altered enzyme levels were the result of altered levels in the plasma albumin to which the enzyme is bound or were the result of abnormal neuronal or neuromuscular activity. No comparable histochemical or microchemical analyses of tissues have been reported.

Many large muscles in rheumatoid arthritis can be shown at biopsy to contain groups of 50 or more lymphocytes termed lymphorrhages (Cruickshank, 1952b). These lesions (Fig. 12.21) are not specific for rheumatoid arthritis but may be encountered in other wasting diseases and in myasthenia gravis. Atrophy and loss of muscle cells are commonplace in longstanding disease but replacement of muscle protein by collagen is not evident. Those muscle samples which contain

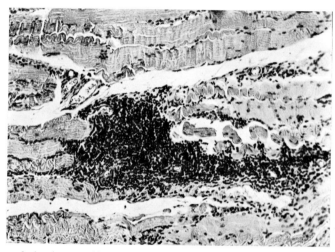

Fig. 12.21 Skeletal muscle in rheumatoid arthritis. Clusters of more than 50 lymphocytes may be defined as a lymphorrhage. The cells lie commonly near peripheral nerves and arteries. Their presence is characteristic but not pathognomonic of rheumatoid arthritis. (From Gardner, D. L., *Pathology of the Connective Tissue Diseases*, London, Arnold, 1965.)

(×120)

lymphorrhages not uncommonly include small arteries which show acute or subacute arteritis. Similar vascular changes are encountered in the peripheral nerves. The focal muscular lesions are not correlated with age, duration or activity of the disease or with the extent of lymphoreticular changes in regional nodes.

The lymphorrhages encountered in skeletal muscle in rheumatoid arthritis and in myasthenia gravis are not the only links between these two conditions, in both of which an autoallergic mechanism has been invoked to explain pathogenesis. A familial concurrence of the 2 disorders has been reported (Namba and Grob, 1970). Both diseases were identified in a brother and a sister while a further brother had rheumatoid arthritis but not myasthenia gravis. Rheumatoid factor, it was claimed, is found in 8·4% of patients with myasthenia compared with 1–5% of the general population. However, the incidence of rheumatoid arthritis in myasthenic patients is only 2·6% and the siblings described by these authors represent the only familial concordance known.

On the basis of the interosseous muscle biopsy of the hands of patients with rheumatoid arthritis, Riley and Harrison (1968) were unable to define any consistent histological change. They concluded that muscle weakness in rheumatoid arthritis probably does not contribute significantly to hand deformities. The validity of this conclusion, in the absence of detailed histochemical and electrophysiological studies, seems open to doubt.

TABLE 12.9. *Nature of amyloid*

Electron microscopy:	
(Shirahama and Cohen, 1967)	Fine fibrils composed of $7\cdot5 \pm 0\cdot9$ nm diameter beaded filaments with definitive subunit structure showing $10\cdot0$ nm periodicity.
(Glenner *et al.*, 1971)	$10\cdot0$ nm diameter fibril composed of 2 twisted $3\cdot5$–$4\cdot0$ nm filaments.
Immunological characteristics:	
(Cathcart, Wollheim and Cohen, 1967; Glenner *et al.*, 1971)	Immunologically distinct; associated with plasma immuno-globulin G.
Biochemical structure:	
(Cohen, 1966, 1967)	Protein containing $14\cdot6\%$ nitrogen and up to $4\cdot6\%$ of a carbohydrate component; no glycosaminoglycan; dissimilar to known fibrous extracellular substances; not susceptible to collagenase or hyaluronidase.
(Glenner *et al.*, 1971)	A unique glycoprotein
X-ray spectroscopy:	
(Schmueli *et al.*, 1969)	(1) Equatorial reflections corresponding to $9\cdot4$ nm.
	(2) Series of near-meridional reflections with spacings ranging from $0\cdot61$ to $0\cdot255$ nm.
	(3) Two broad diffuse reflections centred at $1\cdot0$ nm (near meridional) and at $0\cdot46$ nm (near equatorial) respectively.
(Glenner *et al.*, 1971)	Backbone $0\cdot47$ nm spacing with side-chain $1\cdot1$ nm spacing indicating a β-pleated sheet structure.
Biological properties:	
(Wright *et al.*, 1969)	Some evidence to show cellular production of amyloid by endothelial cells in culture.

Amyloidosis

The widespread deposition of amyloid, a fibrillar glycoprotein, is known to be a common feature of longstanding rheumatoid arthritis. Whether amyloidosis is a 'complication' of rheumatoid disease or whether the presence of recognisable amyloid in some cases but not in others is a quantitative distinction, remains a matter for debate. The biochemical features of amyloid (Cohen, 1966, 1967), its fine structure (Shirahama and Cohen, 1967), biophysical (Shmueli *et al.*, 1969) and immunological characteristics (Cathcart, Wollheim and Cohen, 1967; Glenner *et al.*, 1970) have been analysed in detail in recent years and these features are summarised in Table 12.9. There is a view that amyloid synthesis is a property of the ageing cell (Wright *et al.*, 1969) and that the change detected morphologically as 'amyloidosis' represents only a quantitatively different state from 'normal'. These problems and the whole literature have been admirably reviewed in recent years by Mandema *et al.* (1968) and the reader is referred to this account for detailed descriptions of the biology of amyloidosis and to the papers of Glenner *et al.* (1971) and of Harada *et al.* (1971).

The frequency of amyloidosis in rheumatoid arthritis and its significance were the subjects of a full review by Missen and Taylor (1956) (Table 12.9). The first reported examples of amyloidosis in rheumatoid arthritis, according to these authors, were those of Spitzy (1903) and Whitman (1903) although Stewart (1860–61) mentioned rheumatoid arthritis as one possible underlying cause of amyloid nephritis, then regarded as a form of Bright's disease. Cornil (1864) raised the possibility of amyloid as a cause of persistent albuminuria in 'chronic articular rheumatism' and

TABLE 12.10. *Incidence of amyloidosis in reported* post mortem *series of rheumatoid arthritis cases*

	No. of cases of R.A.	Amyloid found in	Percentage incidence of amyloid		Remarks
			Overall	Conservative	
Fingerman and Andrus (1942–43)	61	13	21·3	17·2	Active tuberculosis in 3 of the 13 amyloid cases.
Baggenstoss and Rosenberg (1943)	30	2	6·7	3·4	Chronic suppurative prostatitis in 1 amyloid case.
Bayles (1943)	23	3	13·0	9·1	1 of the 3 amyloid cases had ankylosing spondylitis (not R.A.).
Bennett (1943)	48	0	0	0	—
Solomon (1943)	7	1	14·3	14·3	Amyloid case treated for 3 years with coccal vaccine.
Young and Schwedel (1944)	38	5	13·2	11·4	2 (without amyloid) were cases of ankylosing spondylitis. Pulmonary tuberculosis in 1 amyloid case.
Unger *et al.* (1948)	58	4	6·9	6·9	—
Teilum and Lindahl (1954)	28	17	60·7	59·3	1 amyloid case (A.S., not R.A.) Histological examination in every case of methyl violet-stained sections.
Gedda (1955)	45	11	24·4	24·4	9 of the 11 died of renal amyloidosis: 'amyloid-shrunken' kidneys in 7.
Missen and Taylor (1956)	47	8	17·0	13·3	Alternative possible cause for amyloid in 2 cases.
Totals	385*	64†	Mean 17·8	Mean 15·9	Total acceptable cases with amyloid and no cause found other than R.A.: 55

A.S. = ankylosing spondylitis   R.A. = rheumatoid arthritis

* Includes 4 cases of ankylosing spondylitis.   † Includes 2 cases of ankylosing spondylitis.

(From Missen, G. A. K. and Taylor, J. D. (1956). *J. Path. Bact.* **71**, 179–192.)

Charcot (1881) also referred to albuminous nephritis, perhaps amyloid in nature, as a reasonably frequent characteristic of 'chronic rheumatism'. Wichmann (1893) again suggested that arthritis was a possible provocative agent for amyloidosis and this view, although debated, is now very generally accepted. The association was not admitted by Reimann and Eklund (1935) or by Moschowitz (1936–37). By 1942–1943 however the high frequency with which the two disorders coexisted was agreed (Fingerman and Andrus, 1943).

Missen and Taylor (1956) collected the principal papers published before that date and found (Table 12.9) 64 instances of amyloidosis, including 2 cases with ankylosing spondylitis, in 381 cases of rheumatoid arthritis and 4 of ankylosing spondylitis, an incidence in the former disease of between 15·9 and 17·8% depending on how strictly diagnostic criteria were applied. In the series of 145 cases of rheumatoid arthritis collected by the present author and briefly summarised in the Appendix (p. 212) there were 17 cases of amyloidosis, an incidence of 11.7%.

Arapakis and Tribe (1963) turned to biopsy material in an attempt to determine the overall incidence of amyloidosis in a group of 115 patients with classical or definite disease according to the American Rheumatism Association (Table 1.1) criteria. Using the convenient technique of rectal biopsy (p. 206), they detected 6 cases with amyloidosis. The condition was more common in longstanding, severe rheumatoid arthritis but in 3 patients it was found in the absence of proteinuria or raised blood urea levels. They concluded that amyloidosis detectable by current *in vivo* diagnostic techniques could be assumed to be present in 5–10% of all cases of rheumatoid arthritis. A more recent view suggests that the presence of amyloid is related to the severity but not to the duration of rheumatoid arthritis (Wolf, 1970) but this opinion would not find universal acceptance.

Amyloid in rheumatoid arthritis was at one time diagnosed during life by uncertain procedures such as the Congo red test with which false negative results were common. Tissue deposits could be detected by lingual biopsy but the tongue is less often the site for amyloidosis secondary to inflammatory disorders than it is for deposits of amyloid in which no underlying cause can be shown ('primary' amyloidosis). The advent of renal biopsy proved of great value in diagnosis (Heptinstall and Joekes, 1960) but more recently it has been shown that rectal biopsy (Gafni and Sohar, 1960; Blum and Sohar, 1962) can be both a simpler and more certain procedure and one of greater diagnostic sensitivity (Arapakis and Tribe, 1963; Maldyk, Piotrowska, Drecka and Maldyk, 1967).

At rectal biopsy, the presence of amyloid is suspected when the small arteries or arterioles of the rectal submucosa are found to contain ill-defined, amorphous, eosinophilic mural deposits that displace medial smooth muscle nuclei and form a uniform zone apparently devoid of cells. Under these circumstances, and also in cases where renal biopsy is made, the faintly eosinophilic amyloid deposits are found in relation to the basement membrane of small blood vessels including glomerular capillaries.

Although the examination of a conventional, haematoxylin and eosin-stained section may be sufficient to suggest the diagnosis of amyloidosis, precision and sensitivity of diagnosis are much improved if special staining methods are adopted. The bright pink colour obtained with Congo red is not specific for amyloid—elastic material stains well—but the demonstration with polarised light that these pink-stained zones display an apple green dichroism was thought, until recently, to be diagnostic of amyloid. Some doubt has been cast on the specificity of the method. Amyloid displays brilliant metachromasia with methyl violet applied to a frozen or cryostat section but the coloration soon fades to the background blue. The fluorescent dye, thioflavine T, is also of value; blue light of short wavelength can excite fluorescence with this chemical. A more sensitive technique may be the use of polarised ultraviolet light to study sections stained with a fluorescent dye.

It has been suspected since the early experimental studies of Teilum (1952) and of Latvalahti (1953) that cortisone promotes amyloid formation. There is no clear evidence that corticosteroids in the much smaller doses used clinically in the treatment of rheumatoid arthritis, have the same effect. Parkins and Bywaters (1959) detected no clinical increase in the signs of amyloidosis in patients with rheumatoid arthritis treated with corticosteroids. Gardner (1962) compared the frequency of amyloid in 54 fatal cases of rheumatoid arthritis dying in hospital prior to 1950, with that in 54 cases dying subsequent to that date, i.e. after the clinical introduction of cortico- steroid treatment (Table 12.3). The numbers of patients receiving corticosteroids and the num- bers with amyloidosis were both small. There was no satisfactory evidence that these factors were associated. In the series reported by Enervaara and Oka (1964) a higher proportion of the patients with amyloidosis and rheumatoid arthritis had been treated with corticosteroids but there was no control population for comparison.

The cause(s) of amyloidosis remain speculative and the high frequency of the condition in rheumatoid arthritis in which it is encountered as a late feature of both the adult and the juvenile disease, is unexplained. Amyloid is an occasional but less common feature of analogous diseases such as ankylosing spondylitis. Amyloid has also been known, since the early days of pathological anatomy, to be commonplace in chronic infective processes such as osteomyelitis, bronchiectasis, leishmaniasis and fibrocaseous pulmonary tuberculosis. It is not the occurrence of amyloid in rheumatoid arthritis therefore that is of particular interest but the fact that this association is so common. Analogy with the other known causes of amyloidosis tends to support the view that rheumatoid arthritis, also, may be of an infective origin. This opinion finds support from extensive experimental evidence, reviewed by Sorenson, Heefner and Kirkpatrick (1966); many infective agents, particularly those causing hyperglobulinaemia such as leishmaniasis, have been used successfully to provoke amyloid formation.

It would be quite wrong to assume from this evidence however that there is no other reasonable explanation for amyloid accumulation. Amyloid glycoprotein fibrils may aggregate as part of the 'normal' ageing process (Wright et al., 1969) and their excessive intracellular synthesis may represent a defect in the autoallergic inhibition mechanism. There is, indeed, new evidence that amyloid, after all, comprises immunoglobulin (Glenner et al., 1971). In rheumatoid arthritis, there may be simply an acceleration of normal amyloid synthesis, leading, for physical reasons, to aggregation of the material in nearby extracellular spaces, often beneath basement membranes. Immunoglobulins are found in association with amyloid but were thought not to be part of the glycoprotein macromolecule (Cathcart, Wollheim and Cohen, 1967), a view that is again being raised (Glenner et al., 1971). One difficulty in accepting that cellular ageing alone normally causes amyloid synthesis is the evidence (Kennedy, 1962) that a circulating glycosaminoglycan derived from endothelial cells may be a component of the ultimate fibrillar structure recognised by electron microscopy. By this reckoning, the glycoprotein synthesised in cells such as those of the reticuloendothelial system, represents only a precursor of the mature, insoluble extracellular amyloid fibril.

CHAPTER 13

Associated Syndromes

Sjögren's syndrome

Although Sjögren published his classical monograph in 1933, with the first full acount of the clinical triad of keratoconjunctivitis sicca, xerostomia and rheumatoid arthritis that became known eponymously as the Sjögren syndrome (Sjögren, 1933, 1943, 1951; Heaton, 1959) it is possible to trace records of similar cases, in retrospect, as early as 1888 (Hadden, 1888; Bunim, 1961, 1964; Bloch, 1969).

Salivary gland enlargement is inconstant. More than one half of the affected patients have rheumatoid arthritis but other systemic connective tissue diseases such as systemic lupus erythematosus, systemic sclerosis and polyarteritis nodosa are occasional accompaniments. Splenomegaly and leucopenia, as in Felty's syndrome, and hepatomegaly and eosinophilia are frequent and there is convincing clinical evidence of renal dysfunction. Interstitial nephritis (Tu et al., 1968), nephrocalcinosis, focal glomerulonephritis and interstitial lymphocytic and plasma cell infiltration are described together with tubular atrophy (Talal, Zisman and Schur, 1968; Talal, 1971). Viral-like structures have been found in 2 of 4 cases (Shearn et al., 1970). The renal changes may be analogous with those of the hyperviscosity syndrome of hyperglobulinaemia (Whaley and Buchanan, 1971) but the deposition of immune complexes in relation to the basement membranes of glomerular capillaries has been suggested reasonably as an alternative explanation for the renal disease. Necrotising arteritis may ensue and myopathy is an occasional feature (Denko et al., 1969).

A full account of this strange disorder including a description of 62 cases and necropsy records of 15, has been given by Bloch, Buchanan, Wohl and Bunim (1965) (see also Bunim, 1961), and remains one of the best contemporary reports. The immunological features have been outlined by Bloch (1969) and recent advances in understanding of the clinical, immunological and histological aspects of the syndrome by Whaley and Buchanan (1971).

Keratoconjunctivitis sicca is, of course, common in rheumatoid arthritis (Thompson and Eadie, 1956). The diagnosis of keratoconjunctivitis rests on the recognition of punctate or filamentary keratitis. When the first evidence of the triad of Sjögren's syndrome develops, the salivary glands display changes both in stromal and parenchymal structures. There is a diminution in the number of gland acini, which may disappear entirely. Lymphocytic infiltration is widespread, and the intraglandular duct epithelium is hyperplastic. Epi-myoepithelial islands form.

A classical *post mortem* study of a single case of Sjögren's syndrome was described in detail by Ellman, Parkes-Weber and Goodier (1951) and the morbid anatomical features of this variant of rheumatoid arthritis are fully depicted in this paper. The patient was a woman of 35 who had suffered from Raynaud's phenomenon since the age of 13 years. Dryness of the lips and mouth developed 9 years before her death; polyarthritis was only detected 13 months before she died. At necropsy, no visible lacrimal, salivary or thymic gland tissue was detected. The kidneys were normal and no evidence of synovitis or of periarticular disease was found in relation to the knee joints. A further typical single case examined at necropsy was discussed by Kissane (1964) in a report of a clinicopathological conference. The patient was a Caucasian female aged 53 who developed bilateral, painless parotid gland enlargement 13 years before her death; 7 years previously she had had polyarthritis. As in the case described by Ellman and his colleagues, respiratory symptoms were conspicuous. At necropsy, there was a sterile ophthalmitis. The submandibular and parotid salivary glands were severely affected.

The histological characteristics of the salivary glands were outlined by Sjögren (1933); Godwin (1952); Morgan and Castleman (1952); Ellman, Parkes-Weber and Goodier (1951); Cardell and Gurling (1954) and Kissane (1964), among others. Thus, Ellman *et al.* (1951) described replacement of the glandular acini of the lacrimal gland by small round cells in a fibrous matrix of scar tissue. Occasional plasma cells were seen and degenerate serous acini and ducts contained inspissated acidophilic material. The parotid glands comprised mainly fat and fibrous tissue. Collapsed, partly necrotic serous acini were accompanied by dilated ducts containing cellular and amorphous debris; they were surrounded by small round cells. The sublingual gland was recognised with difficulty but microscopically resembled the parotid. No taste buds were seen in the tongue. The glands of the lamina propria of the trachea were scanty and degenerate. Bronchial and oesophageal submucous glands were atrophic as were sweat glands. Kissane (1964) emphasised the presence of lymphocytic infiltration of the parotid gland, with myoepithelial cell proliferation and acinar atrophy. These changes were accompanied by comparable disturbances of the structure of the submandibular glands and of the subepithelial mucous glands of the trachea, oesophagus, breasts and vagina. In addition, a focal pancreatitis was noted and the kidneys displayed cortical atrophy and fibrosis and a mononuclear inflammatory cell infiltration, features suggestive of chronic pyelonephritis.

Bloch *et al.* (1965) confirmed that reductions in salivary secretory tissue and severe lymphocytic cellular infiltration were almost invariable. However, germinal centre formation was inconstant and duct cell hyperplasia variable. Sokoloff (see Bunim *et al.*, 1964) reviewing 20 patients, emphasised that only 9 of these met the original criteria of Morgan and Castleman, the lymphoid infiltrate varying widely in extent, the duct hyperplasia being sometimes absent. Investigations by Waterhouse (1963) revealed focal *post mortem* lymphocytic and histiocytic infiltrates in a large proportion of non-rheumatoid patients, particularly women over the age of 45. He suggested that a focal form of Sjögren's syndrome may be much more prevalent than is suspected and Waterhouse and Doniach (1966) proposed that a subclinical form of the syndrome was the common consequence of the frequent salivary and lacrimal histological changes encountered in elderly females.

In spite of conflicting views, it is still widely held that an autoallergic reaction against salivary, lacrimal and possibly thyroid tissue, indicated by local 'immunocyte' infiltration, accounts for the clinical manifestations. The evidence of Waterhouse (1963) and of Waterhouse and Doniach (1966) does little to simplify this analysis. Waterhouse's evidence can be used to support the argument that the lymphocytic 'infiltrates' in Sjögren's syndrome are incidental to the acinar and duct changes rather than causally related, a view indicated by Whaley *et al.* (1969) and by Font, Yanoff and Zimmerman (1967). These authors reviewed the lacrimal glandular changes in Sjögren's syndrome and in unexplained benign, lymphoepithelial lesions. They demonstrated that, in 2 of 4 cases, follow-up of the local, lymphoepithelial swellings revealed the subsequent development of at least one other major 'symptom' of those diagnostic of the Sjögren triad.

In recent years it has been recognised that there are also lymphocytic infiltrates of the minor, buccal salivary glands. Because of their accessibility for biopsy, valuable additional information has come from histological and immunological analyses of these glands. Diffuse lymphocytic infiltrates may be present in the absence of clinical signs of Sjögren's syndrome (Chisholm, Waterhouse and Mason, 1970) but focal infiltration is said to be recognised almost exclusively in Sjögren's syndrome and in rheumatoid arthritis (Whaley et al., 1969; Whaley and Buchanan, 1971). Chisholm and Mason (1968) have identified focal lymphocytic sialoadenitis in 61·9% of patients with the sicca syndrome, in 70% of patients with rheumatoid arthritis and Sjögren's syndrome and in 19·2% only of patients with uncomplicated rheumatoid arthritis without the sicca or Sjögren's syndromes.

The immunological features of Sjögren's syndrome have attracted growing interest. Rheumatoid factor is commonly detectable in the serum (Bloch, 1969). Thyroid autoantibodies (Beck et al., 1965; Bloch et al., 1965), a raised incidence of gastric parietal cell autoantibodies (Anderson et al., 1965), antibodies to smooth muscle (Feltkamp and van Rossum, 1968) and autoimmune complement fixation tests have been reported (Duthie, 1969; Whaley and Buchanan, 1971). Many patients have hypergammaglobulinaemia; some have antibodies against nuclear and various cytoplasmic antigens (Beck et al., 1965); but anti-lacrimal and -salivary gland antibodies were not at first demonstrable. An autoantibody against the cytoplasm of the duct epithelial cells of small salivary glands has, nevertheless, been recognised more recently by indirect immunofluorescence (Bertram and Halberg, 1964) and antibodies to salivary duct cells and other autoantibodies, one third of which were complement fixing, have been found in 53% of cases by Feltkamp and van Rossum (1968). However, a survey of 10 patients with keratoconjunctivitis sicca, 27 with Sjögren's syndrome and 47 with rheumatoid arthritis alone, revealed no correlation between the occurrence of salivary duct autoantibody and focal lymphocytic 'sialoadenitis' of the small glands of the labial mucosa, the prevalence of which at biopsy of the lower lip was 63% (Whaley et al., 1969).

At first sight, these conflicting results, which accord with Waterhouse's report (p. 169), support the suggestion that lymphocytic sialoadenitis is an incidental or secondary consequence of the glandular and duct cell changes in Sjögren's syndrome. Whaley et al. (1969), searching for an explanation, suggest that the salivary duct autoantibody shown by Bertram and Halberg and subsequently by themselves and others, is an epiphenomenon of rheumatoid arthritis and not a manifestation of Sjögren's syndrome.

The thyroid gland may be implicated in Sjögren's syndrome—the prevalence of thyroglobulin autoantibodies is increased—and Hashimoto (1912) drew attention to the similarity in the histological structure of the thyroid gland in autoallergic and Hashimoto thyroiditis, and in spontaneous myxoedema, and of the lacrimal and salivary glands in Sjögren's syndrome (Williamson et al., 1967). In a survey made of patients with autoallergic thyroid disease, the prevalence of keratoconjunctivitis sicca was, however, no higher than in a matched control series.

Information about the nature and pathogenesis of Sjögren's syndrome has come from experimental investigations. It is interesting to read the claim of Kessler (1968) that mice of the NZB and NZB × BZW F_1 strains spontaneously develop signs of Sjögren's syndrome and a deficiency of salivary amylase. The changes arose in the 4th month after birth and became more severe with age: there were mononuclear cell infiltrates and glandular lesions which were more severe in females than in males, and more pronounced in NZB/BZW F_1 hybrids than in the pure NZB line. Salivary duct autoantibody was not found. Sialoadenitis has also been caused by the immunisation of guinea-pigs with homologous salivary gland tissue emulsified in Freund's complete adjuvant (Chan, 1964). Chronic lacrimal and salivary adenitis has been reported (Follis, 1961) as the result of the experimental administration of serotonin and of iodide but there is little to suggest that these procedures are relevant to the origin of the human Sjögren syndrome.

In spite of the immunological evidence, and notwithstanding the experimental data, it still appears possible that the origins of the Sjögren syndrome should be sought in a systemic disorder of glandular 'mucin' synthesis and secretion. To the histologist, descriptions of the tissue changes in this disorder bring to mind those of cystic fibrosis. If the anomaly of protein–polysaccharide synthesis were found to include a defect in synovial protein hyaluronate, it appears possible that the entire syndrome could be explained on the basis of a defect in cell protein-polysaccharide secretion. The glandular changes could then be derived from faulty drainage and the immuno-logical disorders could be viewed as phenomena secondary to glandular inflammation and atrophy.

Felty's syndrome (Editorial, 1970)

The lymphoreticular changes in rheumatoid arthritis may come to dominate the clinical picture. Obvious splenic, and, occasionally, widespread lymph node enlargement are accompanied by leucopenia and anaemia (Fleischhaker and Lachnit, 1940; Hume et al., 1964; Gibberd, Gilbertson and Jepson, 1965) and the term Felty's syndrome can be applied (Felty, 1924). However, there is no good reason to suppose that cases with unusually severe lymphoreticular disease are quali-tatively distinct from those with less marked splenomegaly and lymphadenopathy.

Thymic enlargement is very rare. Evidence of liver dysfunction, secondary to splenic disease, has been described (Blendis et al., 1970). Some writers broaden the term 'Felty's syndrome' to include cases in which hypersplenism accompanies other connective tissue diseases such as systemic lupus erythematosus (Denko and Zumpft, 1962) but this is a minority view. Antinuclear antibodies may be detected: thus Barnett, Ruderman, Jeannet and Bloch (1966) found γ-G anti-nuclear antibodies in 11 of 14 patients, and γ-A and γ-M antinuclear antibodies in 10 of 14 cases each. Lupus cells were not detected nor were anti-DNA antibodies recognised. Four of the 12 cases tested by these authors revealed agglutination of 2 or more white blood cell suspensions by the serum of cases of Felty's syndrome. In another study (Bienenstock and Bloch, 1967), 12 of 13 cases (92%) were found to have serum immunoconglutinin titres of more than 1 in 16. A further series of 27 cases was analysed in the same way (Ruderman, Miller and Pinals, 1968) in a fully annotated paper.

The bone marrow contains a relative excess of plasma cells; there is active erythroid and myeloid haemopoiesis (Price and Schoenfeld, 1934; Curtis and Pollard, 1940; Ekelund, 1943) and abundant megakaryocytes (Williams, 1936). The large spleen shows the features characteristic of rheumatoid arthritis (p. 148) (Table 13.1) but in time, splenic fibrosis ensues. Splenectomy (Bach and Jacobs, 1951) can lead to remission. Portal hypertension and late evidence of liver dysfunction are encountered (Blendis et al., 1970) and at this stage the portal tract lymphocytic infiltrates that occur in rheumatoid arthritis are prominent.

The literature contains only small numbers of reports of full post mortem studies of Felty's syndrome. Curtis and Pollard (1940) and Price and Schoenfeld (1934) described the details of single cases and I have examined one. The results of persistent leucopenia include a tendency to recurrent bacterial infection, particularly of the respiratory tract. Bronchopneumonia is therefore a common cause of death in the Felty syndrome. In other cases bronchiectasis supervenes and death from systemic infections such as subacute bacterial endocarditis is not unusual (Singer and Levy, 1936; Williams, 1936). Reviewing the treatment of 3 cases of Felty's syndrome, Ellman, Cudkowicz and Elwood (1955) described one case in which death was apparently caused by systemic staphylococcal infection: purulent pericarditis and meningitis followed 4 months after palliative splenectomy. Barnes et al. (1971) have recently surveyed 21 collected cases, 10 of whom had had splenectomy, with particular reference to the relationship between the clinical and histological features (Table 13.1) of the disease. All cases had definite or classical rheumatoid arthritis: 19 were seropositive. The mean weight of 12 of the spleens was 911 g. Antiinflammatory and immunosuppressive drugs had been given frequently and there was common evidence of infection. By comparison with control cases of rheumatoid arthritis without signs of Felty's syndrome, the follicular arteries often displayed an increase in elastic tissue with endothelial hyperplasia. Lymphoid tissue was hyperplastic and sinus cell hyperplasia common. Extra-medullary erythropoiesis was an unusually frequent sign of Felty's syndrome and erythro-phagocytosis was more common than in the control series.

TABLE 13.1. *Frequency of histological abnormalities in the spleen in Felty's syndrome*

	Cases of Felty's Syndrome (13)	Rheumatoid control cases (22)
White pulp		
Follicular arteries		
amyloid	0	2
hyaline	13	13
endothelial hyperplasia	13	6
increased elastic	11	0
perivascular fibrosis	0	0
Lymphoid tissue		
hyperplasia	7	0
germinal centre hyperplasia	7	0
'active' germinal centres	4	1
hyaline	10	5
amyloid	0	2
Red pulp		
Venous sinusoids		
congestion	10	17
sinus cell hyperplasia	13	8
erythrophagocytosis	13	10
excess iron	7	13
non-iron pigment	12	22
amyloid	0	1
Splenic cords		
reticulin increase	7	3
plasma cell hyperplasia	13	9
reticulum cell hyperplasia	6	1
excess iron	7	13
non-iron pigment	13	22
extramedullary haemopoiesis	13	3
amyloid	0	1

(From Barnes, Turnbull and Vernon-Roberts, 1971, *Ann. rheum. Dis.*, **30**, 359–374.)

The differential pathological diagnosis of the lymphoreticular features of Felty's syndrome must include causes of lymph node enlargement such as the reticuloses, leukaemia and Hodgkin's disease; causes of splenomegaly such as malaria; portal hypertension due to primary liver disease; subacute bacterial endocarditis (Singer and Levy, 1936); and causes of unexplained anaemia such as haemolysis, undetected bleeding and malabsorption. Therapeutic considerations centre around the need for splenectomy (Hutt, Richardson and Staffurth, 1951) which, as Hume *et al.* (1964) reiterate, may be curative.

Psoriatic arthropathy (Bourdillon, 1888)

Psoriasis occurs in 3–5% of patients with rheumatoid arthritis, i.e. 2–3 times more often than in the general population (Baker, 1966a, b). The occasional association of psoriasis with sero-positive rheumatoid arthritis appears to be due to chance; the association with sero-negative polyarthritis is highly significant. One of the factors determining this association may be genetic. Clinical and radiological studies of the disease are numerous, pathological investigations rare. Very occasionally, psoriasis may accompany Felty's syndrome (Pakula and Artiucha, 1965).

Previously, great stress was placed on the occurrence in psoriasis of a severely destructive form of arthritis (arthritis mutilans) (Bauer, Bennett and Zeller, 1941; Sherman, 1952; Wright, 1969). This is now believed to be very uncommon, and the usual pattern is for psoriasis to accompany sero-negative arthritis of a histological nature closely resembling classical rheumatoid arthritis.

There is evidence of active chronic synovitis of the distal joints of hands and feet with progressive fibrosis, loss of articular cartilage but little pannus formation. Other joints, such as the temporomandibular, may be affected (Lundberg et al., 1967). There is little microscopic similarity between the lesions of the skin in psoriasis and those of the synovia in psoriatic arthropathy. In the latter, widespread periarticular inflammation is found together with loss of cortical bone in the distal phalanx. Bone loss is apparently due to the cellular activity of adjacent granulation tissue but osteoclastic reabsorption may be recognised. The factor provoking arthritis in psoriasis is not known but local trauma could, in theory, precipitate a granulomatous reaction with bone destruction in much the same way as a pin-prick in a psoriatic patient may lead to a new skin lesion at the site of pricking (Koebner phenomenon) (Buckley and Raleigh, 1959). Some authors have emphasised differences between rheumatoid arthritis and psoriatic arthropathy (Coste and Solnica, 1966) but the features they stress—fewer round cell synovial aggregates, increased fibrous tissue formation and thick-walled small blood vessels—may all be seen periodically in classical rheumatoid arthritis.

The disease progresses slowly. Pain and disability tend to be less than in rheumatoid arthritis (Wright, 1969). The severely destructive lesions seen in a minority of cases recall the neurogenic arthropathies of syringomyelia and Charcot's syndrome but, so far as I am aware, the central and peripheral nervous systems have not been investigated histologically in psoriatic arthropathy. Approximately 10% of patients dying with psoriatic arthritis have amyloidosis (Reed and Wright, 1966), an incidence rather less than in those dying with classical rheumatoid arthritis (Missen and Taylor, 1956). Synovial leucocytes may contain non-specific inclusions as in rheumatoid arthritis (Hollander et al., 1965; Rawson et al., 1965). There is anaemia (Gusev et al., 1969), possibly hyperuricaemia (Beveridge, 1967), and changes in uric acid metabolism the pathological significance of which remains quite uncertain.

Juvenile chronic polyarthritis (Still's disease)

'Arthritis starting before the age of 16 (manifest by 2 of the following: pain, swelling and limitation of movement) in four or more joints reliably observed over a period of at least 3 months or in one joint for a similar period with biopsy confirmation, other diseases being excluded' is a very uncommon condition, usually named Still's disease (Cornil, 1864; Still, 1896–7; Ansell and Bywaters, 1969). Tests for rheumatoid factor are almost always negative. Still's original description of fever (Calabro and Marchesano, 1967a, b), arthritis, lymphadenopathy and splenomegaly, may not be specific (Ansell and Bywaters, 1969).

Histologically, there may be transient erythema with a mild mononuclear perivascular cell aggregation of the dermal connective tissue (Sokoloff, 1966). The relatively thick juvenile articular cartilage is destroyed more slowly than is the case in adult rheumatoid arthritis. Synovial inflammatory changes are indistinguishable from those of the adult but may only be mild. The synovial fluid shows no consistent variation from the adult disease (Ropes and Bauer, 1953) (p. 84). Synovitis appears to be most frequent in the wrist joint (Chaplin et al., 1969). Endarterial fibrosis is rare and subcutaneous nodules uncommon. The nodules resemble the rheumatic nodule more closely than the adult granuloma (p. 122) and contain small numbers of proliferating fibroblasts and irregular zones of fibrinous exudation (Sokoloff, 1966); by contrast, areas of necrosis and marginal pallisade formation are unusual.

Tenosynovitis may occur. Pericarditis is encountered but does not indicate a serious prognosis (Ansell and Bywaters, 1969) and does not progress to become constrictive. Iridocyclitis is found sometimes with band keratopathy and complicated cataract, an oculo-articular triad (Hingpeter, Naumann and Bartelheimer, 1971). These authors stress that the complete diagnostic syndrome described by Still is found in only 7% of cases, of whom only 5·5–21% have eye complications. Histologically, they found the disorder in Still's disease to be quite different from the granulomatous scleritis commonly present in adult cases. There are multiple epithelioid cell granulomas in the ciliary body, vitreous, choroid, retina and around scleral emissary vessels. Secondary glaucoma may be present with rubeosis iridis, intercalary staphyloma and band-shaped keratopathy. Complicated anterior, capsular, partially calcified cataract is recognised. Pulmonary fibrosis has been described and, as in the adult disease, amyloidosis (p. 164) may develop (Rostropowicz-Denisiewicz et al., 1969). Joint biopsy (p. 206) is valuable and may help to exclude traumatic synovitis and tuberculosis.

One characteristic change encountered in the juvenile disease is an interference, by the presence of subchondral granulation tissue, with normal epiphyseal bone growth. The resultant 'rheumatic dwarfism' must be distinguished from the influence of therapeutic corticosteroids on growth, effects which also arrest endochondral ossification.

Of 33 cases presenting with monarticular synovitis 8, at biopsy, showed the changes of classical rheumatoid arthritis, 8 showed less marked but similar changes and in 12 the histological features were atypical, the cellular infiltrates slight (Bywaters and Ansell, 1965). Sclerodactylia and calcinosis are rare complications (Ellman and Parkes Weber, 1948) and occasionally the process of calcification may involve the peripheral and visceral arteries, leading to coronary artery occlusion, a combination of circumstances that Reid (1968) observed in a case with amyloidosis. Debré, Milhit and Lamy (1938) and Schlesinger and Cathie (1951) reported the bone marrow findings. In 32 cases, Schlesinger confirmed that the marrow was hyperplastic, with a shift to the left in maturation.

The disease often persists into adult life (Jeremy et al., 1968). In 4 cases studied personally at necropsy the mean age at death was 26 years.

Relationship between rheumatoid arthritis and ankylosing spondylitis

For many years the close similarity between the synovitis of rheumatoid arthritis and that of ankylosing spondylitis encouraged the idea that these were two manifestations of a single disease. The confusing term 'rheumatoid spondylitis' was used but, by common consent, has now been relegated to the proper description of the spondylitis of rheumatoid arthritis. The conspicuous involvement of cartilaginous and fibrocartilaginous, as well as synovial, joints in ankylosing spondylitis, the male preponderance and low age of onset, and the nature and distribution of the extraarticular and visceral lesions, all indicate that this must be regarded as a distinct disease entity.

The pathological distinction of ankylosing spondylitis from rheumatoid arthritis is not readily made if examination is confined to a single diarthrodial joint. In the former, as in the latter, there is a low grade subacute or chronic synovitis in which synovial villi, with synovial cell hyperplasia, become enlarged, adhere to and spread across articular cartilaginous surfaces. The opposing cartilages, progressively covered by granulation tissue, become united. Fibrous ankylosis develops and, in ankylosing spondylitis, advances to bone formation. As Cruickshank (1951) points out, all phases of the ankylosing spondylitic synovitis can be matched to lesions encountered in rheumatoid arthritis, in which, however, the apparent activity of the inflammatory reaction tends to be greater. Differences are, nevertheless, detectable. They include the more common occurrence of haemorrhage in ankylosing spondylitic synovitis, the greater frequency, in non-irradiated cases, of endarterial fibrosis, and a tendency to earlier fibrosis, followed by bony ankylosis. Finally, it is salutary to recall that synovial lesions attributable to either rheumatoid arthritis or ankylosing spondylitis, have been encountered in the absence of either disease.

When the cartilaginous joints are considered (Cruickshank, 1956), it appears that there is considerable overlap in the nature of the changes seen. The lesions of the manubriosternal joint, for example, are not specific for ankylosing spondylitis. There is an early, low-grade osteitis accompanied by granulation tissue formation and followed by destruction of adjacent bone. Fibrous ankylosis ensues and advances to complete bony ankylosis. Closely similar changes have been encountered in rheumatoid arthritis by the small number of authors who have examined this joint. So far as has been determined, very similar disorders affect other cartilaginous or fibrocartilaginous joints such as the symphysis pubis but there is little published evidence on the state of these joints in rheumatoid arthritis.

The main invertebral joints in ankylosing spondylitis are the sites for changes that are distinct from those of rheumatoid arthritis (van Swaay, 1950; Cruickshank, 1956). The changes observed are largely confined within the anatomical outlines of the disc and adjacent vertebral bodies. The annulus margins, and the adjacent portions of the anterior ligament are infiltrated by inflammatory cells and progressively replaced by fibrous tissue. Ossification follows and is ultimately extensive, binding the vertebral bodies together in rigid fusion.

In rheumatoid arthritis by contrast, when the cervical vertebrae are found to be subluxated or dislocated, the disease process can be traced to marginal synovitis of the neurocentral joints, with secondary destruction of the main articulations (Ball and Sharp, 1971). Fibrous ankylosis is ill-defined and not restricted to the disc margins; bony ankylosis is most exceptional. The lumbar and thoracic vertebrae, devoid of synovial neurocentral joints, are spared (p. 83).

Relationship between rheumatoid arthritis and systemic lupus erythematosus

Both clinically and pathologically (Pagel and Treip, 1955) an overlap between the features of rheumatoid arthritis and those of systemic lupus erythematosus (S.L.E.) has long been recognised.

Clinically, patients with S.L.E. very commonly present with arthralgia or frank arthritis. In a typical series, Black, Goldin, Poske and Malmed (1959) found positive sheep cell agglutination tests in 71% of 35 rheumatoid sera and 54% of 28 S.L.E. sera using an euglobulin test, and 51% and 14% respectively when using a cold precipitation variant of the test on the same sera. Depending on the sensitivity of the test system used, L.E. cells have been found in preparations made from 3 to 27% of rheumatoid bloods.

Histologically, the arthritis of S.L.E. can be distinguished from that of rheumatoid arthritis by criteria detailed by Gritsman and Rogov (1965) and by Cruickshank (1966). In S.L.E., fibrin is deposited on the synovial surface and within the synovial membrane: occasionally, synovial cells are absent from significant areas of the synovial surface and fibrin lies directly upon subsynovial connective tissue. Basophilic bodies are often present but the cellular infiltrates, characteristically

seen in rheumatoid arthritis, are slight. Pannus formation is uncommon and adhesions and ankylosis rare. Vascular lesions are occasionally encountered and affect veins rather than arteries, as in
rheumatoid arthritis.

Cruickshank regarded the collective lesions in S.L.E. as diagnostic but he described them as
individually 'non-specific', a view which cannot, of course, be applied to the pathognomonic
basophilic bodies. Tendon sheath synovitis was encountered and the cellular infiltrates were more
marked here than those in the joint synovium; basophilic bodies were present (Cruickshank, 1966).
The specificity of the synovial lesion in S.L.E. was also questioned by Zevely *et al.* (1956) and by
Rodnan, Yunis and Totten (1960) on the basis of punch biopsy material; neither group of authors,
however, mentioned the presence of the basophilic bodies described by Klemperer *et al.* (1950).
Using open biopsy (Orabona and Semeraro, 1961) or multiple tissue blocks obtained at necropsy
(Cruickshank, 1959*b*), the presence of the diagnostic basophilic bodies was commonly confirmed
and the distinction of lupus from rheumatoid synovitis readily effected.

'Rheumatoid-like' subcutaneous nodules may occasionally be encountered in systemic lupus
erythematosus. Hahn, Yardley and Stevens (1970) described 6 patients with S.L.E. in whom
such periarticular nodules developed. Three of the nodules, on biopsy, were found to resemble
those of rheumatoid arthritis microscopically. In each of the 6 cases, there was polyarthritis,
decreased synovial fluid complement, positive serum L.E. cell tests and the presence of circulating
antinuclear factor. Glomerulonephritis was encountered in 5 cases.

In my own series, the histological evidence suggests that long-standing lupus-like renal injury
in patients with clinical rheumatoid arthritis is very uncommon. However the mean survival time
in acute S.L.E. with glomerular disease was not in excess of 5 years before the therapeutic introduction of corticosteroids. It is difficult, therefore, to rule out the role of selection in a series
where case records have been collected over a period of years dating back to 1929 (Appendix). In
one of my cases (Case 148), the diagnosis of S.L.E. was made 7 years before death. The patient
was treated with corticosteroids. L.E. cells were recognised in appropriate preparations. Later,
arthritis developed, followed by peripheral circulatory insufficiency and Raynaud's phenomenon.
Signs of right-sided heart disease appeared. Pulmonary hypertension was diagnosed and the
patient died from cor pulmonale and congestive cardiac failure. Necropsy revealed severe pulmonary changes (Figs. 12.6, 12.10) that mimicked those of systemic sclerosis and which emphasised the possibility that 3 or more systemic connective tissue diseases might have coexisted. The
kidneys, however, were intact and there was no evidence that there had ever been active proliferative or membranous glomerulonephritis. In making this assessment it is necessary to recall that the
basement membrane changes of the membranous glomerulonephritis of S.L.E. are reversible.
Geidel (1967) clearly regards the presence of the L.E. cell phenomenon in rheumatoid arthritis
as evidence of an association with systemic lupus erythematosus. This is not generally agreed.

CHAPTER 14

Pathological Results of Drug Treatment

Much has been written of the hazards of drug therapy and only selected aspects of the pathological changes caused by treatment can be reviewed here (see Dunlop, 1969) (Table 14.1).

TABLE 14.1.   *Instances of drug toxicity in 142 hospital cases of rheumatoid arthritis examined at necropsy*

Gold: aplastic anaemia or thrombocytopenia	9
Phenylbutazone	2
Iron	1
Colchicine	1
Steroids	Contributory in at least 17 cases.
Salicylates ⎫ Phenacetin ⎭	11 cases of necrotising papillitis, 7 of which had active pyelonephritis.

The present tendency for small doses of *gold* to find favour in the treatment of rheumatoid arthritis (Empire Rheumatism Council, 1960) does not alter the accumulated evidence which shows that larger, uncontrolled doses are hazardous. In the 145 fatal cases that I have investigated there were 9 examples of aplastic anaemia or thrombocytopenia following gold treatment. Three other cases had been treated without hazard. Gold has been given intraarticularly, with success, to avoid these systemic effects (Lewis and Ziff, 1966) and more recently experimental studies have confirmed the efficacy of intraarticular injections of radioactive ^{90}Y-yttrium in the suppression of fibrin arthritis due to hypersensitivity (Webb, Lowe and Bluestone, 1969). ^{198}Au-gold has, in the same way, been exclaimed clinically and experimentally as a means of administering ionising radiation locally following injection. It is not yet certain whether synovial ^{198}Au can be distributed systemically via synovial lymphatics, constituting a serious hazard.

Phenylbutazone may induce bone marrow changes, including arrested maturation, agranulocytosis, and thrombotic microangiopathy with thrombocytopenia (Thomson and Gardner, 1969). *Colchicine* poisoning was also recorded among my cases (Case 11). It has been shown that *phenacetin* may cause desquamation of epithelial cells from the urinary tract even in normal persons and it is suspected that this action may be related to the high incidence of necrotising papillitis found in patients dying with rheumatoid arthritis (Lawson and Maclean, 1966) (p. 145). In the present series, necrotising papillitis was recognised in 11 cases. It is important to note that 7 of these patients also suffered from pyelonephritis suggesting that, as in diabetes mellitus, the occurrence of papillary necrosis is attributable to a dual mechanism.

The toxic effects of *corticosteroids* are often suspected at necropsy in rheumatoid arthritis but are difficult to assess. Systemic corticosteroids have been invoked as a cause for posterior, subcapsular cataracts (Black *et al.*, 1960). After treatment with large doses of corticosteroids for prolonged periods, peptic ulcers perforate or bleed, infection is exacerbated, intestinal perforation occurs and osteoporosis is exaggerated. To *prove* that these disorders are caused by corticosteroid therapy remains practically impossible in the majority of retrospective pathological studies. Case 45 of my series exemplifies that problem. A male aged 54 had undergone gastrojejunostomy for peptic ulcer 20 years previously. He had received corticosteroid treatment for rheumatoid arthritis before admission to hospital for hip arthroplasty. Following operation, signs of peritonitis developed. In spite of laparotomy the patient died and was found to have very large, paired stomal ulcers one of which had perforated. The ulcers had given no signs or symptoms during the period of corticosteroid treatment before operation.

Excessive use of a joint with rheumatoid arthritis while under local treatment with hydrocortisone may induce a Charcot-like arthropathy (Alarçon-Segovia and Ward, 1965).

The theory that rheumatoid factor, which circulates as an IgG/IgM (7S/19S) complex, may be a result of decreased protein-SH content with an impaired mechanism for regenerating and maintaining such groups, led to the therapeutic trial of *penicillamine* (Lorber, 1966), a thiol compound known to dissociate polymeric proteins by cleaving disulphide bonds (p. 117). Rheumatoid lung disease which is often associated with sero-positivity, responded well but the drug caused side effects including nephrosis and bone marrow depression. The role of the *salicylates* in provoking gastrointestinal bleeding has been clearly recognised (Duthie, 1969); since 8 of the 145 patients in my *post mortem* series had gastric ulcers and 7 duodenal, the hazards of this form of treatment do not require additional emphasis.

Septic arthritis complicating rheumatoid arthritis

The incidence of infection among patients with rheumatoid arthritis is higher than in the general hospital population (Parker, 1965) and it is not surprising therefore to find that septic and suppurative arthritis may be superimposed on the longstanding proliferative joint changes of rheumatoid synovitis (Kellgren *et al.*, 1958). Kellgren's cases accounted for half of the admissions for suppurative arthritis in a busy general hospital. Karten (1969) reviewing 102 cases, reported septic arthritis in 3 of those not subjected to surgery. That this proportion was greater than among the cases reviewed by de Andrade and Tribe (1962), by Gaulhofer-de Klerck and van Dam (1963) and by Gibberd (1965) they attributed, rightly or wrongly, to a larger proportion of old, debilitated persons among those treated. The infecting organisms are particularly *Staphylococcus aureus, Streptococcus haemolyticus, Haemophilus, Escherichia coli,* other coliforms, *Proteus* (Norden and Sellers, 1964; Hoagland and Lord, 1967), *Pasteurella,* and a variety of microaerophilic fungi (Gardner *et al.*, 1962; Gardner, 1969).

CHAPTER 15

Pathological Consequences of Surgery

Synovectomy

Renewed interest has developed in recent years in the procedure of synovectomy for rheumatoid arthritis (Lipscomb, 1965; Wilkinson and Lowry, 1965; Gariepy *et al.*, 1966; Mohing, 1967; Gschwend, 1970). The operation was recommended by Stockman (1920) but first performed, apparently, by Schüller (1887). The historical development of synovectomy, the surgical techniques and the early results have recently been surveyed fully by Laine (1967), by Geens (1969) and by Geens *et al.* (1969).

The rationale for the operation has varied in different decades according to prevailing views on the nature of the disease. Early workers sought to alleviate mechanical difficulties and in 2 such operations Ropes and Bauer (1953) refer to patients from whom synovial fluid had been obtained before and after synovectomy of a knee joint. In the first case, of $3\frac{1}{2}$ years duration, no effusion developed in the joint following operation but 1·5 ml. was obtained at aspiration 2 years later. Following this a small effusion was found and 10 ml. was obtained at that time and 15 ml. four months later. In the second case, a slight persistent effusion developed six months post-operatively and 25 ml. of fluid was obtained at aspiration 3 years later. Ropes and Bauer emphasised that the analyses of the fluids were fundamentally the same before and after operation with the exception of the 'mucin' content which was markedly decreased. There was also evidence of a diminished viscosity. They deduced from evidence derived from experimental synovectomy that the connective tissue which reforms the lining of the joint after operation is not capable of producing 'mucin' in large quantities. There does not appear to be any work with synovial cell culture (p. 39) after synovectomy to confirm or refute this view.

More recently (Bastow, 1964) the removal of local sites of immunoglobulin synthesis, of activated lysosomal enzymes or of foci of infection have been advocated. Thus, synovectomy causes a reduction in the content of synovial fluid rheumatoid factor and IgG, IgA and IgM immunoglobulins but no reduction in the already relatively low complementary activity or in $\beta_1 C$ ($C'3$) levels (Cracchiolo and Barnett, 1969). However, the correlation between synovial serological changes and clinical improvement is not always good although levels of rheumatoid factor fall more often in patients with good surgical results. Early measurements of synovial rheumatoid factor (Goldie, 1970) may be misleading. Hollander justified the operation by invoking the theories with which his name is now associated (p. 103). Glynn (p. 203) would presumably attribute the beneficial results of synovectomy to the removal of the altered fibrin which he believes to account for the chronic nature of the disease. His view finds support in the demonstration that fibrinolytic agents injected into the joint benefit the patient but is not substantiated by recent studies with Arvin in experimental arthritis (Holt *et al.*, 1969).

Until now, insufficient time has elapsed to allow substantial numbers of cases treated by contemporary techniques to be assessed pathologically. The surgical philosophy tends to be misleading and Laine (1967) draws inappropriate analogies between the behaviour of the granulation tissue in rheumatoid arthritis and the growth of benign or malignant tumours.

Synovial tissue has considerable capacity for regeneration (Key, 1925; Currey, Moore and Prentice, 1970) and hemisynovectomy in rabbits is followed by almost complete synovial regeneration within 60 days. In man, regeneration follows even the most complete excision. The newly-formed tissue appears capable of secreting synovial fluid but has a diminished capacity for synthesising and secreting protein-polysaccharides and collagen. Within limits, the ultrastructure of the A(M) and B(F) cells of the reformed tissue is closely similar to that of the original synovium (Wassilev, 1970). Synovial tissue seems, however, to be more fibrous and less vascular than normal 6 years after synovectomy (for synovial chondromata) (Hosford, 1937) in spite of a normal radiological appearance at arthrography. Whether the vasculature remains normal after rheumatoid synovectomy or reverts to an abnormal structure (Lindström, 1966) appears to depend on whether the periosteum is injured at operation. The reformed synovium is susceptible to rheumatoid synovitis (Teleszyński and Patroś, 1970) but the response is modified by the fibrotic nature of the new tissue (Geens et al., 1969). When recurrence occurs it is not known whether the primary cause of the rheumatoid arthritis persists in residual tissue or is conveyed from distant foci. There is often persistent effusion but the fluid is of changed quality. Attempts are being made to measure the inflammatory response in regenerated synovium and to compare this reaction with untreated rheumatoid synovia. In one such study, Granda, Ranawat and Posner (1971) were able to show that of 3 enzyme activities measured, β-glucuronidase, acid phosphatase and cathepsin D, only determinations of the last provided a valuable index of inflammation. Levels approximating to those found in untreated rheumatoid synovium were found after $3\frac{1}{2}$ years.

In one series, recurrence was reported in 6·5% of cases (Brown, 1969). The biologist would not be surprised that grossly intact joints form new lining synovial layers. After all, continued movement at the site of fractures leads to pseudoarthrosis formation and is presumed to be a stimulus to joint formation in the mammalian embryo, although the main morphological features of the joint are determined by genetic factors (Gardner and O'Rahilly, 1968). There is, of course, no way of establishing that the whole of the synovial surface of any particular joint has been removed and the possibility always remains that the synovial tissue found if a subsequent operation such as arthroplasty or arthrodesis becomes necessary, is no more than a new lining formed in continuity with a residual island of synovial cells. Aidem and Baker (1964) suggest that if regeneration of the excised synovium is widespread, recurrence of the disease is likely. But this, again, is an extremely difficult point to establish: how to tell when regeneration is complete is particularly uncertain. Stereoscopic microscopy of the living, opened joint would appear to be the only possible technique.

'Chemical' synovectomy

Chemical 'synovectomy' can be substituted for surgical operation. The hyperplastic synovium of rheumatoid arthritis has been the object of attack by cytotoxic drugs, externally applied X-irradiation and locally instilled radioactive isotopes. Obviously, if a material could be found which, injected locally, would safely and efficiently deplete joints of inflamed, enlarged synovial villi, the main reason for elective early synovectomy would be removed. Various techniques have been attempted. Gold (Lewis and Ziff, 1966), radium (Louyot et al., 1970), nitrogen mustards (Scherbel, Schuchter and Harrison, 1957; Scherbel, Schuchter and Weyman, 1957; Vainio and Julkunen, 1960; Gross, 1963) thio-tepa (Flatt, 1962; Howes and Jarnis, 1965; Wenley and Glick, 1964), thorotrast (Sutro, 1961); and osmic acid (Hurri, Sievers and Oka, 1963) have been used in the human disease; osmic acid in rabbit caragheenin arthritis (Dazziano, Gagnon and Laurin, 1969) and radioactive ^{90}Y-yttrium in rabbit fibrin arthritis (Webb, Lowe and Bluestone, 1969).

Most of the agents employed cause direct injury to, and death of synovial cells. For example, in one investigation, the synthesis of DNA and of RNA was shown to be inhibited (Greiling, Kisters and Vojtisek, 1970). In the majority of reported studies, synovial ablation by chemical or physical means has been followed by regeneration. As in surgical synovectomy, it is not clear whether regeneration is from residual uninjured synovial cells, or whether an entirely new lining cell layer forms *ab initio*, the capacity to form spaces lined by these cells being, apparently, a genetic characteristic inherent in synovial mechanocytes.

Whole joint X-irradiation, it is appreciated, is liable to cause bone necrosis, sometimes necessitating subsequent radical palliative surgery. In theory, radioactive isotopes may be carried by the lymphatic circulation to the regional lymph nodes and thence, systemically. However, the local experimental use of ^{198}Au and ^{90}Y have not been shown to cause lymphoreticular or haemopoietic disease, possibly because the capacity of synovial phagocytes to retain particulate material near the site of injection is great. Nevertheless, the opportunity to make autoradiographs of regional lymphoid tissues and to subject them to radiation counting procedures would be welcomed as a means of assessing the safety of this form of treatment.

Although 'immunosuppressive' treatment may be held to ablate lymphoreticular tissues as well as to diminish immunoglobulin secretion, the effects are not always clear or easily explained. For example, Vojtisek *et al.* (1970), after treatment with intraarticular podophyllin and ethyl hydrazide, or with prednisolone, recognised a diminished number of synovial fluid cells and granulocytes but an increase in the lymphocyte and monocyte count. In some cases there was a decrease in synovial fluid and serum immunoglobulin levels but this effect was not consistent.

Post-operative death

Even more frequent in hospital than the cases where death can be attributed to medical treatment for rheumatoid arthritis are those where there has been a recent surgical operation (Table 15.1). The relative importance of surgery and of drug therapy in terms of the whole rheumatoid

TABLE 15.1. *Postoperative deaths among 142 hospital cases of rheumatoid arthritis examined at necropsy*

F	33	Mandibular condylectomy	Respiratory failure
F	61	Gastrectomy	Fungal septicaemia
M	44	Excision of rheumatoid nodule	Fungal septicaemia
F	57	Arthroplasty for hallus valgus	Pulmonary atelectasis
M	55	Hip arthroplasty	Perforated stomal ulcer
F	67	Fractured femur; operative fixation	Gas gangrene
M	73	Hip arthroplasty	Pulmonary abscesses
M	53	Enucleation of eye for malignant tumour	Metastatic spread
F	57	Hip arthroplasty	β-haemolytic streptococcal septicaemia
F	72	Tear of infected uterus during D and C	Pulmonary atelectasis

population is however difficult to estimate. Drug therapy may contribute to surgical difficulties. In a personal series of 142 fatal hospital cases, generalised infection caused postoperative death in 4 of 10 patients; of these, 2 had been treated with corticosteroids. A patient who developed gas gangrene displayed methaemoglobinaemia produced by phenacetin (case 48).

There remain a small number of cases in which postoperative death is the direct result of one of the pathological changes of rheumatoid arthritis. Case 46 of my series is an example. A young woman aged 33, wholly crippled with Still's disease, had undergone right mandibular condy-lectomy for relief of mandibular ankylosis. At a second, left, operation, difficulty with intubation was experienced. Pulmonary atelectasis developed and the patient died. Necropsy revealed active rheumatoid arthritis of the intrinsic laryngeal joints, disease of which could therefore be held to be the factor directly responsible for death.

CHAPTER 16

Causes of Death

Hollingsworth (1968), writing of the mortality associated with rheumatoid arthritis, says, 'No really representative figures are available. All surveys are based on clinic populations . . . not representative of the disease . . . in a general population.' Subject to bias and selection as are the Registrar-General's records, they surely do something to answer Hollingsworth's strictures. A recent Statistical Appendix (1969), the first of a series of annual digests of statistics from the Report of the Ministry of Pensions and National Insurance (1963) and from the Registrar General's Statistical Review of England and Wales (1963) and the Annual Report of the Registrar General for Scotland for the year 1963, summarises the morbidity and mortality for the main groups of rheumatic diseases and compares the morbidity from rheumatism with that from the other main causes of incapacity. The crude death rates (1963) were: males—8·5/1,000,000 living (England and Wales), 13·6/1,000,000 (Scotland); females—30·8 (E and W), 48·4 (Scotland). 763 males and 1607 females were certified as having died from 'rheumatism'; 54·6% of this total for women was attributed to rheumatoid arthritis. In addition, Uddin, Kraus and Kelly (1970) reviewed 475 patients with rheumatoid arthritis first seen between 1954 and 1966. The cumulative survival rate was determined in each year for up to 10 years, compared to that of a normal matched population. The evidence shows that the observed cumulative survival rate in rheumatoid arthritis is lower than normal for each sex at each year of follow-up, particularly in the later years. The cumulative survival rate is lower in rheumatoid males than in rheumatoid females and an unexpectedly high incidence of death from infection is encountered.

There are, however, surprisingly few reports in which the pathological details of substantial numbers of fatal cases of rheumatoid arthritis are critically examined and few, with the exception of that of Ball (1968) in which an attempt is made to contrast the frequency of pathological lesions

TABLE 16.1. *Evidence supporting suggestion that cerebral haemorrhage and myocardial infarction may be less prevalent in Rheumatoid Arthritis than in control cases.*

	Numbers observed			MRI*			Numbers expected	England and Wales
	M	F	T	M	F	T		T
Cerebral haemorrhage	2	0	2†	3·0	5·3	8·3†		6·2
Cerebral infarction	0	5	5	2·3	3·2	5·5		4·5
Myocardial infarction	4	2	6‡	5·7	4·5	10·2		17·4‡
Cancer (excluding leukaemia and Hodgkin's disease)	6	4	10‡	11·9	15·2	27·1‡		24·5§

* Manchester Royal Infirmary.   † P<0·05   ‡ P<&0·01.   § P<0·001.

(From Ball, J., 1968, In: *Rheumatic Diseases: Pfizer Medical Monograph Number 3*. Edited by Duthie, J. J. R. and Alexander, W. R. M. University Press, Edinburgh.)

at death with those encountered in an unselected control population, matched for age, sex or physical characteristics or on an arbitrary basis.

TABLE 16.2. *Diseases significantly more frequent in group of cases of Rheumatoid Arthritis*

	Numbers observed			Numbers expected (MRI)*		
	M	F	T	M	F	T
Chronic peptic ulcer	15	11	26†	3·90	1·31	5·21
Chronic peptic ulcer (active only)	9	6	15†	2·80	0·49	3·29
Polyarteritis nodosa	7	7	14†	0·58	0·31	0·89
Septicaemia	10	5	15†	1·01	2·24	3·25
Amyloidosis	6	2	8†	0·33	0·13	0·46
Chronic pyelonephritis	1	10	11‡	1·20	3·84	5·04
Renal papillary necrosis	1	1	2	0·25	0·75	1·00

    * Manchester Royal Infirmary.   † P < 0·001.   ‡ P < 0·05.

(From Ball, J., 1968, In: *Rheumatic Diseases: Pfizer Medical Monograph Number 3*. Edited by Duthie, J. J. R. and Alexander, W. R. M. University Press, Edinburgh.)

Rosenberg, Baggenstoss and Hench (1943) referred briefly to the 30 fatal cases of rheumatoid arthritis collected in the Mayo Clinic files over a 25-year period. Bennett (1943) summarised his more extensive findings in 48 *post mortem* examinations, with particular reference to the incidence of heart disease (Table 16.8). Missen and Taylor (1956), reviewing the incidence of amyloidosis in rheumatoid arthritis, were able to collect 47 cases from the records of the (Royal) Postgraduate Medical School, London, while Cruickshank (1958), making a comparable study of the nature of the cardiac lesions in this disease, uncovered 100 necropsy records in the files of the Royal Infirmary, Edinburgh.

I have reviewed the necropsy records in the Southeastern region of Scotland for the years 1929–1966. The data are summarised in the Appendix (p. 212). The collection of cases cannot be regarded as complete for the region but the frequency of disease processes encountered at death

TABLE 16.3. *Mean age at death of 142 hospital cases of rheumatoid arthritis examined at necropsy between 1929–1966*

(a) of 142 cases* of rheumatoid arthritis examined *post mortem* 1929–1966	Number	Mean age
Males	44	59·0
Mean age at death of whole male population		67·0†
Females	98	63·0
Mean age at death of whole female population		72·8†
Female/male sex ratio 2·2/1·0		
(b) of 106 cases examined *post mortem* 1950–1966		
Males	31	58·7
Females	75	63·4

    * Includes 4 cases of Still's disease, mean age at death 28 years.   † Registrar-General for Scotland, 1964.

in rheumatoid arthritis is of interest. Unlike Ball (1968), I am not convinced that reliable information is obtainable by comparing the frequency of disease processes at death with those in a selected hospital population during the same period. Nor is the choice of a more appropriate control hospital population easy or necessarily valid: bias is inevitable. Only prospective studies can answer some of the outstanding questions relating to morbidity and mortality.

When my necropsy records were reviewed (Tables 16.4, 16.5, 16.8 and 16.9) an extremely high

TABLE 16.4. *Frequency of pathological changes found at necropsy in 142 cases of rheumatoid arthritis*

Pleural fibrosis	56	(41%)
Bronchopneumonia	54	(40%)
Lymphadenopathy	41	(30%)
Osteoporosis	41	(30%)
Pyelonephritis	39	(29%)
Emphysema	31	(23%)
Purulent bronchitis	30	(22%)
Malignant tumours	24	(18%)
Mitral valve disease	24	(18%)
Pericardial fibrosis	22	(16%)
Thyroiditis or fibrosis	17	(13%)
Amyloidosis	17	(13%)
Acute pericarditis	15	(11%)
Pulmonary embolism	14	(10%)
Venous thrombosis	13	(10%)
Tuberculosis	13	(10%)
Aortic valve disease	13	(10%)
Cystitis	12	(9%)
Peritoneal adhesions	10	(7%)
Renal papillary necrosis	9	(7%)
Postoperative deaths	9	(7%)
Generalised infection	8	(6%)

TABLE 16.5. *Unusual pathological features found at necropsy in 142 hospital cases of rheumatoid arthritis*

Arterial thrombi	8
Fractures	8
cervical	2
Arteritis	7
Fungus infection	3
Septic arthritis	3
Megaloblastic anaemia	2
Retroperitoneal abscess	3
Polymyositis	1
Parathyroid adenoma	1
Pharyngeal nodules	1
Tracheal stenosis	1

incidence of respiratory disease was found (p. 137). The frequency of pleural fibrosis and of emphysema shows that there were longstanding changes other than the terminal bronchopneumonia or purulent bronchitis to which so many of these old people succumb. Interstitial pulmonary fibrosis (Scadding, 1969) with cystic changes was encountered. A generalised enlargement of lymphoid tissue and splenomegaly was frequent (p. 148). Osteoporosis, with or without corticosteroid therapy, was often recognisable macroscopically and the occurrence of fractures was a feature of 8 cases (p. 74). Numbers of these hospital patients suffered from acute or chronic pyelonephritis and renal failure from this cause, and from amyloidosis, was common (p. 164). Thyroid atrophy is common in old age but more cases of thyroid disease than would be expected by chance appear to occur in association with rheumatoid arthritis (p. 158). It is known

TABLE 16.6.   *Frequency of renal disease in 142 hospital cases of rheumatoid arthritis examined at necropsy*

Pyelonephritis	39	(29%)
Papillary necrosis	11	(8%)
Hydronephrosis	4	(3%)
Cystic kidney	3	—
Tubular necrosis	3	—
Calculus	2	—
Pyronephrosis	2	—

TABLE 16.7.   *Syndromes associated with rheumatoid arthritis encountered among 142 hospital cases examined at necropsy*

Still's disease	4
Felty's syndrome	3
Psoriasis	3
Lacrimal ⎱ disease Salivary ⎰	2
Laryngeal arthritis	1
Thrombotic microangiopathy	1

TABLE 16.8.   *Pathological changes at death in 142 cases of rheumatoid arthritis*

Amyloid:	17	*Kidney:*		pneumoconiosis	3
Arteries:		calculus	2	tuberculosis	13
arteritis	7	cystic	3	tumours	7
arterial thrombosis	8	hydronephrosis	4	*Lymph nodes:* enlargement	41
Bladder: cystitis	7	papillary necrosis	11	*Muscle:* polymyositis	1
Blood: anaemia, megalo-		pyelonephritis	39	*Nerve:* polyneuritis	1
blastic	2	pyonephrosis	2	*Operations:* (recent)	9
Bone:		tubular necrosis	3	*Peritoneum:*	
fractures (2 cervical)	8	*Liver:*		adhesions	10
osteoporosis	41	cirrhosis	2	acute peritonitis	8
Bone marrow: hypoplasia	7	extramedullary-		*Psoriasis:*	3
Brain: meningitis	4	haemopoiesis	1	*Retroperitoneal abscess:*	3
Drug toxicity:		haemangioma	1	*Still's disease:*	4
colchicine	1	hepatitis	2	*Stomach:* ulcer	8
gold	12	necrosis	7	*Thyroid:*	
iron	1	pylephlebitis	1	adenoma or nodular	6
phenylbutazone	2	*Lung:*		fibrous or thyroiditis	17
steroids	17	abscess	6	*Tumours:*	
Duodenum: ulcer	7	atelectasis	5	malignant	24
Felty's syndrome:	3	bronchiectasis	6	breast	1
Heart:		bronchitis, purulent	30	bronchus	7
aortic valve disease	13	bronchopneumonia	54	colon	3
failure	12	cystic disease	1	carcinoid	2
endocarditis	9	pulmonary embolism	14	ovary	1
infarction	9	emphysema	31	rectum	1
mitral valve disease	24	empyema	3	stomach	1
myocardial fibrosis	12	pulmonary hypertension	9	uterus	2
pericarditis		infarction	8	gall bladder	1
(subacute)	6	interstitial fibrosis	4	oesophagus	1
(chronic)	22	lobar pneumonia	2	sarcoma	1
Infection: generalised	8	nodules	1	liver	1
Joints: septic arthritis	3	pleuritis		mesothelioma	1
		(acute)	8	basal cell carcinoma	1
		(fibrous)	56	*Veins:* thrombosis	13

that some forms of thyroid fibrosis are of immunological origin and it is therefore particularly interesting that thyroid auto-antibodies and autoallergic thyroiditis may be more prevalent in rheumatoid arthritis than in normal persons (Buchanan *et al.*, 1961) although this has not been confirmed (Hijmans *et al.*, 1961).

It has been suggested, in analogy with dermatomyositis and usually on the basis of the study of small numbers of cases, that malignant tumours coexist with rheumatoid arthritis more often than would be expected by chance, and that there may be an association between the two states. The finding of malignant tumours (Table 16.9) in 18% of the present series of cases represents an

TABLE *16.9. Frequency of malignant tumours in 142 hospital cases of rheumatoid arthritis examined at necropsy*

Alimentary	10	(7%)
carcinoids	2	—
Bronchus	7	(5%)
Female genital	4	—
Sarcoma	1	—
Mesothelioma	1	—
Basal cell tumour	1	—

incidence that may be higher than would be expected in a random hospital population of comparable age and sex. There is no reason to link rheumatoid arthritis with any particular form of tumour although the occurrence of 2 cases of carcinoid tumour in the present series is noteworthy. However, Moesmann (1969) encountered malignant disease in 14% and 43% of series of 85 and 28 rheumatoid patients respectively, figures which he says, are 2·0–2·2 times those expected to occur in a random, matched population. There was no correlation between malignancy and sex, disease class, rheumatoid factor titres, X-ray changes, serum α_2-globulin or serum alkaline phosphatase levels. Mortality, in the two series, was 2·6 and 1·3 times that expected, an observation precisely the converse of that of Ball (1968). Finally, Owen, Waller and Toone (1970), in a retrospective survey, identified malignant disease in 4% of rheumatoid arthritics and in 4% of controls. In their age range (50–74 years) malignancy was more closely associated with steroid treatment than with arthritis.

Five per cent of the general hospital population die from pulmonary embolism. The frequency of pulmonary embolism and infarction in rheumatoid arthritis appears somewhat higher although the episodes of venous thrombosis recorded after complete immobilisation in the treatment of rheumatoid arthritis were not followed by pulmonary disease (Partridge and Duthie, 1963*b*). When venous thrombosis affects the renal vein, amyloidosis may be present simultaneously but it is not clear whether amyloid predisposes to renal vein thrombosis or *vice versa*. However, renal vein thrombosis can accelerate amyloid deposition.

Cardiac valve disease (p. 127) was recognised commonly. The mitral valve was abnormal in approximately twice as many cases as the aortic. Occasionally a history of rheumatic fever was obtained but very often the valvular disease was of the calcific variety.

The occurrence of three cases of unexplained retroperitoneal infection raises the question of the relationship between rheumatoid arthritis and retroperitoneal fibrosis (Saxton *et al.*, 1969). No systematic search has been made for this condition in rheumatoid arthritis but Mitchinson (1970), who surveyed 40 collected cases of the syndrome, considered that connective tissue diseases were possible agencies for retroperitoneal fibrosis. He substituted the term 'systemic idiopathic fibrosis' for 'retroperitoneal fibrosis' and showed that fibrosis was predominantly periaortic.

CHAPTER 17

Aetiology and Pathogenesis

That the 'target' organ in rheumatoid arthritis is the synovial tissue is considered highly probable; a minority view suggests that there may be a primary insult to articular cartilage (Janis and Hamerman, 1969). However, speculation is rife as to the precise origin and nature of the disease. Much is now known of the way in which polyarthritis leads to clinical deformity; but the exact cause for the initial synovitis, and the explanation for its remarkable persistence, remain obscure (Gardner, 1971).

During the past 70 years, views on the aetiology of rheumatoid arthritis have undergone curious cyclic modifications. These periodic changes of view can be traced through the writings of Bannatyne (1896); Stockman (1920); Fisher (1929); Collins (1949); Dresner (1955); Sokoloff (1961, 1966); Hamerman (1966); and Hamerman, Rosenberg and Schubert (1970). In 1906 rheumatoid arthritis was 'probably an infectious disease' (Bannatyne, 1896). Klinge's work on rheumatic fever (1929–1934) suggested that hypersensitivity might also play a part. Disturbances of connective tissue components such as collagen, it was subsequently thought, could explain the pathogenesis, not only of systemic lupus erythematosus and systemic sclerosis but also of rheumatoid arthritis (Klemperer, Pollack and Baehr, 1942; Klemperer, 1955). These views merged with controversial theories on 'Stress' and the 'Adaptation Syndrome' (Selye, 1950). The significance of stress and the role of the adreno-hypophyseal axis in rheumatoid arthritis gained support from the discovery of the therapeutic action of the corticosteroids. Later it became clear that cortisone was little more beneficial than salicylates; and opinion reverted to the earlier view that infective and immunological mechanisms were probable aetiological agents.

Heredity

No adequate evidence has emerged to show that a predisposition to rheumatoid arthritis is inherited or that heredity is a major predisposing state but it remains reasonable to assume that, as in all infectious diseases, inheritance plays some part in determining the nature and severity of the response (Schull and Cobb, 1969; Lawrence, 1970). Investigations of identical twins have yielded conflicting results. The apparent predisposition of females to rheumatoid arthritis and the common onset of the disease in the young to middle-aged, remain unexplained.

Infection

The role of infection in rheumatoid arthritis has recently been surveyed by Walton (1968a) and by Duthie (1971).

Rheumatoid arthritis, in the absence of incidental secondary bacterial infection (Gaulhofer-de Klerck and van Dam, 1963), is clearly not a straightforward bacterial infection. The synovial fluid is sterile by conventional aerobic and anaerobic cultural techniques and no virus has yet been isolated. However, when the synovial tissue or its component cells are cultured, reports have indicated that mycoplasmas, Bedsoniae, pleomorphic corynebacteria and bacterial 'L' forms, can be isolated. Recent evidence implicating viral infection has also been obtained by the study of antibody titres in blood and synovial fluids (Marin *et al.*, 1969).

If a microbial agent were demonstrable as *the* exogenous agent initiating rheumatoid arthritis then this agent could be supposed to act *directly*, causing tissue damage, or indirectly. An *indirect* action could be exerted by the release of toxins or by a variety of possible immunological mechanisms. Thus, a microbial agent sharing common antigenic determinants with components of synovial cells could (1) start a chain of reactions such as those believed to operate in rheumatic fever in which Lancefield group A, β-haemolytic streptococci share such determinants with components of heart muscle cells. There is at present no evidence for such a view. The microbial agent could (2) alter, or degrade normal antigenic determinants in synovial tissue, thus causing the immunological mechanism to respond as though these antigens were foreign. It is in this way that rheumatoid factors are believed to be produced. Such a reaction could be termed an auto-allergic process. In the same way (3) clones of immunologically competent cells normally suppressed at or shortly after birth or held latent, could emerge as a result of infection and react with and damage synovial tissue by a breakdown in immune tolerance. These hypothetical immunological mechanisms are discussed more fully on p. 195.

(a) *Mycoplasmas*

Mycoplasmas can cause arthritis in other species than man (da Silva and Adler, 1969; Piercy, 1970; Sharp, 1970). Bartholomew (1965) used tissue culture methods in a study of rheumatoid arthritis and found mycoplasmas in 14 of 17 patients with this disease, with systemic lupus erythematosus or with Reiter's syndrome. The infective agents were obtained from synovial fluid, bone marrow, kidney or serum. All isolated strains were found to be sensitive to tetracycline; the infective agent haemolysed sheep red blood cells. Antigenic relationships, examined by complement fixation and by growth inhibition, showed, with the exception of one strain, only minor differences; growth inhibition against several recognised human mycoplasma strains was confirmed. Similar results were obtained by Marcolongo *et al.* (1969) and by Fraser, Shirodaria, Haire and Middleton (1971). Fraser and his colleagues identified 10 mycoplasma strains of 2 main-serological types after observing that rheumatoid synovium introduced into culture tended to induce acidity. They concluded that the rheumatoid tissue is apt to carry small numbers of practically non-antigenic mycoplasmas.

Jansson *et al.* (1971) isolated mycoplasmas from 4 of 33 rheumatoid synovial fluids by direct culture on cell-free media, and a further 7 after preliminary passage into 6–8 day embryonated hen eggs. Subsequently, a few patients were found to have antibody against one strain of mycoplasma and the highest titres by complement fixation, haemagglutination or leucocyte migration inhibition tests, were from patients from whom mycoplasmas had been grown.

TABLE 17.1. *Isolation of mycoplasma from synovial fluid*

Specimen	Total No. of specimens	No. of mycoplasma isolates	No. negative for mycoplasma
All rheumatoid arthritics	90	36	54
R.A. seropositive	79	31	48
R.A. seronegative	11	5	6
Controls	26	5	21
Various arthritides	11	3	8
Totals	127	44 (35%)	83 (65%)

(From Williams, M. H., 1968, Pfizer Medical Monograph Number 3, Edited by Duthie, J.J.R. and Alexander, W.R.M., University Press, Edinburgh.)

The significance of these findings has been considered in detail by Decker (1966), by Walton (1968a) and by Morton (1970). At the present time the majority view emphasises that mycoplasmas isolated from rheumatoid tissues are probably contaminants (Editorials, 1967, 1970). This is contrary to the evidence of Williams (1968) (Tables 17.1 and 17.2) who was able to

TABLE 17.2.   *Identification of mycoplasma isolated from synovial fluids*

| Specimen | No. of mycoplasma isolates serologically related to: | | |
	M. fermentans	*M. hominis*	*Unidentified*
All rheumatoid arthritics			
R.A. seropositive	31	—	—
R.A. seronegative	5	—	—
Controls	1	2	2
Various arthritides	2	1	—
Totals	39	3	2

(From Williams, M. H., 1968, Pfizer Medical Monograph Number 3.)

identify mycoplasma strains in 45% of 11 cases of seronegative rheumatoid arthritis and in 39% of 79 cases of seropositive cases. This evidence was followed by the demonstration that membrane preparations from *Mycoplasma fermentans* inhibited leucocyte migration in 29 (67%) of 45 patients with rheumatoid arthritis (Fig. 9.4). No inhibition was shown with osteoarthrotic cases or with controls (Williams, Brostoff and Roitt, 1970). Since *Mycoplasma fermentans* is often present in the affected joints it was suggested that the chronic course of the disease, if not its initiation, could be due to the persistence of this organism. Immunoglobulin, present in the surrounding synovial fluid and bound firmly to the mycoplasmal membrane, it was held, could be the stimulus for the production of rheumatoid factor. Evidence for the role of a cellular-immune mechanism was gained when the leucocyte migration inhibition test was found to be positive in the presence of *M. fermentans*, in 10 of 17 rheumatoid cases.

(b) *Bacterial 'L' forms*

The evidence of Pease (1969) in respect of bacterial 'L' forms remains highly controversial. Pease recognised bacterial 'L' forms in disorders as diverse as the decidua in spontaneous abortion and the tumour tissue in certain carcinomata. She examined blood and joint fluid from 24 cases of rheumatoid arthritis, 4 of osteoarthrosis and 12 of miscellaneous arthritis. All the samples examined after 2–6 weeks incubation gave positive cultures. Reversion to the bacterial phase of *Listeria* was variable and 'rather unpredictable'. Pease (1969) believes that her evidence supports the view that the bacterial 'L' forms isolated from rheumatoid arthritis may be able to cause an allergic disturbance. She emphasises the hazard of misinterpreting the 'L' forms as mycoplasmas, Bedsonia or corynebacteria, and the morphological variability of these organisms. The significance of her results remains quite uncertain.

(c) *Diphtheroids*

Cadham (1932) recovered diphtheroid organisms from 27 of 34 rheumatoid nodes. He suggested that the organisms isolated by Schueller (1906) from patients with arthritis and by Rosenow (1914) from 35 of 38 lymph nodes draining inflamed joints, were also diphtheroids, a view supported by Cadham (1942) who found these organisms in 87 of 131 patients with rheumatoid arthritis.

These observations were confirmed and extended by Duthie *et al.* (1967) in a series of meticulous microbiological studies that have been reviewed (Duthie, 1971). Diphtheroid bacilli were recovered from 9 of 36 samples of rheumatoid synovial tissue and from 7 of 48 specimens of synovial fluid. Although a positive culture was obtained in 1 of 2 patients with Reiter's syndrome, 10 control synovial tissue samples and 10 control synovial fluids were negative. Alexander, Stewart and Duthie (1968) reported additional observations and demonstrated that 12 of 47 synovial tissue samples but only 10 of 89 synovial fluids contained diphtheroid organisms. At this time, Duthie and his colleagues were able to show a correlation between recovery of the diphtheroids and positivity of the sheep cell agglutination test for rheumatoid factor. In studies of the response of synovial cells in culture to diphtheroids it was further recognised that the organisms could be recovered for up to 12 days after inoculation in spite of the sterility of the culture medium. There was a loss of bacterial cell walls leading to a suggestion that antigens, exposed in this way, might be capable of causing a cell-mediated immunological response, a view that has not been substantiated but which may be considered in the light of Pease's (1969) work on bacterial 'L' forms (p. 190). In the most recent published work, diphtheroids have been identified from 27% of 78 rheumatoid synovial tissue samples by contrast with a recovery of *nil* from 20 non-rheumatoid cases (Table 17.3) (Stewart, Alexander and Duthie, 1969). The isolation of staphylococci and of other organisms was found to be of similar frequency in rheumatoid and non-rheumatoid tissue samples.

TABLE 17.3.　*Isolation rate of diphtheroid bacilli from synovial membranes*

Diagnosis	No. of patients	Diphtheroids Isolated	Diphtheroids Not isolated	Total no. of membranes examined
Rheumatoid arthritis	71	21 (27%)	57	78
Other conditions*	20	0	20	20
Total	91	21	77	98

(P < 0·05)

* Diagnosis: Torn menisci and other internal derangements of the knee　15
Osteoarthrosis　4
Osteochondritis　1

(From Stewart, Alexander and Duthie, 1969, *Ann. rheum. Dis.*, **28** 477–487.)

Hill *et al.* (1967) also recovered diphtheroids from 15 of 30 rheumatoid patients. However, 4 of 11 patients with osteoarthrosis gave positive cultures. A recovery rate for diphtheroids almost identical to that of Duthie and his colleagues was obtained by Clasener and Biersteker (1969) in a small series, using extremely careful isolation techniques that eliminated contaminants such as staphylococci.

The significance of the diphtheroids found in rheumatoid synovia remains entirely open to question. They may exert an adjuvant action (White and Gordon, 1970). A particular difficulty is that the organisms have been isolated from cases ranging up to 20 years in duration. No local or systemic immunological reaction against these organisms has been shown and there is nothing to prove that they are not incidental commensals or 'passengers', taken up by susceptible macrophage-like synovial cells during the long course of a chronic disease in which phagocytosis is active, in which the host resistance to infection is impaired and in which all manner of immunosuppressive and cytotoxic drugs have been used in treatment. In supplementary studies, Maini,

Stewart and Dumonde (1970) tested peripheral leucocytes from 12 rheumatoid and from 9 non-rheumatoid patients with a strain of diphtheroid previously isolated from a case of rheumatoid arthritis and with another non-pathogenic strain, *C. bovis*. Both strains inhibited leucocyte migration and the rheumatoid white cells might, in a sense, be supposed to have developed some form of cell-mediated immunological response to both bacterial strains. The results do not clarify the position of the diphtheroids as tissue-damaging agents in rheumatoid arthritis. In more recent studies, Maini and his colleagues have extended their observations to include mycoplasma strains and herpes-virus.

(d) *Protozoa and Metazoa*

There is no evidence that other organisms such as protozoa are capable of initiating rheumatoid arthritis. However, less attention has been paid to the immunological characteristics of agents such as leishmania in this context than is desirable. It is always salutary to compare a rheumatoid granuloma with the skin lesions of onchocerciasis. Fungi have been isolated as incidental invaders from cases of the disease under treatment with broad spectrum antibiotics or corticosteroids but their presence is clearly of secondary importance: fungi are recognised primary causes of human and animal pyogenic arthritis (Gardner, 1965; Cutlip, 1970).

Greenwood (1969*a*, *b*, *c*) made a careful survey of arthritis in a Western Nigerian population. His evidence suggested that this population had a distinct form of chronic arthritis, in addition to rheumatoid arthritis, in which nodules, neuritis and vascular lesions were infrequent. Rheumatoid factor was not more common than in control cases, X-ray changes were mild and the prognosis good. Still's disease in Nigerians was apparently identical with the condition in Europeans. This evidence raised the possibility that some agent in the tropical environment, perhaps protozoal, possibly nutritional or genetic, determines a different response in a tropical African population to that seen in temperate climates among Caucasians.

The importance of searching for the causal agent of rheumatoid arthritis in a variety of populations is shown by Greenwood's additional finding of a distinctive acute tropical polyarthritis. It appears possible that this may be a viral arthritis analogous with O'nyong O'nyong or the tic-borne arthritides of the Northern Territories of Australia and of South-East Asia.

(e) *Viruses*

In the early days of virology when the presence of virus could only be shown indirectly by techniques such as differential filtration, particles with virus-like properties were identified in 'atrophic' arthritis, rheumatic fever and chorea (Eagles, Evans, Fisher and Keith, 1937). The infective nature of the virus particles was not established by innoculation but virus agglutination by patients' serum was demonstrated. Since that time, there has been growing recognition that rubella, mumps, variola and other virus infections in Europe, America, Africa and Australia may be accompanied by polyarthritis. There is no *a priori* reason therefore why viral infection should not account for other disorders of unknown origin such as rheumatoid arthritis. Synovial tissue is clearly susceptible to a wide variety of viral infections. It may seem justifiable to consider the use of the term 'arthrotropic' virus since, in rubella for example, synovitis is such a common feature among adult women, in selected epidemics, that it seems that some virus strains have a particular predilection for synovial tissue. It could be said, under these circumstances, that the metabolic pathways essential to viral survival, were peculiarly available in synovial mechanocytes.

During the past 6 years considerable evidence has accumulated to show that viral bodies persist in synovial tissues. Thus, Highton, Caughey and Rayns (1966) (p. 47) reported the finding of rod-shaped inclusions in capillary endothelial cells in rheumatoid synovia. However, similar structures were identified in the capillary endothelium of synovia from non-rheumatoid patients (Ghadially and Roy, 1967; Roy and Ghadially, 1967; Brånemark, Ekholm and Goldie, 1969) and comparable structures had in fact been reported previously in arterial endothelial cells both in rats and in unaffected men (Weibel and Palade, 1964). More recently there have been a number of descriptions of single-stranded RNA myxovirus-like structures in the endothelial cells of patients with diseases related to rheumatoid arthritis such as polymyositis (Chou, 1967), systemic lupus erythematosus (Fresco, 1968; Györkey, Min, Sincovics and Györkey, 1968; Hashimoto, 1969; Norton, 1969; Hurd, Eigenbrodt, Ziff and Strunk, 1969; Kawano, Miller and Kimmelstiel, 1969; Haas, 1970; Norton, Velayos and Robison, 1970; and Schumacher, 1970), dermatomyositis (Hashimoto, 1969) and related disorders including idiopathic thrombocytopenic purpura (Norton, 1969). There is, as yet, no evidence that any of these virus-like structures can be isolated from the tissues in which they have been found. There are still good reasons for suspecting that the intracellular inclusions may be microtubules, phagocytosed material or incidental viral invaders. It is important to recall that Schumacher (1970) found synovial vascular endothelial inclusions in only 2 of many specimens examined.

Techniques are available for the culture of a considerable number of suspected viral agents: the way has therefore been paved for direct attempts to isolate virus from synovial tissues in early rheumatoid arthritis. Such work has not yet been reported although studies of the herpes simplex virus and of the attachment of herpes virus/antiviral antibody complexes to rheumatoid factor in rheumatoid arthritis are being made (Ashe, 1971). Indirect evidence of previous or current viral infection can of course be obtained by the demonstration of anti-viral serum antibodies. However, the virus infections that are most frequently accompanied or followed by arthritis in this country are diseases of young people and antiviral antibodies are therefore normally detectable in early adult life whether or not arthritis has been known to occur. Nevertheless, Marin et al. (1969) have detected interesting titres of antibodies against R. burneti, the Bedsoniae, adenoviruses and enteroviruses in patients with rheumatoid arthritis and comparable diseases; the blood and synovial fluid antibody titres were parallel in 90% of instances.

Some negative evidence is available. Rheumatoid factor is not detectable within 1 month of the onset of rubella synovitis (Gupta and Peterson, 1970; Barfield, 1969) and patients with rheumatoid arthritis do not display titres of anti-rubella antibody greater than normal (Kacaki et al. 1970). The interpretation of raised antibody titres is, of course, difficult and an analysis of titres at the onset of rheumatoid arthritis unlikely to be helpful unless some indirect early diagnostic technique such as that of Cohen et al. (1968) is used. The meaning of the polyarthritis which complicates 17% of rubella vaccinations (Thompson et al., 1971) is not yet known.

In any hypothesis that supports the viral aetiology of rheumatoid arthritis the role of the synovial cell as 'target organ' is critical (Ford, 1969). The earlier work of Ford and Oh (1965) had shown that no evidence suggestive of latent viral infection was recognisable in cell cultures of rheumatoid and non-rheumatoid synovial cells maintained for up to 5 weeks and examined for signs of 'spontaneous degeneration' (but see p. 43). The rheumatoid and control cultures were tested with Newcastle disease virus: no difference in the capacity of the virus to multiply in the two groups was detected. Further, no virus-interfering or -inactivating property was shown by fluid taken from the cultures of rheumatoid cells. In similar work, Barnett, Balduzzi, Vaughan and Morgan (1966) searched without success for the presence of viral agents and mycoplasmas in cell lines inoculated with rheumatoid synovial fluid or tissue extracts. In one instance a mycoplasma was cultured but was regarded as a contaminant. With patient's serum as a presumptive source of antibodies, Barnett et al. (1966) used an immunofluorescent technique to test the cultured specimens for new antigen. None was found.

This work contrasts with the interesting demonstration by Grayzel and Beck (1970) that 28 non-rheumatoid synovial cell cultures could be readily induced to show cytopathic effects when infected by rubella virus; none of 21 rheumatoid cultures tested were susceptible to the virus. It is known that rheumatoid sera show no higher titres of rubella haemagglutination antibody than do sera of patients with comparable diseases (Kacaki *et al.*, 1970). Grayzel and Beck, however, also showed that the apparent lack of susceptibility of rheumatoid synovial cells to rubella virus was not due to interferon production. Their evidence, which has not been confirmed, is the first in which a conclusive demonstration of some kind of viral interference phenomenon in relation to rheumatoid synovial cells has been possible. The nature of the interfering agent is not yet known, nor is the relationship of this observation to the complications of rubella immunization understood (Kilroy *et al.* 1970).

The persistence of a 'slow' virus in joint tissue in rheumatoid arthritis has been proposed (Hamerman, Rosenberg and Schubert, 1970) and some evidence in favour of this view has come from recent work by Warren and his colleagues. These workers (Warren, Marmor, Liebes and Hollins, 1969*a*, *b*; Warren *et al.*, 1970) injected an homogenate of pooled rheumatoid synovial tissue into inbred Swiss mice and demonstrated the presence of a transmissible agent. The agent was recovered (but not identified) from inoculated mice that developed a periarthritis* after intraperitoneal injection: the homogenised foot material conveyed the transmissible agent to further inbred animals. It was demonstrated that the agent was transmissible spontaneously through 3 generations, apparently by some form of congenital mechanism, and that the transmissible agent could remain latent for a year or more within infected females.

There appear to be a number of explanations for the phenomenon discovered by Warren *et al.*; the role of mycoplasmas cannot for example be excluded—but the observations have offered an important direct approach to the problem of infection in rheumatoid arthritis. Thus, it has already been found that the transmissible mouse 'agent' can be transferred to the cultured synovial cells of rabbits (Smith *et al.*, 1970). The role of the genetic mechanism remains to be investigated; a viral agent associated with synovial cell nucleoprotein may be implicated. A similar explanation may account for the transmissible agent demonstrated in rheumatoid blood (Dmochowski and Tyrawska-Spychal, 1968). Like the agent found by Warren and his colleagues, that of Dmochowski and Tyrawska-Spychal could be shown only by the use of inbred mouse strains.

At least one further hypothesis may be considered. It is possible that a causative viral agent is extremely widespread and, perhaps, a universal component of human cells: it could bear a similarity to, be part of or be associated with, the genetic material of the mechanocyte. The incidence of the disease could perhaps be explained if it were supposed that in late middle age resistance was reduced and the virus encouraged to escape from a 'latent' state to one of parasitism. The reader may be reminded of the effect of neonatal infections with LCM (a RNA virus) or polyoma (a DNA virus) in aggravating immune complex glomerulonephritis (Tonietti, Oldstone and Dixon, 1970). If it were further supposed that the metabolism of synovial cells offers particularly favourable conditions for this 'escape', then any local injury to joints or any systemic disturbance such as, for example, severe anaemia, could perhaps account for the development of the first clinical signs of the disease. The occasional premature onset of rheumatoid arthritis in childhood (Still's disease) would, under these circumstances, become less difficult to explain. The normal delayed onset of the disease would represent, not a late infection of older women, but more simply, the influence of a reduction in an hypothetical 'resistance' to viral multiplication provoked by environmental factors.

* The lesions described in the mouse foot did not correspond closely with those found in human rheumatoid arthritis. They were recognised principally by the vascular pattern seen on transillumination of the whole foot.

Immunological changes

There is extensive evidence that immunological phenomena are characteristic of rheumatoid arthritis (Chapter 12). It is now very generally believed that these disturbances are secondary features of the disease rather than prime causes. Nevertheless, some of the immunological reactions that develop in the course of rheumatoid arthritis contribute materially to the natural history of the disease and to its chronic character. They may be of a protective type (Muirden, 1971).

For the sake of the present discussion it may be accepted that the cause of rheumatoid arthritis is an exogenous microbial antigen. Infection is likely to provoke one or more immune responses, both to the infective agent itself and, perhaps, to toxins formed by the infecting agent. There is little to show that these immune reactions contribute to the tissue injuries of rheumatoid arthritis. They may however account for the secretion of rheumatoid-like factors, as in subacute bacterial endocarditis, and they may determine amyloid synthesis. More important, in analogy with evidence obtained from comparable diseases such as rheumatic fever and polyarteritis nodosa, is the likelihood that allergic responses to microbial infection cause or exacerbate synovial and cartilage destruction. Both immediate (humoral antibody-mediated) and delayed (cell-mediated) allergic responses are probable. In addition, the possibility has been raised, and is supported both by direct and circumstantial evidence, that autoallergic reactions may develop in rheumatoid arthritis in response to infection. These reactions may also contribute significantly to tissue damage and to the progressive, chronic course of the disease.

Although humoral antibodies are often formed in rheumatoid arthritis, they are secreted incidentally and there is no reason to believe that they contribute to the course of the disease. Thus, approximately one-third of patients develop anti-streptococcal agglutinating and precipitating antibodies together with raised anti-streptolysin O titres. The union of precipitating antibody and antigen can cause connective tissue injury (p. 202) but there is no adequate direct evidence of such injury in the course of the human disease. The studies of lymphoreticular and bone marrow tissues described in Chapter 12 also suggest the common presence of cellular reactions to regional antigens of a kind known to occur experimentally during humoral antibody synthesis; and lymph follicle formation in the inflamed synovia is reasonably common. But there is no evidence that these changes influence connective tissue injury directly. Those cells that infiltrate the synovia in rheumatoid arthritis and that morphologically resemble plasmablasts and plasma cells often contain or bind humoral IgG and IgM immunoglobulins. But the presence of these proteins, and of the cells that appear to be engaged in their synthesis, are apparently indirect consequences of the disease just as they are in sarcoidosis and hepatic cirrhosis.

Immune complexes circulate in the blood of seropositive patients as aggregates with a sedimentation constant of approximately 22S. The presence of similar IgG/IgM complexes in the polymorphs of rheumatoid synovial fluid and in the synovial cells themselves, is also commonplace. Synovial fluid complement levels, by contrast, are relatively low. The polymorph reaction, which is not pathognomonic of rheumatoid arthritis and which is influenced by the genetic characteristics of the IgG antigen, may be one mechanism by which lysosomal proteases are activated in rheumatoid arthritis. That inherited antigenic determinants influence the response to autologous IgG suggests that immunological reactivity may be fundamentally disordered as is the case in systemic lupus erythematosus. Immune complexes in rheumatoid arthritis, it is also suspected, contribute to the visceral lesions of arteritis, pneumonitis and nodule formation. Although some rheumatoid factors are IgG immunoglobulins, the origin of the majority of these complexes has been traced, with reasonable certainty, to the formation of anti-IgG, IgM immunoglobulins. It is supposed that the configurational changes in the tertiary structure of autologous IgG that lead to the synthesis of anti-IgG immunoglobulin M, are the result of an interaction between native immunoglobulin and microbial antigen. But there is no certain knowledge of the nature of the hypothetical antigen and no proof to validate this suggestion.

Autoallergy then, in so far as rheumatoid factor secretion is concerned, is a common feature of rheumatoid arthritis. The response, by contrast with the autoallergic reactions encountered in many other comparable diseases such as experimental allergic encephalomyelitis and lymphadenoid goitre, is not organ- or tissue-specific. But there are reasons for suspecting that autoallergy may be an important factor contributing to the pathogenesis of the disease.

In general terms, autoallergy can appear when immunological tolerance fails to develop, when segregated antigens to which there is no immunological tolerance gain access to the lymphoreticular tissues, when the tertiary structure of autologous antigens is distorted as, for example, by the enzymes of infective microorganisms, or when the specific tolerance acquired during immunological immaturity is lost. Undoubtedly the suspicion that rheumatoid factor is an autoantibody has stimulated interest in the possible role of other autoallergic antigens in the pathogenesis of rheumatoid arthritis.

There is no reason in rheumatoid arthritis to suspect a failure of development of immunological tolerance. However, the frequent association or coexistence of rheumatoid arthritis, Sjögren's syndrome, thyroid disease and systemic lupus erythematosus raises the possibility that immunological tolerance can be lost. In a more direct way, it seems reasonable to suppose that distortion of autologous synovial and cartilage antigens could provoke an autoallergic reaction to mature but changed autologous antigens. This mechanism, together with the proposed loss of tolerance, are the most likely ways in which the surveillance—and the autoallergic inhibition—mechanisms may break down in rheumatoid arthritis and exacerbate the probably slight initial, inflammatory lesions caused by the hypothetical microbial agent.

Lysosomes (Figs. 17.1, 17.2)

The role of lysosomes in the articular injuries of rheumatoid arthritis is also apparently secondary. The capacity of chondrocyte lysosomal hydrolases to degrade cartilage matrix under a variety of physiological and pathological circumstances is not in doubt (Coombs and Fell, 1969; Lack, 1969; Page Thomas, 1969; Reynolds, 1969). The knowledge that acid phosphatase activity is high in rheumatoid synovial cells (Hamerman, Stephens and Barland, 1961; Smith and Hamerman, 1962), that the synovial fluid displays high lysosomal enzyme activity (Jacox and Feldmahn, 1955; Smith and Hamerman, 1962) and that intracellular organelles with the morphological characteristics of lysosomes and cytolysosomes are abnormally frequent in type A(M) synovial cells (Barland, Novikoff and Hamerman, 1964; Hirohata and Kobayashi, 1964; Wyllie et al., 1966; Ghadially and Roy, 1967a, b, 1969) strongly supports the hypothesis that cartilage lysis by synovial lysosomal enzyme activity may be an important part of the process of pannus formation (p. 27). This view receives indirect support from the demonstration that agents such as streptolysin S, non-antigenic but known to be effective activators of lysosomal hydrolases, are capable of causing cartilage protein-polysaccharide breakdown and of eliciting arthritis experimentally (Weissman and Spilberg, 1965).

The role of the synovial fluid enzymes in rheumatoid pannus formation, enzymes apparently derived from the numerous synovial polymorphs containing immune complexes, is uncertain: it might be expected that their presence would cause widespread rather than marginal cartilage lysis (Ball, 1968). Since the synovial tissue itself is apparently the 'target' in rheumatoid arthritis

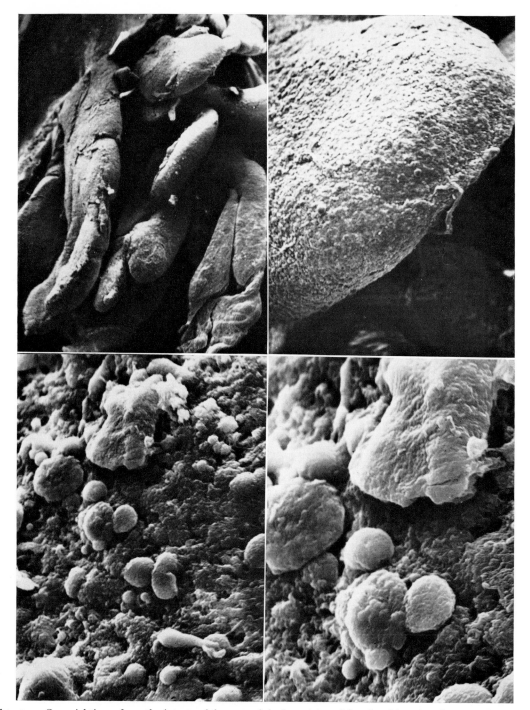

Fig. 17.1 Synovial tissue from the intercondylar area of the knee joint of female with active rheumatoid arthritis. Each Figure represents an enlargement of a selected area of the previous illustration. (*Top left*) The synovial villi are enlarged and prominent. (*Top right*) The surface of a single villus showing irregular appearance and recognisable secondary and tertiary irregularities. (*Bottom left*) Single polymorphs, red cells, cell debris and unidentified particles seen resting on the surface of synovial cells. (*Bottom right*) Individual polymorphs and cell debris seen at higher magnification upon the surface of discrete synovial cells.

(*Top left* ×24; *right* ×120; *bottom left* ×1,245; *right* ×2,720)

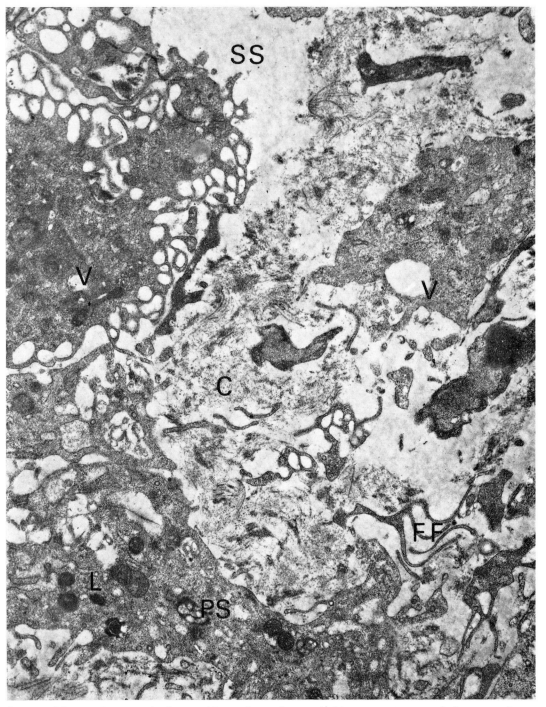

Fig. 17.2 Many surface zones in rheumatoid synovia are characterised by an arrangement of plasma membranes, demonstrated in this Figure, that recalls the surface structure of phagocytes actively engaged in endocytosis. Part of the material seen between the cells is debris, the product of the surface cell injury that is common in this disease; part comprises the tangential and obliquely-sectioned processes of cells that lie beyond the plane of the thin section. (From a micrograph of Dr. A. J. Palfrey.) (× 12,000)

and since the biological characteristics of the synovium appear to be the principal determinants of the natural history of rheumatoid arthritis, it is the lysosomal enzymes of synovial cells rather than of synovial fluid or of cartilage cells that are the objects of greatest interest in considering the pathogenesis of this disease.

Although the precise identification of the free and intravacuolar material seen by electron microscopy in rheumatoid synovial cells remains a matter for debate, immunofluorescent surveys have indicated the presence of immune complexes and of components of complement (Kinsella, Baum and Ziff, 1970). There are reasons for suspecting that the activation of complement can lead to changes in lysosomal membrane permeability and hydrolytic enzyme activity. For example, Dumonde et al. (1965) showed that ascites tumour cells treated with antibody and exposed to the action of complement displayed greatly increased manifest lysosomal enzyme activity and Dingle, Fell and Coombs (1967) and Lachman, Coombs, Fell and Dingle (1969) found that anti-plasma membrane antiserum degraded cartilage, provided complement was present, by the action of a lysosomal protease. It appears therefore that one action of complement is to increase the permeability of lysosomal membranes, leading to the injury of other nearby cells. This hypothesis can be correlated with the view of Humphrey and Dourmashkin (1969) who demonstrated that the combination of complement with the surface of sensitised cells leads to holes being 'punched' in the plasma membrane, a mechanism probably responsible for immediate cell injury, and perhaps determined by C'2 esterase activity. It therefore appears reasonable to propose that the binding of complement to intracellular immune complexes in rheumatoid synovial cells is one explanation for the increased lysosomal enzyme activity detectable in this tissue particularly since it has been known for some years that the phagocytosis of immune complexes by leucocytes can liberate lysosomal hydrolases (Astorga and Bollet, 1965; Williamson and Ling, 1965) (p. 102).

This sequence, the magnitude of which has been assessed by the measurement of acid phosphatase and of arylamidase activities in synovial lining cells (Chayen et al., 1969), is presumably initiated by the hypothetical infective agent which, in turn, causes a series of immunological phenomena including immune complex formation. It appears improbable that lysosomal enzyme activity is provoked by a *primary* immunological change of autoallergic character (Glynn and Holborow, 1965). But the synovial lysosomal enzymes liberated between marginal cartilage cells by this hypothetical mechanism may themselves so alter the antigenicity of articular cell components that this has been suggested as a way in which *secondary* autoallergic responses could be caused (Weissman, 1964). As Lack (1969) points out, there are additional alternative causes for autoallergic responses such as defective or perverted synovial cell phagocytosis; these defects may encourage the persistence of altered, antigenically reactive cell debris and inflammatory products. Among such material that can be identified within synovial A(M) cells is a fibrin-like constituent (p. 203).

Changes in the permeability of synovial lysosomal membranes, lysosomal enzymic activation, the access of these enzymes to adjacent intercellular cartilage matrix (Dingle, 1969a) and the progressive degradation of cartilage as a preliminary to replacement by vascular granulation tissue, are therefore probable consequences of the early synovial cell injury of rheumatoid arthritis. They offer an attractive explanation linking (1) the early inflammatory reaction to an exogenous microbiological agent; (2) the immunological responses to this agent, and (3) the long-continued sequence of progressive cartilage destruction that follows these responses and that is responsible for the morphological features of the clinical disease (Fig. 17.3). Although lysosomal enzyme activation can only be accepted as an incidental, secondary feature of the disease, it remains possible that control or suppression of this activity by agents that diminish

Genetic predisposition →

Premature response

(Still's disease)

? increased effectiveness of genetic factor

? early, severe infection

? early activation, by external stress

Cellular immunological response to infective agent: cytotoxic injury by sensitised lymphocytes.

Intraarticular accumulation of mediators of inflammation and proteins.

Fibrin polymerisation and denaturation.

Hypothetical exogenous infective agent

? slow or latent virus

? mycoplasma

? diphtheroid

Synovitis

Reticuloendothelial hyperactivity, exaggerated in Felty's syndrome: leucopenia.

Diminished resistance to generalised infection.

Phagocytosis of incidental bacterial parasites, e.g. *Haemophilus*, by synovial cells.

Synovial fluid and synovial cell phagocytosis of IgG/IgM complexes.

Synovial cells or subsynovial connective tissue injured by complement-mediated chemotactic and inflammatory properties of immune complexes: Synovitis: venulitis. Further accumulation of fibrin. Plasmatic vasculosis.

Humoral antibody (IgG) response by synovial plasma cells to infective agents.

Bone marrow plasmacytosis.

Local (synovial) and systemic secretion of macroglobulin IgM (rheumatoid factors, antibodies to IgG antibodies formed against infective agents, altered by union with antigen).

Endocrine
Age } Factors

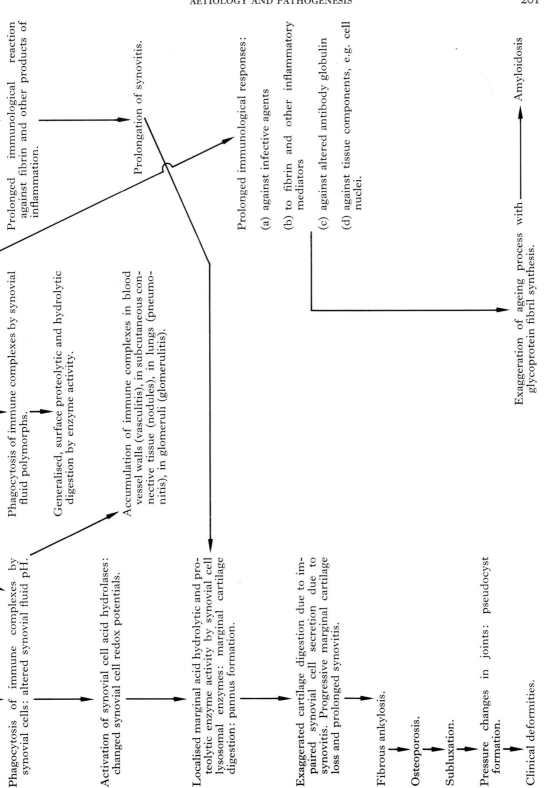

Fig. 17.3 Hypothetical scheme of present views of pathogenesis of rheumatoid arthritis

lysosomal membrane permeability such as the corticosteroids (Weissman and Thomas, 1963; Weissman, 1967) or that suppress protease activity immunologically (Barnett, 1969, 1970) may prove to be effective in the treatment of the clinical disorder.

Collagen injury

Rheumatoid arthritis has many pathological features in common with systemic lupus erythematosus and systemic sclerosis. It therefore seemed possible that in rheumatoid arthritis there might be a widespread, primary disturbance of collagen. Collagen destruction certainly appears to be a necessary preliminary to cartilage breakdown in infective arthritis (Curtis and Klein, 1963) and this may be the case in rheumatoid arthritis. Collagen (Ramachandran, 1968) is, however, a remarkably stable material with a low turnover rate (Gould, 1968) and it has proved difficult to obtain direct evidence to refute or confirm this hypothesis. A number of investigations have consequently approached this matter indirectly. Beginning with the premise that important characteristics of the 'diffuse diseases of collagen' (Klemperer, Pollack and Baehr, 1942) including rheumatoid arthritis, are determined by immunological mechanisms, it was assumed that evidence of injury to collagen in other immunological experiments would provide support for the role of collagen injury in rheumatoid arthritis. Some aspects of this work have been surveyed by Wagner (1967) and Mohos and Wagner (1969) while the antigenicity of connective tissue components has attracted attention (Hamerman and Sandson, 1970).

Wagner and his colleagues (Mohos and Wagner, 1969) used as an experimental model the interesting technique of Germuth et al. (1962) in which a soluble antigen was encouraged to react with precipitating antibody in the avascular rabbit cornea. Germuth et al. (1962) had shown that corneal collagen damage occurred where an immune precipitate formed. Although Movat et al. (1963) found by electron microscopy that collagen in the area of the precipitate remained intact, this view did not coincide with that of Rich, Voisin and Bang (1953) who believed that the fibrinoid of experimental hypersensitivity vasculitis contained damaged collagen. Their opinion was quite distinct from the more recent electron microscope evidence on the nature of 'fibrinoid' in other comparable disorders such as experimental hypertensive vascular injury (Gardner and Matthews, 1969). These various investigations may be compared with electron microscopic studies (Cochrane et al., 1964) of the rheumatoid subcutaneous nodule in which the integrity of collagen rather than its disruption is a conspicuous feature and with the observations of Chang and Houck, 1970 (p. 76).

Mohos and Wagner (1969) undertook light, ultraviolet and electron microscopic studies of zones of corneal precipitation and of antigen excess. In the latter region, there was lysosomal degranulation and polymorphs in the precipitation line area were engorged with phagocytosed immune precipitate. Where this precipitate was extracellular, it enclosed or surrounded collagen fibres and the fibres displayed reduced spacing and variable calibre. The altered collagen lay near phagocyte pseudopods in which microvesicles were numerous; there was a tendency for shedding of the superficial collagen layers. Mohos and Wagner concluded that in areas where immune precipitate had provoked phagocytosis and lysosomal activity, the appearance of 'fibrinoid' corresponded to sites of altered collagen in relation to the precipitate. It could be deduced from this evidence that immune complex formation and, possibly, the local adsorption and activation of components of complement, can cause direct injury to collagen.

Vascular injury

Although necrotising vasculitis and plasmatic vasculosis are uncommon features of rheumatoid arthritis synovitis, Kulka (1959, 1966) made out a convincing case for the early involvement of smaller vessels, particularly the venules, in the pathogenesis of the joint lesions. A similar sequence of vascular changes has been demonstrated in experimental immune complex arthritis (Bakowska and Gardner, 1971). The accumulation of fibrin, γ-globulin and complement in the walls of injured synovial vessels in rheumatoid arthritis shown simultaneously by immuno-fluorescence microscopy, would favour an immunological origin for the occasional arterial in-juries that are identified (Paronetto, 1969); polymorph infiltration in such circumstances would support the case for an Arthus reaction as an explanation for synovial injury. However, the infrequency in rheumatoid arthritis of the classical synovial lesions associated with the Arthus phenomenon suggests that vascular disease in rheumatoid synovia is a secondary disturbance. Vascular involvement appears to be part of the inflammatory reaction rather than a primary explanation for the characteristic synovitis.

There remains the interesting possibility that pharmacological agents, enzymes and permea-bility factors liberated by the early rheumatoid synovitis, may play a part in perpetuating and exaggerating joint injury. The role of Hageman factor activator in crystal synovitis is appreciated and this factor and other chemical mediators are undoubtedly important in the pathogenesis of rheumatoid synovitis if not in its causation. Both may be liberated as a result of the local activity of lysosomal hydrolases.

Chronicity

The chronic nature of rheumatoid arthritis has led to much speculation on possible reasons for the prolonged inflammatory response. It is questionable, however, whether it is any more justi-fiable to consider the chronicity of the disease as an isolated question than it is to debate the long course of fibrocaseous tuberculosis without considering the properties of the tubercle bacillus. This has not prevented attempts to explain the extended nature of the disease. Glynn (1968), for example, following the work of Riddle, Bluhm and Barnhart (1965) suggested that the chronicity of rheumatoid arthritis may be due to (1) prolonged immunological phenomena, (2) the retention of inflammatory products locally in the synovial tissues, (3) the longstanding production of irritant metabolites such as those seen in gout, (4) poor drainage of the inflamed tissues, (5) an inter-ference with the local circulation, (6) excessive movement, (7) exaggerated local cellular responses leading to the proliferation of sensitised lymphoid cells, or, as has been discussed above, (8) the longstanding persistence locally of intracellular symbiotic microorganisms.

Glynn favours the view that, whatever the initial agent, a major factor in prolonging rheumatoid arthritis is a persistent immunological response. His evidence is derived from extensive experi-mental studies that lead him to support the suggestion that the immunological reaction is of an autoallergic character. The antigen may therefore be, not the aetiological agent causing rheu-matoid arthritis but one of the mediators or products of the inflammatory reaction. Thus, the responsible antigen may be an immune complex formed locally, an altered plasma protein such as fibrin, or the degraded products of cell injury.

Glynn has examined the experimental response to the local injection of fibrin, a protein normally polymerised after the soluble precursor fibrinogen has escaped through blood vessels into the nearby extracellular spaces during acute inflammation. When the fibrin of a rabbit is injected into its own knee joint the fibrin is rapidly removed. When the fibrin of another species is injected into such a joint the response is very much slower and a chronic inflammatory reaction persists for as long as 16 weeks with the presence of plasma cells, lymphocytes and abundant new granulation tissue. The difference between the response to autologous and heterologous fibrin is apparently of an immunological character and may, Glynn supposes, throw some light on the natural history of rheumatoid arthritis. Factors that modify the response to fibrin may include a change in the antigenicity of the native fibrin or the presence of other, foreign antigens.

Thus when another antigen is incorporated in the implanted autologous fibrin placed in the rabbit synovial joint no difference in the local response is observed; the fibrin is quickly removed. When, however, the animal has previously been sensitised to this additional antigen, organisation is grossly impaired and a prolonged local reaction is produced that may persist for more than 30 weeks. However, the degree of the response is closely determined by the mechanism used to produce the original sensitisation; it is particularly severe when a local skin reaction, following the injection of Freund's complete adjuvant, precedes the development of delayed hypersensitivity, confirmed by skin testing. The prolonged response is not apparently due to local persistence of the original antigen (although this is debated) but is likely to be caused by an immunological reaction against autologous products of the local inflammatory response.

These views are supported by the experiments of Phillips, Kaklamanis and Glynn (1966). Rabbit joints were injected with the autologous products of a subcutaneous inflammatory reaction produced by the irritant action of croton oil. The inflammatory products occasionally caused a synovitis. When, however, the rabbit was first sensitised with the inflammatory material and later injected locally into the joint with the same substances, then the frequency and persistence of the inflammation were greatly increased. Finally, when such animals were subjected to physical exercise the arthritis tended to become polyarticular, supporting the view that a widespread autoallergic reaction had been caused.

The evidence that suggests that experimental fibrin arthritis is of an autoallergic character is derived first, from the experiments of Phillips *et al.* (1966) referred to above, and second, from the demonstration in the reacting animals of IgM rheumatoid factor-like antiglobulins. Both pieces of evidence are open to criticism, that of Phillips *et al.* (1966) because the reactions described are by no means consistent, and that derived from the demonstration of rheumatoid factors because the secretion of these factors can be found as a non-specific response in inflammatory disorders other than those of autoallergic character.

The role of fibrin in maintaining the chronicity of rheumatoid arthritis is therefore still uncertain. Direct attempts to test the significance of fibrin have been made. In one such study treatment of animals with a defibrinating drug, Arvin, had no influence on the progress and extent of experimental Arthus-type arthritis (P. M. Ford *et al.*, 1970). However, this particular experiment was conducted for a limited period of 28 days and it remains possible that an autoallergic reaction to autologous intraarticular fibrin develops only at a much later stage of the human disease. Willoughby and Ryan (1970) have carried Glynn's hypotheses a stage further in a study in which cotton pellets were implanted in rats, causing a typical chronic inflammatory response. These animals, it was found, could be sensitised either by injecting an extract of the cotton-pellet granuloma or lymph node permeability factor (LNPF), both necessarily in Freund's complete adjuvant. The severity of the chronic inflammatory reaction could be much reduced by neonatal treatment of the rats with similar extracts, a hyporesponsive state that could be transferred to radiation-immunosuppressed normal adult recipients by bone marrow and lymphoid cells.

Summary

The tissue changes in rheumatoid arthritis have been described. It is still not certain whether the synovial cells or the subsynovial connective tissue is the site first disturbed in this disease. Many viscera are affected but this diversity is perhaps less interesting than the observation that collagenous connective tissue *outside* synovial joints, with the exception of tendons, ligaments and subcutaneous tissue, is, for the most part, spared.

Genetic, endocrine, chemical, physical, infective and immunological factors probably contribute to the origin of rheumatoid arthritis but most recent views favour a sequence of disturbances *initiated* by an infective agent, *mediated* by lysosomal hydrolases and *promoted* by secondary immunological phenomena (Fig. 17.3). The available evidence supports the view that an exogenous factor such as a slow or latent virus survives within synovial connective tissues. The synovia may be universally infected. Manifest, parasitic, inflammatory disease develops more commonly in older women than in other age groups. The disease appears therefore to follow some form of predisposing physical or mental stress that brings the latent infection to light.

The causal 'virus' belongs to a class of microorganism that finds the enzyme systems it needs for survival and multiplication in the connective tissues components of synovial joints. Searches for organisms with these characteristics are now being conducted; they could be extended by testing known viruses in pure cultures of synovial cells or by defining the individual metabolic peculiarities of rheumatoid mechanocytes. The delineation of a specific metabolic pathway within synovial cells would then permit a test of known viruses under controlled conditions in which the characteristic metabolic path was facilitated or inhibited.

In considering the later factors that may contribute to the longstanding nature of human rheumatoid arthritis, insufficient importance has been attached to the operation of the mechanical and physical factors reviewed on p. 70. Once secondary osteoarthrosis has developed, once osteoporosis has permitted pseudocyst formation, once tendon and ligament laxity has encouraged subluxation, then mechanical changes, altered alignments and impaired lubrication may all be expected to cause or prolong inflammatory joint disease. It is also important to recall that the histological features that indicate active arthritis ('fibrinoid', mononuclear cell synovial infiltration, synovial hypertrophy, vasculosis) may all be found in the absence of many of the clinical criteria of active rheumatoid synovitis, namely anaemia, a raised erythrocyte sedimentation rate, and significant titres of rheumatoid factor. Clinical disease 'activity' cannot therefore be equated, necessarily, with the signs by which active synovitis is recognised microscopically.

A further agency that may maintain chronic inflammation is the occurrence of secondary infection. The possible role of infective agents in the aetiology of rheumatoid arthritis has been considered earlier in this Chapter. It is clear, from the work of Kellgren, Ball, Fairbrother and Barnes (1958) that subclinical bacterial infection is surprisingly common in the joint tissues of patients with longstanding rheumatoid arthritis. Staphylococci, haemophilus and other bacteria have been isolated. It is likely that the intracellular corynebacteria discovered by Duthie and his colleagues are similar agents. The incidence of secondary, latent infection has almost certainly been underestimated. It remains probable that the persistent presence of microorganisms contributes to the inflammatory response.

The factors that regulate and influence *remission* in rheumatoid arthritis are not well understood. The classical observations that demonstrated the beneficial effects of pregnancy and of jaundice and which led to studies of the action of the corticosteroids may be held to be exceptions to this generalisation: but the reasons why the clinical, histological and serological features of the disease fluctuate so much, in individuals, remains quite uncertain. That, occasionally, cases of rheumatoid arthritis remit wholly and permanently is not disputed. Why this is so, and the sequence of tissue changes leading to this phenomenon, are obscure.

CHAPTER 18

Tissue Laboratory Diagnosis

(a) **Biopsy**

The criteria laid down for the clinical diagnosis of rheumatoid arthritis, by common international agreement, represent a compromise (Tables 1.1, 1.2). There is no single clinical feature, by the recognition of which it is possible to say that a patient with non-suppurative inflammatory joint disease has rheumatoid arthritis. When arthritis affects only one joint, when the radiological appearances are not conclusive, when the immunological criteria are uncertain, and when there are signs or symptoms of some other disorder such as systemic lupus erythematosus, brucellosis or sarcoidosis, then it is necessary to turn for diagnostic help to the examination of samples of tissues obtained by open- or by needle-biopsy. Punch biopsy has certain advantages for the operator (Stroesen and Leahun, 1969) but the sampling errors in open joint biopsy, already considerable (Cruickshank, 1952a), are compounded when blind needle biopsy is attempted. The re-introduction of arthroscopy into clinical practice and the development of arthroscopes with optical systems of high quality and fibre-optic illumination (p. 208) has done much to overcome this objection. Small samples of synovial tissue or cartilage can now therefore be taken under direct vision with the reasonable certainty that the material chosen is representative of the state of the whole joint. The systematic comparison of open and needle biopsy made by Dabrowski and Jakubowski (1970) is instructive.

The diagnosis of early rheumatoid arthritis rests upon the recognition of the microscopic features described on p. 14. Synovitis, with an early polymorph, later lymphocyte and, finally, a plasma cell accumulation is characteristic. Synovial cell hyperplasia is common, multinucleated giant cells and haemosiderin deposits frequent. Fibrin often lies on the free synovial surface or beneath the surface cell layer; the venules and capillaries are congested, the lymphatics inconspicuous.

A common problem is to establish the significance of monoarticular arthritis in a teenager or young adult. In one series of 91 children with persistent inflammatory monoarticular arthritis suspected to be tuberculous, 34 were shown to have confirmed rheumatoid arthritis and 24 more were suspected to be rheumatoid (Kozicka-Polak et al., 1970). Early rheumatoid synovitis is rarely accompanied by sero-positivity but it is, nevertheless, worth testing cryostat sections of the synovial tissue removed at biopsy, for the presence of rheumatoid factor and for immunoglobulins. IgG immunoglobulin accumulates early, IgM macroglobulins including rheumatoid factor, later. The presence of IgG and of rheumatoid factor IgM in, or in relation to a synovial aggregate of plasma cells in a joint with active synovitis and fibrin exudate, may be regarded as strongly suggestive evidence in support of the diagnosis of rheumatoid arthritis. Failure to demonstrate the presence of these immunoglobulins does not, of course, exclude the diagnosis and may only be a reflection of the early stage of the disease. Equally, at a much later stage, synovial fibrosis and a subsidence of the acute inflammatory response, are likely to be accompanied by an absence of demonstrable immunoglobulin G or rheumatoid factor.

To exclude the diagnosis of *rheumatic* synovitis is generally not difficult. The transient, flitting arthritis with oedema, the sparse fibrinous exudate, the polymorphs, including eosinophils, the few lymphocytes or macrophages and the plasma cells, are characteristic. Mast cells are no more common than normal.

In early *systemic lupus erythematosus* the synovitis may resemble rheumatoid arthritis closely: joint signs and symptoms are common features of the initial disease. Fibrin may be less abundant than in rheumatoid synovitis. Whether this reflects the integrity of the synovial fibrinolytic systems or a lower grade of inflammatory reaction is not certain—and pannus (granulation tissue) formation is neither so considerable nor so extensive. The cytology of the synovitis, with a predominance of lymphocytes and pyroninophilic plasma cells, is such that differentiation from rheumatoid arthritis by virtue of this feature is unreliable.

Synovitis in *polyarteritis nodosa* is very uncommon. Plasmatic vasculosis is occasionally encountered in rheumatoid synovitis but the other features of this disease are distinctive. A lamina of faintly eosinophilic collagenous material deposited beneath the synovial intima in *systemic sclerosis* is now clearly recognised as a feature of the not uncommon joint involvement in this disease (Rodnan, 1962). Little is known, by contrast, of the occasional mild synovitis which accompanies the constant muscular and occasional skin lesions of *dermatomyositis*.

Particularly among immigrants to the United Kingdom and in countries where bovine tuberculosis has not been eradicated, it is of particular importance to exclude the diagnosis of early *tuberculous synovitis*. The synovial fluid should be analysed (Table 8.1) and the fluid, or synovial biopsy material, cultured. The presence of tubercle-like structures, with central zones of eosinophilic caseous necrosis, marginal histiocytes and a surrounding lymphocytic infiltrate is suggestive evidence of tuberculosis, and the presence, in Ziehl–Neelsen stained preparations, of acid and alcohol-fast bacilli, diagnostic. Synovial joints are quite commonly implicated in active *brucellosis*, the tissue reactions in which commonly include the formation of epithelioid cell follicles indistinguishable from those encountered in synovial *sarcoidosis*. The presence, in follicular accumulations, of small zones of necrosis nevertheless strongly suggests that mycobacterial infection should be excluded before the histological diagnosis of sarcoidosis can be seriously entertained. The joints in established, longstanding rheumatoid arthritis are susceptible to secondary infections such as those caused by *Staphylococcus aureus* and *Haemophilus*; there may be no good clinical reason to suspect this infection which may only be recognised on aspiration, arthrotomy or arthroscopy. In young persons with monoarticular arthritis, pyogenic infection, whether staphylococcal, gonococcal, streptococcal or meningococcal, usually presents an acute or fulminating character. The clinical signs, together with the persistent synovitis, the abundance of polymorphs in the synovial fluid and the positive cultures, allow the diagnosis of rheumatoid synovitis to be excluded.

Surprisingly active and acute synovial reactions may follow *traumatic injury*, particularly if, as occasionally happens, the synovial tissue is struck directly. An intense synovitis ensues: the clinical features recall those of acute gouty arthritis—and it appears that a form of fat necrosis may have provoked an abrupt inflammatory reaction. There is an extensive plasma cell infiltration, recalling that seen in plasma cell mastitis; there are moderate numbers of polymorphs and of multinucleated giant cells. The reaction is sterile.

Monoarticular *gouty* arthritis in young persons is, of course, rare. The presence of biurate crystals, distinguished by polarisation microscopy from calcium pyrophosphate, is diagnostic and the acute synovial response polymorphonuclear. Plasma cells and lymphocytes are sparse. Again, examination of the synovial fluid, without the need for biopsy, is sufficient to permit a diagnosis in most instances.

The joint is infiltrated by neoplastic white cells in *leukaemia* but *metaplastic carcinomatosis* of synovial tissue is very rare. Occasionally, however, *synovial sarcoma, liposarcoma* or *reticulum cell sarcoma* originates sufficiently near a single synovial joint to cause clinical diagnostic difficulty. In these circumstances, biopsy of the tumour mass, if recognisable, or of the apparently inflamed joint, permits the histological diagnosis to be made and rheumatoid arthritis to be excluded. The distribution of *villonodular synovitis* and the heavy haemosiderin deposits of this disease contrast with the synovial changes in rheumatoid arthritis in which synovial iron in the form of ferritin is abundant but haemosiderin iron extremely variable in amount. In advanced rheumatoid arthritis with amyloidosis, amyloid nephrosclerosis and uraemia, bleeding into a single large joint is not infrequent and the microscopic distinction between rheumatoid and villonodular synovitis difficult.

The differential diagnosis of the histopathology of rheumatoid arthritis and its variants is considered in synoptic tabular form by Hamerman, Barland and Janis (1969).

The biopsy study of lymph nodes, lung, pericardium, muscle, blood vessels, skin and other tissues is referred to in the relevant sections of the present text.

(b) Diagnostic arthroscopy

A very full, illustrated account of the technique of arthroscopy has recently been published (Watanabe, Takeda and Ikeuchi, 1969). These authors trace the history of the technique, introduced by Takagi in 1920 and perfected in 1931 (Takagi, 1933). With the aid of numerous coloured plates, they depict the internal surfaces both of normal joints and of joints from patients and animals with a wide variety of articular diseases. For observation, the joint, normally the knee, is distended with warm, physiological saline. Photographic records are made and with this technique Watanabe and his colleagues have recorded the selected appearances of 800 joints observed since the time at which the first edition of their Atlas was published (1957). Among these cases are 90 of rheumatoid arthritis.

In detailing the appearances of the synovia in 51 cases of rheumatoid arthritis Watanabe *et al.* (1969) emphasise that redness, oedema, irregular swelling and opacity are the features first recognised. With time, longer, yellow-white opaque villi stand out from nearby congested hyperaemic structures. The union of such long villi may lead to the formation of arches across the synovial surface, an appearance which is characteristic but not diagnostic of rheumatoid arthritis. Later, polypoid synovial structures form. Alternatively, granulation tissue with an incomplete fibrinous covering may be conspicuous but the presence of abundant fibrin in the opaque synovial fluid may render identification of synovial and cartilaginous surface structure very difficult.

Watanabe *et al.* (1969) emphasise that the arthroscopic appearances in rheumatoid arthritis are not diagnostic and that a close resemblance to mild tuberculous, syphilitic and suppurative arthritis is usual. In this context, it is not clear what is intended by the term 'syphilitic arthritis'.

The tissue viewed with the arthroscope may be sampled by blind biopsy or by biopsy under direct vision. The sample obtained by the former technique is, in my experience, often unsatisfactory: either representative tissue is not collected or the source of the tissue is so uncertain that no satisfactory analysis of its state is possible. Biopsy by direct observation via the arthroscope is a very much more valuable procedure and the closest correlation is often possible between the observed surface structure and the microscopic appearances found when the chosen tissue is examined by cryostat or paraffin section.

It is usually valuable to examine the sample gained through arthroscopic biopsy, by stereoscopic binocular microscopy. This expedites orientation and permits photography of the sample should this be wished. Blocks can be selected with the aid of an operating or stereomicroscope.

The size of the specimens obtained in this way is such that the final embedding prior to sectioning may also require microscopic aid.

Among the complications that may accompany or follow arthroscopy are, (1) infection (none observed in more than 1,000 cases by Watanabe *et al.* 1969); (2) injury to the joint cartilage and capsule; (3) haemarthrosis and trauma; (4) exacerbation of the underlying disease; (5) quadriceps inhibition; (6) loss of bulbs, instruments or other foreign bodies into the joint during arthroscopy; and (7) electrical injury.

(c) Necropsy

It is not infrequent in this country for the diagnosis of rheumatoid arthritis to be omitted from the summary of the clinical case notes that is transmitted to the pathologist conducting a necropsy. Cases of renal failure due to amyloidosis, of cardiac valvular disease, of death following ortho-paedic procedures such as pinning of a hip fracture, of interstitial pneumonitis or of postoperative pulmonary atelectasis, may not be immediately associated with the coexistent and, possibly fundamental condition of rheumatoid disease. I have generally made it a rule therefore to examine in all cases the whole of one femur including a knee and hip joint, to bisect the lumbar vertebrae, to examine the costochondral junctions and skull, and in any case where the diagnosis of rheumatoid arthritis is suspected, to prepare blocks, not only of these tissues, but of not less than 3 finger joints.

Where the clinical diagnosis of rheumatoid disease is already suspected, tissue from the joints thought to be clinically abnormal should be taken. Not infrequently the extent of the synovial disease, pathologically, may far exceed the scale of the clinical assessment. Large, adventitious bursae filled with 'rice bodies', knee joints distended with blood-stained or haemosiderin-laden synovial villi, subluxated, dislocated or fractured phalanges and fractured vertebrae all may escape clinical notice but can be recognised by careful necropsy study. Because of the growing recognition of the frequency of laryngeal arthritis, the whole of the larynx should be taken for subsequent semi-serial, longitudinal section.

The lacrimal gland, readily accessible after deflecting the skin of the scalp laterally from the orbit, and the salivary glands, should be examined and blocks made for paraffin and for cryostat section. The application of fluorescein-conjugated sera to these tissues and to synovial sections may be necessary. Bone marrow, examined during division of the vertebrae and of the shaft of a femur, is kept for cytological examination. Small amounts of marrow are suspended in a protective medium such as egg albumin. After gentle centrifugation, smears can be made from the deposited cells. The cells are protected from lysis by an albumin coating which does not, however, interfere with subsequent differential staining by the Giemsa or Leishman methods. The state of bone marrow haemopoiesis can then be assessed and correlated with the information available concerning the peripheral blood picture and the clinical state of the patient.

CHAPTER 19

Technical Problems in Tissue Studies

Much is now known of the technical difficulties which have hindered the study of the connective tissue diseases. For example, in 1955, Klemperer published a series of excellent colour photographs of the ground substance in his authoritative review of the significance of the intercellular matrix. His photographs were presumably derived from stained, paraffin-embedded sections of tissue fixed in formalin. Yet, it is now suspected that immersion in 10% aqueous formaldehyde (Engfeldt and Hjertquist, 1967) for as little as 4 hours, or a corresponding exposure to glutaraldehyde and alcohol (Engfeldt and Hjertquist, 1968) can lead to the loss of up to 70% of the component glycosaminoglycans of epiphyseal cartilage. In the same way, the newer biochemical knowledge of the inherited mucopolysaccharidoses (Muir, 1969) has shown how the erroneous interpretation of these diseases as disturbances of lipid metabolism arose: much of the microscopically demonstrable glycosaminoglycan is lost during fixation in aqueous formaldehyde. Any microscopic work on the pathology of the connective tissue matrix must take account of these findings. Tissue studies must be based on the use of fixatives containing additives such as cetyl pyridinium chloride which retain proteoglycans *in situ*, or, preferably, on rapidly-frozen, unfixed or freeze-dried sections. An additional method of considerable value is the immersion of fresh tissue samples in glutaraldehyde containing ruthenium red. Ruthenium (Luft, 1966) simultaneously 'fixes' and 'stains' proteoglycan material: the 'stained' components can be identified by electron microscopy with considerable precision. Highton and Donaldson (1970) have used a similar preparative technique with advantage prior to scanning electron microscopy.

There is a particular need to link the chemical and physical analysis of tissue samples in rheumatoid arthritis directly with classical microscopic observations. The gap between molecular and microscopic analysis has been partially bridged by a number of recent approaches which employ the techniques of cell and organ culture (p. 117), autoradiography, physical and microchemical analysis. The use of scanning electron microscopy is discussed on p. 54. As an example of the integrated studies now in progress it has been shown that 2-stage replicas can be made of the articular surface after enzymatic digestion or immunological injury. The replicas can then be surveyed in the transmission electron microscope. Commercial hyaluronidase (the commercially available enzyme preparations display proteolytic activity) has been shown by this technique to 'unmask' the surface layers of collagen, and to do this more quickly in the joints of small animals with experimental, immunological arthritis than in the normal joint (Gardner and Woodward, 1969). Other enzymes, including collagenase, papain, trypsin, muramidase and cathepsin D, have also been employed in surface analyses (Inone and Gardner, 1971).

It has been found possible to analyse freeze-dried sections of cartilage mounted on quartz slides by means of the electron microprobe. Individual cells or fields can be selected under direct vision, and point analyses or line scans made for the quantities of any element with an atomic weight greater than 5. Early results with normal material, using sections stained by the von Kossa method, have shown that this silver technique defines the site of bone mineral calcium exactly and that epiphyseal and articular cartilage contains a surprisingly large amount of non-apatitic calcium (Gardner and Hall, 1969).

It may be possible to use microprobe analysis to measure sulphate *in situ* in zones of rheumatoid arthritic articular cartilage and thus to obtain, by inference, a measure of the cartilage content of component glycosaminoglycans. Maroudas (1970) has suggested that calcium chloride, allowed to diffuse through small blocks of excised cartilage, quickly equilibrates with the free anionic radicals. She believes that calcium, binding to anionic radicals of the matrix proteoglycans, can be used as a marker for recognising glycosaminoglycans. The electron microprobe analysis of cartilage can consequently be expected to provide data on the distribution of cartilage glycosaminoglycans in rheumatoid arthritis; thus, it may be anticipated that the microprobe will be used to analyse the matrix of marginal cartilage lysis in rheumatoid pannus formation. In time, it may prove possible to measure the concentration of individual polysaccharides in relation to zones of cartilage no larger than individual chondrocytes.

Microscopic techniques can be used with some assurance in the identification of components of the cartilage matrix (Curran, 1964). The Alcian blue technique, at selected pH, in the presence of 0·6 M $MgCl_2$, with the PAS reaction as a counterstain, allows cartilage matrix glycosaminoglycans to be identified (Scott, Quintarelli and Dellovo, 1964; Quintarelli, Scott and Dellovo, 1965). The application of this method to the analysis of tissues in rheumatoid arthritis can be helped by scanning microspectrophotometry, in which the absorption of light of a chosen wavelength can be measured and integrated over selected small areas. The percentage absorption can be used, against a baseline calculated from conventional biochemical measurements of cartilage proteoglycans, to give an indirect measurement of cartilage polysaccharide content. The need for repeated (and cumbersome) point determinations can be avoided by using a scanning system such as that employed in the Vickers M85 microscope. The value of the Alcian blue technique can be further extended by taking advantage of the copper moiety of the dye and submitting stained sections to electron probe microanalysis (Scott, 1971). It seems probable that cartilage, simultaneously 'stained' and 'fixed' with ruthenium red, can be analysed in the same way.

Provided that problems of fixation are met, it is possible also to show the two-dimensional location of the sulphated glycosaminoglycans, although not very precisely, with autoradiography after labelling with radioactive $^{35}So_4$ and to make counts of samples so labelled (Collins and McElligott, 1960; Collins and Meachim, 1961). In the same way, it is to be expected that light will be thrown on the relationship between the mineral content of cartilage and the location of component glycosaminoglycans by comparable autoradiographic studies using ^{45}C (Vaughan, 1970). The autoradiographic and fluorescent investigation of joint tissues in human and in experimental arthritis will be aided by the bone cryostat (Pearse and Gardner, 1972).

Appendix

Diseases encountered during a survey of 148 fatal cases of rheumatoid arthritis dying in hospital, classified for the most part anatomically.

Tissue	Case Number
Adrenal	
atrophy	53, 59, 90, 115, 133, 142
haemorrhage	50
tumours	38, 44, 45, 101
Amyloidosis: (17)	16, 29, 38, 42, 44, 45, 60, 75, 83, 97, 105, 108, 121, 128, 136, 140, 143
Aorta:	
thrombosis	14
Arteries:	
aneurysms	12, 101 (aorta)
arteritis (7)	36, 85 (coronary), 96 (breast), 111 (coronary), 125 (pulmonary), 131 (poly), 144 (poly)
thrombosis (8)	30, 38, 44, 55, (superior mesenteric), 90 (iliac, femoral), 118 (fingers, legs), 131 (polyarteritis), 142 (superior mesenteric)
Bladder:	
cystitis (12)	24, 31, 60, 74, 75, 76, 85, 103, 123, 111, 129, 143
Blood:	
megaloblastic anaemia	111, 129
Bone:	
fracture (8)	10, 17, 24, 48, 63, 66, 94*, 122*
	* cervical dislocation
hyperostosis	143 (+large odontoid)
osteoporosis (41)	54, 56, 57, 58, 62, 63, 65, 67, 74, 76, 78, 90, 100, 103, 104, 106, 108, 110, 111, 112 (osteomalacia), 116, 117, 120, 121, 122, 124, 125, 127, 128, 129, 132, 133, 136, 137, 138, 140, 141, 142, 143, 144, 145
Paget's disease	99
Bone marrow:	
hypoplasia (7)	14, 25*, 62, 71, 110, 126, 136†
	* thrombocytopenia, active marrow; † erythrophagocytosis
Brain:	
encephalititis	15, 20
haemorrhage	12, 25, 26, 81
hydrocephalus	90
infarction	21, 36, 63, 144
meningitis	2, 39, 51, 90 (old), 130
Parkinson's disease	66, 80
subdural haemorrhage	14

Tissue	Case Number

Breast:

   mammary dysplasia   56

   tumours   29

Bronchus:

   purulent bronchitis (30)   1, 2, 12, 24, 36, 40, 41 (bronchiolitis), 43, 45, 47, 48, 50, 53, 54, 55, 60, 63, 69, 80, 82, 86, 119, 113, 115 (early), 116, 121, 124, 128, 129 (bronchiolitis), 136

   stenosis   65

Drugs:*

   colchicine   11

   gold (12)   4, 8, 14, 16, 25, 27, 49, 71, 76, 78 108, 110,

   iron   100

   phenylbutazone   49, 62

   steroids (17)   43, 49, 63, 108, 109, 110, 112, 113, 124, 125, 126, 130, 131, 133, 134, 137, 144

Duodenum:

   ulcer (7)   10, 50, 51, 57, 77, 90, 93

Ear:

   otitis media   39

Eye:

   episcleritis   78

   tumour   92

Gall bladder:

   cholelithiasis (18)   8, 10, 15, 19, 24, 30, 50, 54, 55, 77, 80, 84, 94, 114, 115, 129, 133, 140

   tumours   84

Heart:

   aortic valve disease (13)   24, 31, 54, 58, 65, 82, 86, 92, 94, 96, 100, 136, 139

   atrial thrombus   37, 106

   cardiac failure (12)   7, 13, 18, 21, 23, 37, 39, 47, 88, 104, 109, 133

   congenital anomalies   138

   cor pulmonale   10, 12, 133

   endocarditis (22)   17, 26, 44, 78, 80*, 81, 82, 83, 86, 88, 92, 94, 96, 97, 98, 105*, 106, 111, 119*, 133, 136, 139

                     * round cell infiltration;

   infarction (9)   55, 66*, 73‡, 83‡, 95, 109, 115, 131, 144

                     * old + recent; ‡ old

   mitral valve disease (24)   12, 13, 23, 54, 65, 66, 80*, 81, 82, 83, 86, 88, 92, 94, 96, 97, 98, 105*, 106, 111, 119*, 133, 136, 139

                     * round cell infiltration;

   myocarditis   21

   myocardial fibrosis (12)   31, 53, 57, 66, 67, 76, 80, 83, 86, 94, 134 (focal), 135 (focal)

   nodule   78

   pericarditis, acute (15)   16, 30, 44, 49, 50, 52, 56 (staphylococcal), 59, 67, 79, 87, 101 (carcinomatous), 105, 121, 140

   pericarditis, chronic (22)   23, 27, 35, 50, 55, 61, 75, 76, 77, 80*, 86, 92, 94*, 96* 106, 107*, 112, 116, 118*, 139*, 142, 146

                     * subacute

   tumours   93, 112

Hypertension (34)   16, 19, 21, 26, 29, 38, 42 (? renal), 43, 47, 50, 58, 60, 63, 67, 86, 96, 100, 102, 104, 106, 107, 108, 109, 113, 116, 124, 130, 134, 137, 138, 141, 143, 144, 146

* As a major factor causing death

Tissue	Case Number

Infection, generalised:

gas gangrene   48
staphylococcal   56
postoperative β-haemolytic streptococcal   103, 116, 117
candida   123
pyaemia   125
perisplenic abscess   137

Intestine:

diverticulosis (9)   19, 35, 50, 57, 58 (perforation), 63, 86, 107 (Meckel's), 115
infarction   7, 30
strangulation   74
tuberculosis   77
tumours (8)   3, 20, 30, 32, 35, 81, 93, 115
ulcerative colitis   54

Joints:

septic arthritis   125, 130 (coliform), 133

Kidney:

calculus   90, 142
cystic   138 (single large), 141 (isolated), 146 (multiple)
diabetic glomerulosclerosis 28
focal 'embolic' nephritis   98
hydronephrosis (4)   12, 40 (R), 67 (L) (nephrocalcinosis + R. nephrectomy), 137 (slight)
hypoplastic   126
infarct   106, 144
papillary necrosis (11)   7, 28, 49, 52, 85, 97, 121, 129, 130, 141, 142
pyelonephritis (39)   1, 16, 17, 18, 24, 40, 46, 47, 49, 50, 51, 53, 54, 60, 63, 76, 80, 81, 83, 94, 95, 97, 98, 103, 108, 111, 113, 115, 121, 123, 129, 130, 134, 136, 137, 138, 141, 142, 143
pyonephrosis   68, 142
tubular necrosis   14, 20, 48

Lacrimal adenitis   35, 38, 54, 56, 101, 102, 103, 104, 105, 107, 108

Leukaemia   102, 134

Liver

cirrhosis   1, 81
extramedullary haemopoiesis 126
haemangioma   87
hepatitis   20, 81 (subacute)
necrosis (7)   14, 27, 48 (honeycomb), 55 (infarcts), 121 (centrilobular), 124 (zonal), 139 (centrilobular)
pylephlebitis   116

Lung:

abscess (6)   7, 37, 50, 99, 103, 141
atelectasis (5)   41, 102, 103 (R), 106, 112
bronchiectasis (6)   57, 85, 87, 99, 103, 123
bronchopneumonia (54)   8, 13, 20, 23, 26, 27, 28, 31, 33, 35, 36, 37, 39, 40*, 42, 43, 49, 50*, 51*, 57, 60*, 61, 65, 66, 67, 72, 76, 81*, 82, 83, 90, 91, 94*, 95, 98, 99, 100, 101, 102, 105, 107, 108, 110 (haemorrhagic), 111*, 113*, 114, 119*, 120, 121, 127, 136, 140, 144, 145 (aspiration)
    * resolving or organising
cystic disease   138
pulmonary embolism (14)   5, 22, 24, 29, 45, 59, 65, 66, 70, 80, 97, 112, 124, 140

Tissue	Case Number
emphysema (31)	2, 5, 11, 16, 31, 32, 34, 35, 38, 48, 53, 54, 58, 65, 74, 78, 84, 85, 90, 91, 95, 98, 105, 119, 124, 128, 129, 135, 138, 140, 144
empyema	37, 87, 101
hypertension (9)	47, 58, 86, 87, 99, 106, 118, 119, 129, 148
infarction (8)	5, 29, 30, 44, 59, 95, 107, 125
interstitial fibrosis (4)	43, 50, 88, 106
intraalveolar haemorrhage	20
lobar pneumonia	50, 51
nodules	139
pneumoconiosis	36, 81, 134
tuberculosis (13)	1, 15, 37, 54 (inactive), 60 (inactive), 73, 77, 79, 80 (inactive), 84, 85, 92 (inactive), 96 (focal)
tumours (7)	57, 61, 96, 101, 107, 134, 145

Lymph node enlargement: (41) 11, 21, 26, 29, 31, 33, 37, 39, 40, 44, 45, 46, 47, 48, 50 (hilar), 52, 54, 56, 58, 60, 62, 76, 96, 97, 99, 100, 108, 109, 110, 111, 114, 115, 118, 120 (mediastinal), 124, 125, 126, 132, 133, 135, 139

Microangiopathy: 62

Muscle:
arteritis	36
polymyositis	78

Nerve:

polyneuritis	143

Oesophagus:

diverticulum	19, 105
haemorrhage	25, 43, 55
tumours	112
oesophagitis	79

Operations:

(recent) (9) 41, 45, 46, 48 (gas gangrene + methaemoglobinaemia), 50, 93 (enucleation eye), 117 (L. hip arthroplasty), 115 (cervical dilatation), 123 (partial gastrectomy)

Ovary:

tumours	22

Pancreas:

diabetes mellitus	28, 33
pancreatitis	20, 55

Parathyroid: 58, 141 (hyperplasia), 142 (1 large)

Peritoneum:

adhesions (10)	3, 13, 17, 23, 33, 50, 51, 74 (with obstruction), 109, 118
acute peritonitis (8)	30, 34, 44, 45, 58, 72, 116, 144

Pharynx:

nodules	76

Pineal: 65

Pituitary:

abscess	125
focal necrosis	14
hyperplasia	62
tumours	120 (foetal adenoma), 139 (chromophobe)

Tissue	Case Number

Pleura:

tumours — 124 (mesothelioma)

adhesions (55) — 1, 2, 8, 12, 13, 16, 17, 19, 21, 22, 23, 24, 25, 26, 27, 28, 31, 33, 35, 37, 40, 42, 45, 54, 57 (L), 59 (apical), 60, 66, 76, 78, 80, 81, 83, 84, 85, 88, 90, 91, 92, 93, 94, 97, 99, 103 (few), 108 (apical), 109, 118, 120, 125, 126, 132 (L), 135, 138, 139, 142

fibrinous pleuritis (8) — 44, 49, 59, 94, 105, 111, 114, 121

Prostate:

hyperplasia — 31, 50, 81, 92

Pyaemia: — 125

Retroperitoneal abscess: — 105 (paravertebral), 137 (perisplenic), 142

Salivary gland disease: (12) — 54, 56, 57, 101, 102, 103, 104, 105, 107, 108, 111, 113

Skin:

exfoliative dermatitis — 8

dermatitis — 14, 27

nodules — 25*

* It appears unlikely that every case was systematically examined in a search for rheumatoid granulomata.

psoriasis — 60, 102, 140

purpura — 4

sclerodactyly — 86

Spinal cord:

compression — 122

Spleen:

erythrophagocytosis — 136

infarcts — 30, 36, 131

Still's Disease (4) — 46, 82, 113, 138

Stomach:

atrophy — 129 (with pernicious anaemia)

erosions (5) — 43, 62, 93, 124, 131

tumours — 34

ulcer (8) — 45 (stomal), 53, 56, 59, 79, 99, 116 (healed), 141 (old)

Synovium:

metastasis — 93

Testis:

hypoplasia — 57

Thyroid:

adenoma (6) — 38, 40, 51, 52*, 120, 129* (with pernicious anaemia)
* nodular

thyroglossal cyst — 76

thyroiditis (17) — 15, 23, 26*, 48 (fibrosis), 57, 62, 67†, 78, 79, 107, 116, 118 (large round cell foci), 124 (R. lobe), 132†‡, 133, 137, 141
* goitre;   † myxoedema;   ‡ lymphadenoid

thyrotoxicosis — 106, 123

tumours — 134

Trachea:

nodules — 76

stenosis — 65

Tissue	Case Number
Tumours:	
benign	87 (haemangioma liver), 90 (lymphangioma jejunum)
malignant (24)	3 (colon), 20 (ileal carcinoid), 22 (ovary), 29 (breast), 30 (colon), 32 (colon), 34 (stomach), 35 (rectum), 52 (uterus), 57 (bronchus), 61 (bronchus), 81 (carcinoid ileum), 84 (carcinoma gall bladder), 90 (bronchus), 92 (sarcoma ileum), 101 (bronchus), 107 (bronchus), 112 (oesophagus), 116 (cervix), 120 (primary liver), 124 (mesothelioma pleura), 134 (bronchus), 135 (basal cell), 145 (bronchus)
Ureter:	
calculus	27
hydroureter	103
Uterus:	
pyometrium	115
tumours	52, 116
Veins:	
venous thrombosis (13)	5, 29, 39, 48, 59, 65, 66, 83 (renal), 105 (retroperitoneal), 113 (L. renal, portal), 125 (tibial), 136 (iliac), 142 (portal, splenic)

References

Abrams, E. and Sandson, J. (1964). Effects of ascorbic acid on rheumatoid synovial fluid. *Ann. rheum. Dis.* **23**, 295–299.

Abruzzo, J. L., Heimer, R., Giulliano, V. and Martinez, J. (1970). The hyperviscosity syndrome, polysynovitis, polymyositis and an unusual 13S serum IgG component. *Amer. J. Med.* **49**, 258–264.

Adams, R. (1857a). In: *Illustrations of the Effects of Rheumatic Gout or Chronic Rheumatic Arthritis on all the Articulations: with descriptive and explanatory statements.* John Churchill, London.

— (1857b). In: *A Treatise on Rheumatic Gout or Chronic Rheumatic Arthritis of all the Joints.* John Churchill, London.

Aidem, H. P. and Baker, L. D. (1964). Synovectomy of the knee joint in rheumatoid arthritis. *J. Amer. med. Ass.* **187**, 4–6.

Akers, W. A. and Miller, D. A. (1965). Rheumatoid nodules in adults without rheumatoid arthritis. *Arch. Derm.* **93**, 428–431.

Alarçon-Segovia, D. and Ward, L. E. (1965). Charcot-like arthropathy in rheumatoid arthritis. Consequence of overuse of a joint repeatedly injected with hydrocortisone. *J. Amer. med. Ass.* **193**, 1052–1054.

Albrecht, M., Marinette, G. V., Jacox, R. F. and Vaughan, J. H. (1965). A biochemical and electron microscopy study of rice bodies from rheumatoid patients. *Arthr. and Rheum.* **8**, 1053–1063.

Alexander, K., (1967). Rheuma und Hautdurchblutung. *Ztschr. Rheumaforsch.* **26**, 214–223.

Alexander, W. R. M., Stewart, S. M. and Duthie, J. J. R. (1968). Aetiological factors in rheumatoid arthritis. In: *Rheumatic Diseases.* Pfizer Medical Monograph Number 3, pp. 156–164. Edited by Duthie, J. J. R. and Alexander, W. R. M. University Press, Edinburgh.

Allander, E., Bucht, H., Lövgren, O. and Wehle, B. (1963). Renal function in rheumatoid arthritis. *Acta rheum. scand.* **9**, 116–121.

Allison, A. C. (1968). Lysosomes. In: *The Biological Basis of Medicine*, Vol. I, p. 209. Edited by Bittar, E. E. and Bittar, N. Academic Press, New York and London.

Allison, N. and Ghormley, R. K. (1931). *Diagnosis in Joint Disease. A Clinical and Pathological Study of Arthritis.* Wm. Wood, New York.

Altman, F. P. (1971). The use of a recording microdensitometer for the quantitative measurement of enzyme activities inside tissue sections. *Histochemie*, **27**, 125–136.

Andersen, R. B. and Gormsen, J. (1970). Fibrinolytic and fibrin-stabilizing activity of synovial membranes. *Ann. rheum. Dis.* **29**, 287–293.

Andersen, R. B. and Winther, O. (1969). Blood fibrinolysis and activity of rheumatoid arthritis. *Acta rheum. Scand.* **15**, 178–184.

Andersen, S. B. and Jensen, K. B. (1965). Metabolism of γ-globulin in collagen disease. *Clin. Sci.* **29**, 533–539.

Anderson, A. E. and Foraker, A. G. (1960). Morphologic aspects of interstitial pulmonary fibrosis. *Arch. Path.* **70**, 79–93.

Anderson, J. R., Beck, J. S., Bloch, K., Buchanan, W. W. and Bunim, J. J. (1965). In: *Autoimmunity Symposium, 5th Congress of the International Academy of Pathology.* Blackwell, Oxford.

Ansell, B. M. and Bywaters, E. G. L. (1969). Juvenile chronic polyarthritis or Still's disease. In: *Textbook of the Rheumatic Diseases*, pp. 323–343. Edited by Copeman, W. S. C. Livingstone, Edinburgh and London.

Arapakis, G. and Tribe, C. R. (1963). Amyloidosis in rheumatoid arthritis investigated by means of rectal biopsy. *Ann. rheum. Dis.* **22**, 256–262.

Aronoff, A., Bywaters, E. G. L. and Fearnley, G. R. (1955). Lung lesions in rheumatoid arthritis. *Brit. med. J.* **2**, 228–232.

Ashe, W. K., Daniels, C. A., Scott, G. S. and Notlein, A. L. (1971). Interaction of rheumatoid factor with infectious herpes simplex virus-antibody complexes. *Science*, **172**, 176–177.

Astorga, G. P. and Bollet, A. J. (1964). Diagnostic specificity and possible pathogenic significance of inclusion-body cells in synovial fluid. *Arthr. and Rheum.* (abstract) **7**, 288.

Astorga, G. P. and Bollet, A. J. (1965). Diagnostic specificity and possible pathogenetic significance of inclusions in synovial leucocytes. *Arthr. and Rheum.* **8**, 511–523.

Astorga, G. P. and Williams, R. C. (1969). Altered reactivity in mixed lymphocyte culture of lymphocytes from patients with rheumatoid arthritis. *Arthr. and Rheum.* **12**, 547–554.

Atwater, E. C., Mongan, E. S., Wieche, D. R. and Jacox, R. F. (1965). Peptic ulcer and rheumatoid arthritis. *Arch. intern. Med.* **115**, 184–189.

Bach, F. and Jacobs, J. H. (1951). Splenectomy in rheumatoid arthritis. *Ann. rheum. Dis.* **10**, 320–327.

Bach, J.-F. and Delbarre, F. (1968). Nouvelle méthode de détection du facteur rhumatoide au niveau cellulaire. *C.R. Acad. Sci. (D) (Paris)*, **267**, 134–136.

Bach, J.-F., Delrieu, F. and Delbarre, F. (1970*a*), The rheumatoid rosette phenomenon—I. A new method of detecting the rheumatoid factor at the cellular level. *Presse méd.* **78**, 301–306.

— (1970*b*). The rheumatoid rosette. A diagnostic test unifying seropositive and seronegative rheumatoid arthritis. *Amer. J. Med.* **49**, 213–222.

Baggenstoss, A. H. and Rosenberg, E. F. (1941). Cardiac lesions associated with chronic infectious arthritis. *Arch. intern. Med.* **67**, 241–258.

— (1943). Visceral lesions associated with chronic infectious (rheumatoid) arthritis. *Arch. Path.* **35**, 503–516.

— (1944). Unusual cardiac lesions associated with chronic multiple rheumatoid arthritis. *Arch. Path.* **37**, 54–60.

Baillie, M. (1793). *The Morbid Anatomy of Some of the Most Important Parts of the Human Body.* J. Johnson, London.

— (1799–1802). *A Series of Engravings, Accompanied with Explanations, to Illustrate the Morbid Anatomy of the Human Body.* Nichol, London.

Baker, H. (1966*a*). Prevalence of psoriasis in polyarthritic patients and their relatives. *Ann. rheum. Dis.* **25**, 229–234.

— (1966*b*). Epidemiological aspects of psoriasis and arthritis. *Brit. J. Dermat.* **78**, 249–261.

Bakowska, A. and Gardner, D. L. (1971). Microvascular aspects of immunological tissue injury. Proceedings of the VII European Rheumatology Congress (abstract).

Balazs, E. A., Watson, D., Duff, I. F. and Roseman, S. (1967). Hyaluronic acid in synovial fluid. I. Molecular parameters of hyaluronic acid in normal and arthritic human fluids. *Arthr. and Rheum.* **10**, 357–376.

Ball, J. (1954). Rheumatoid arthritis and polyarteritis nodosa. *Ann. rheum. Dis.* **13**, 277–290.

— (1968). Postmortem findings and articular pathology in rheumatoid arthritis. In: *Rheumatic Diseases: Pfizer Medical Monograph Number 3*, pp. 124–126. Edited by Duthie, J. J. R. and Alexander, W. R. M. University Press, Edinburgh.

— (1971). Enthesopathy of rheumatoid and ankylosing spondylitis. *Ann. rheum. Dis.* **30**, 213–223.

Ball, J., Bahgat, N. E. D. and Taylor, G. (1964). Effect of aldehyde fixation on cellular rheumatoid factor and certain tissue antigens. *J. Histochem.* **12**, 737–739.

Ball, J. and Sharp, J. (1971). Rheumatoid arthritis of the cervical spine. In: *Modern Trends in Rheumatology* Vol. 2, pp. 117–138. Edited by Hill, A. G. S. Butterworths, London.

Bannatyne, G. A. (1896). *Rheumatoid Arthritis: its Pathology, Morbid Anatomy and Treatment* (1st edition). Wright, Bristol.

Barfield, H. (1969). Distribution of rheumatoid factor activity in nonrheumatoid states. *Ann. N.Y. Acad. Sci.*, **168**, 30–40.

Barland, P., Janis, R. and Sandson, J. (1966). Immunofluorescent studies of human articular cartilage. *Ann. rheum. Dis.* **25**, 156–164.

Barland, P., Novikoff, A. B. and Hamerman, D. (1964*a*). Fine structure and cytochemistry of the rheumatoid synovial membrane, with special reference to lysosomes. *Amer. J. Path.* **44**, 853–866.

— (1964*b*). Lysosomes in the synovial membrane in rheumatoid arthritis: a mechanism for cartilage erosion. *Trans. Ass. Amer. Phycns.* **77**, 239–247.

Barnes, C. G., Turnbull, A. L. and Vernon-Roberts, B. (1971). Felty's syndrome. A clinical and pathological survey of 21 patients and their response to treatment. *Ann. rheum. Dis.* **30**, 359–374.

Barnett, E. V., Balduzzi, P., Vaughan, J. H. and Morgan, H. R. (1966). Search for infectious agents in rheumatoid arthritis. *Arthr. and Rheum.* **9**, 720–724.

Barnett, E. V., Bienenstock, J. and Bloch, K. J. (1966). Antinuclear factors in synovia. *J. Amer. med. Ass.* **198**, 143–148.

Barnett, E. V., Ruderman, M., Jeannet, M. and Bloch, K. J. (1966). Felty's syndrome: occurrence of antinuclear antibodies and leucocyte agglutinins in 14 patients. *Arthr. and Rheum.* **9**, 846 (abstract).

Barnhart, M. I., Riddle, J. M., Bluhm, G. B. and Quintana, C. (1967). Fibrin promotion and lysis in arthritic joints. *Ann. rheum. Dis.* **26**, 206–218.

Barrett, A. J. (1969*a*). Properties of lysosomal enzymes. In: *Lysosomes in Biology and Pathology* Vol. 2, pp. 245–312. Edited by Dingle, J. T. and Fell, H. B. North Holland Publishing Co.

— (1969*b*). Cathepsins in pathology: an immunoenzymic study. *Biochem. J.* **115**, 36–37P.

Barrett, A. J. and Poole, A. R. (1970). Unsuitability of leucine naphthylamide for the histochemical demonstration of lysosomal proteolytic activity. *Nature* **224**, 279–280.

Bartfield, H. (1965). Rheumatoid arthritic and non-rheumatoid synovium in cell culture. Morphological observations, acridine orange, and fluorescent fraction II studies. *Ann. rheum. Dis.* **24**, 31–39.

Bartholomew, L. E. (1965a). Isolation of mycoplasma (PPLO) from patients with rheumatoid arthritis, systemic lupus erythematosus and Reiter's syndrome. *Arthr. and Rheum.* **7**, 291.

— (1965b). Isolation and characterization of mycoplasmas (PPLO) from patients with rheumatoid arthritis, systemic lupus erythematosus and Reiter's syndrome. *Arthr. and Rheum.* **8**, 376–388.

Bastow, J. (1964). The place of surgery in rheumatoid arthritis. *Proc. Roy. soc. Med.* **57**, 64–65.

Batley, W. J., Uddin, J. and Kelly, H. G. (1969). Rheumatoid arthritis complicated by constrictive pericarditis: Report of a case treated successfully by periocardiectomy. *Canad. Med. Ass. J.* **100**, 863–866.

Bauer, W., Bennett, G. A. and Zeller, J. W. (1941). The pathology of joint lesions in patients with psoriasis and arthritis. *Trans. Ass. Amer. Phycns.* **56**, 349–352.

Bauer, W., Short, C. L. and Bennett, G. A. (1933). The manner of removal of proteins from normal joints. *J. exp.Med.* **57**, 419–433.

Bayles, T. B. (1943). Rheumatic heart disease in autopsied cases of rheumatoid arthritis. *Ann. intern. Med.* **19**, 113–114. (abstract).

Bayles, T. B. (1943). Rheumatoid Arthritis and Rheumatic Heart Disease in Autopsy Cases. *Amer. J. med. Sci.* **205**, 42–48.

Beck, J. S., Anderson, J. R., Bloch, K. J., Buchanan, W. W. and Bunim, J. J. (1965). Antinuclear and precipitating autoantibodies in Sjögren's syndrome. *Ann. rheum. Dis.* **24**, 16–22.

Bedi, S. S. and Ellis, W. (1970). Spontaneous rupture of the calcaneal tendon in rheumatoid arthritis after local steroid injection. *Ann. rheum. Dis.* **29**, 494–495.

Bendixen, G. and Søborg, M. (1969). A leucocyte migration technique for *in vitro* detection of cellular (delayed type) hypersensitivity in man. *Dan. med. Bull.* **16**, 1–6.

Bennett, G. A. (1943). Comparison of the pathology of rheumatic fever and rheumatoid arthritis. *Ann. intern. Med.* **19**, 111–113.

Bennett, G. A., Waine, H. and Bauer, W. (1942). Changes in the knee joint at various ages with particular reference to the nature and development of degenerative joint disease. The Commonwealth Fund, New York.

Bennett, G. A., Zeller, J. W. and Bauer, W. (1940). Subcutaneous nodules of rheumatoid arthritis and rheumatic fever. *Arch. Path.* **30**, 70–89.

Bennett, P. H. and Scott, J. T. (1965). Autonomic neuropathy in rheumatoid arthritis. *Ann. rheum. Dis.* **24**, 161–168.

Berge, G., Lundquist, A., Rorsman, H. and Åkerman, M. (1970). Liver biopsy in psoriasis. *Brit. J. Derm.* **82**, 250–253.

Bertram, U. and Halberg, P. (1964). A specific antibody against the epithelium of the salivary ducts in sera from patients with Sjögren's syndrome. *Acta allerg. (Kbh.)* **19**, 458–466.

Bett, I. M. (1962a). Metabolism of tryptophan in rheumatoid arthritis. *Ann. rheum. Dis.* **21**, 63–69.

— (1962b). Effect of pyridoxine on tryptophan metabolism in rheumatoid arthritis. *Ann. rheum. Dis.* **21**, 388–391.

— (1966). Urinary tryptophan metabolites in rheumatoid arthritis and some other diseases. *Ann. rheum. Dis.* **25**, 556–562.

Bevans, M., Nadell, J., Demartini, F. and Ragan, C. (1954). The systemic lesions of malignant rheumatoid arthritis. *Amer. J. Med.* **16**, 197–211.

Beveridge, G. W. and Lawson, A. A. H. (1967). Serum uric acid in psoriasis and arthritis. *Scot. med. J.* **12**, 21–27.

Bienenstock, J. and Bloch, K. J. (1967). Immunoconglutinin in various rheumatic diseases and certain diseases suspected of an autoimmune pathogenesis. *Arthr. and Rheum.* **10**, 187–198.

Bienenstock, H., Ehrlich, G. E. and Freyberg, R. H. (1963). Rheumatoid arthritis of the crico-arytenoid joint: a clinicopathological study. *Arthr. and Rheum.* **6**, 48–63.

Bienenstock, H. and Kilbrick, A. C. (1969). Urinary excretion of prolylhydroxyproline in rheumatic diseases. *Ann. rheum. Dis.* **28**, 28–30.

Bienenstock, H., Minick, C. R. and Rogoff, B. (1967). Mesenteric arteritis and intestinal infarction in rheumatoid disease. *Arch. intern. Med.* **119**, 359–364.

Bierther, M. F. W. amd Wegner, K. W. (1971). Elektronenmikroskopische Untersuchungen synovialer Gefäßveränderungen bei chronischer Polyarthritis. *Z. Rheumaforsch.* **30**, 214–222.

Binette, J. P. and Schmid, K. (1965). The proteins of synovial fluid: a study of the α_1/α_2 globulin ratio. *Arthr. and Rheum.* **8**, 14–28.

Bischoff, M. B., Harrison, M. C., Bucci, T. J. and Nelson, R. A. (1969). Cytoplasmic lamellar inclusions resembling tissue mast cell granules in suspected rheumatoid lung disease. *Amer. J. clin. Path.* **52**, 593–598.

Bitter, T. (1969). Aminoacridine-precipitable polyuronide excretion in rheumatoid arthritis. Preliminary results. *Ann. rheum. Dis.*, **28**, 676–677.

Black, A., Goldin, M., Poske, R. M. and Malmed, L. (1959). Differentiation between rheumatoid arthritis and systemic lupus erythematosus by sheep cell agglutination tests. *Arthr. and Rheum.* **2**, 99–103.

Black, R. L., Oglesby, R. B., von Sallmann, L. and Bunim, J. (1960). Posterior subcapsular cataracts induced by corticosteroids in patients with rheumatoid arthritis. *J. Amer. med. Assoc.* **174**, 166–171.

Bland, J. H. (1967). Rheumatoid arthritis of the cervical spine. *Bull. rheum. Dis.* **18**, 471–476.

Bland, J. H., Davis, P. H., London, M. G., von Buskirk, F. W. and Duarte, C. G. (1963). Rheumatoid arthritis of cervical spine. *Arch. intern. Med.* **112**, 892–898.

Bland, J. H. and Eddy, W. M. (1968). Hemiplegia and rheumatoid arthritis. *Arthr. and Rheum.* **11**, 72–80.

Blendis, L. M., Ansell, I. D., Lloyd Jones, K., Hamilton, E. and Williams, R. (1970). Liver in Felty's syndrome. *Brit. med. J.* **1**, 131–135.

Bloch, K. J. (1969). Sjögrens syndrome. In: *Textbook of Immunopathology*, Vol. II, pp. 745–751. Edited by Miescher, P. A. and Muller-Eberhard, H. J. Grune and Stratton, New York.

Bloch, K. J., Buchanan, W. W., Wohl, M. J. and Bunim, J. J. (1965). Sjögren's syndrome: A clinical, pathological, and serological study of sixty-two cases. *Medicine* **44**, 187–231.

Bluhm, G. B. (1969). Rheumatoid arthritis cells. *Ann. intern. Med.* **71**, 432.

Blum, A. and Sohar, E. (1962). The diagnosis of amyloidosis. *Lancet* **i**, 721–723.

Boas, N. F., Bollet, A. J. and Bunim, J. J. (1955). Effect of acute clinical stress on the levels of hexosamine in serum and its excretion in urine. *J. Clin. Invest.* **34**, 782–789.

Boddington, M. M., Spriggs, A. I., Morton, J. A. and Mowat, A. G. (1971). Cytodiagnosis of rheumatoid pleural effusions. *J. clin. Path.* **24**, 95–106.

Boddy, K. and Will, G. (1969). Iron absorption in rheumatoid arthritis. *Ann. rheum. Dis.* **28**, 537–540.

Bodel, P. T. and Hollingsworth, J. W. (1966). Comparative morphology, respiration, and phagocytic function of leukocytes from blood and joint fluid in rheumatoid arthritis. *J. clin. Invest.* **45**, 580–589.

Bollett, A. J. (1966). Immunologic aspects of rheumatoid arthritis. *Postgrad. Med.* **40**, 391–395.

Bonfiglio, T. and Atwater, E. C. (1969). Heart disease in patients with seropositive rheumatoid arthritis; a controlled autopsy study and review. *Arch. intern. Med.* **124**, 714–719.

Bonomo, L., Tursi, A. and Gillardi, U. (1968). Distribution of the anti-gamma globulin factors in the synovial membrane and other tissues in various diseases. *Ann. rheum. Dis.* **27**, 122–129.

Borden, A. L., Walraff, E. B., Brodie, E. C., Holbrook, W. P., Hill, D. F., Stephens, C. A. L., Kent, L. J. and Kemmerer, A. B. (1950). Plasma levels of free amino acids in normal subjects compared with patients with rheumatoid arthritis. *Proc. Soc. exp. Biol. Med. N.Y.*, **75**, 28–30.

Bourdillon, C. (1888). *Psoriasis et Arthropathies*. Lescrosnier et Babe, Paris.

Bränemark, P.-I., Ekholm, R. and Goldie, I. (1969). To the question of angiopathy in rheumatoid arthritis an electron miscroscopic study. *Acta orthop. scand.* **40**, 153–175.

Bränemark, P.-I., Lindstrøm, J., Jonsson, I., Laine, V. and Vainio, K. (1963). Capillary structure and function in rheumatoid arthritis. A vital miscroscopic study of conjunctival and surgically exposed joint tissue. *Acta rheum. scand.* **9**, 284–292.

Broder, I., Baumal, R., Gordon, D. and Bell, D. (1969). Histamine-releasing activity of rheumatoid and non-rheumatoid serum and synovial fluid. *Ann. N.Y. Acad. Sci.* **168**, 126–139.

Brodie, B. C. (1813). Pathological researches respecting the diseases of joints. *Medico-chir. Trans.* **4**, 207–277.

— (1818). *Pathological and Surgical Observations on the Diseases of the Joints*. Longman, London.

Brown, P. W. (1969). Early recurrence of rheumatoid synovium after early synovectomy in the hand and wrist. In: *Early Synovectomy in Rheumatoid Arthritis*, pp. 201–206. Edited by Hijmans, W., Paul, W. D. and Herschel, H. Excerpta Medica, Amsterdam.

Brun, C., Olsen, T. S., Raaschou, F., Arne, W. S. and Sørenson, A. W. S. (1963). On the kidney in rheumatoid arthritis. A biopsy study. *Second International Congress of Nephrology, Prague*.

Brun, C., Olsen, T. S., Raaschou, F. and Sørensen, A. W. S. (1965). Renal biopsy in rheumatoid arthritis. *Nephron* **2**, 65–81.

Brunk, J. R., Drash, E. C. and Swineford, O. (1966). Rheumatoid pleuritis successfully treated with decortication. Report of a case and review of the literature. *Amer. J. med. Sci.* **251**, 545–551.

Buchanan, W. W. (1965). The relationship of Hashimoto's thyroiditis to rheumatoid arthritis. *Geriatrics* **20**, 941–948.

Buchanan, W. W., Crooks, J., Alexander, W. D., Koutras, D. A., Wayne, E. J. and Gray, K. G. (1961). Association of Hashimoto's thyroiditis and rheumatoid arthritis. *Lancet* **i**, 245–248.

Buckley, W. R. and Raleigh, R. L. (1959). Psoriasis with acro-osteolysis. *New Engl. J. Med.* **261**, 539–541.

Bunim, J. J. (1961). A broader spectrum of Sjögren's syndrome and its pathogenetic implications. *Ann. rheum. Dis.* **20**, 1–10.

— (1964). Clinical, pathologic and serologic studies in Sjögren's syndrome. Combined clinical staff conference at the NIH. *Ann. intern. Med.* **61**, 509–530.

Bunim, J. J., Buchanan, W. W., Wertlake, P. T., Sokoloff, L., Bloch, K. J., Beck, J. S. and Alepa, F. P. (1964). Clinical, pathologic and serologic studies in Sjögren's syndrome. *Ann. intern. Med.* **61**, 509–530.

Burch, P. R. J. (1968). Genetic aspects of rheumatic and arthritic diseases. In: *Rheumatic Diseases. Pfizer Medical Monograph, Number 3*, pp. 30–50. Edited by Duthie, J. J. R. and Alexander, W. R. M. University Press, Edinburgh.

Burkhardt, R. (1967). Histomorphologische Untersuchungen über die Rolle des Knochenmarkes bei rheumatischen Krankheiten. *Z. ges. exp. Med.* **143**, 1–66.

Burnet, F. M. (1969). *Cellular Immunology*, pp. 266–271. University Presses, Melbourne and Cambridge.

Burstone, M. A. (1956). Histochemical demonstration of proteolytic activity in human neoplasms. *J. nat. Cancer Inst.* **16**, 1149–1161.

— (1962). *Enzyme Histochemistry and its Application in the Study of Neoplasms*, p. 409. Academic Press, New York.

Butcher, R. G. and Chayen, J. (1971). Unbalanced production of reduced nicotinamide-adenine dinucleotide phosphate in rheumatoid synovial lining cells. *Biochem. J.* **124**, 19P.

Butler, J. J. (1969). Non-neoplastic lesions of lymph nodes of man to be differentiated from lymphomas. *Nat. Cancer Inst. Monogr.* **32**, 322–355.

Bywaters, E. G. L. (1939). The metabolism of joint tissues. *J. Path. Bact.* **44**, 247–268.

— (1950). The relation between heart and joint disease including 'rheumatoid heart disease' and chronic post-rheumatic arthritis (Type-Jaccoud). *Brit. Heart J.* **12**, 101–131.

— (1957). Peripheral vascular obstruction in rheumatoid arthritis and its relationship to other vascular lesions. *Ann. rheum. Dis.* **16**, 84–103.

Bywaters, E. G. L. and Ansell, B. M. (1965). Monoarticular arthritis in children. *Ann. rheum. Dis.*, **24**, 116–122.

Bywaters, E. G. L. and Glynn, L. E. (1970). Connective tissue disorders. In: *Biochemical Disorders in Human Disease*, pp. 723–750. Edited by Thompson, R. H. A. and Wootton, I. D. P. Churchill, London.

Bywaters, E. G. L., Glynn, L. E. and Zeldis, A. (1958). Subcutaneous nodules of Still's disease. *Ann. rheum. Dis.* **17**, 278–285.

Bywaters, E. G. L., Holborow, E. J. and Keech, M. K. (1951). Reconstitution of the dermal barrier to dye spread after hyaluronidase injection. *Brit. med. J.*, **2**, 1178–1183.

Bywaters, E. G. L. and Scott, J. T. (1963). The natural history of vascular lesions in rheumatoid arthritis. *J. chron. Dis.* **16**, 905–914.

Cadham, F. T. (1932). A discussion on the etiology and specific treatment of arthritis. *Canad. med. Ass. J.*, **26**, 287–293.

— (1942). A method of vaccine therapy in atrophic arthritis. *Canad. med. Ass. J.* **46**, 31–34.

Calabro, J. J. and Marchesano, J. M. (1967a). Fever associated with juvenile rheumatoid arthritis. *New Engl. J. Med.* **276**, 11–18.

— (1967b). Current concepts: juvenile rheumatoid arthritis. *New Engl. J. Med.* **277**, 696–699, 746–749.

Cameron, R. (1952). *Pathology of the Cell*, pp. 36–40. Oliver and Boyd, Edinburgh and London.

Campbell, J. A. (1958). A case of Caplan's syndrome in a boiler-scaler. *Thorax*, **13**, 177–180.

Caplan, A. (1953). Certain unusual radiological appearances in the chests of coal-miners suffering from rheumatoid arthritis. *Thorax* **8**, 29–37.

Caplan, A., Cowen, E. D. H. and Gough, J. (1958). Rheumatoid pneumoconiosis in a foundry worker. *Thorax* **13**, 181–184.

Caplan, A., Payne, R. B. and Withey, J. L. (1962). A broader concept of Caplan's syndrome related to rheumatoid factors. *Thorax* **17**, 205–212.

Cardell, B. S. and Gurling, K. J. (1954). Observations on the pathology of Sjögren's syndrome. *J. Path. Bact.* **68**, 137–146.

Carmichael, D. S. and Golding, D. N. (1967). Rheumatoid pleural effusion with 'RA' cells in the pleural fluid. *Brit. med. J.* **2**, 814.

Carpenter, D. F., Golden, A. and Roberts, W. C. (1967). Quadrivalvular rheumatoid heart disease associated with left bundle branch block. *Amer. J. Med.* **43**, 922–929.

Carr, D. T. and Mayne, J. G. (1962). Pleurisy with effusion in rheumatoid arthritis, with reference to the low concentration of glucose in pleural fluid. *Amer. Rev. resp. Dis.* **85**, 345–350.

Carswell, R. (1838). *Pathological Anatomy. Illustrations of the Elementary Forms of Disease*. Longman, London.

Castenfors, H., Hultman, E. and Lovgren, O. (1964). The bromsulphthalein test (BSP) as a measure of rheumatoid arthritis activity. *Acta rheum. scand.* **10**, 128–132.

Castor, C. W. (1957). Production of mucopolysaccharides by synovial cells in a simplified tissue culture medium. *Proc. Soc. exp. Biol. (N.Y.)* **94**, 51.

— (1960). The microscopic structure of normal human synovial tissue. *Arthr. and Rheum.* **3**, 140–151.

— (1970). Regulation of collagen and hyaluronate formation in human synovial fibroblast cultures. *J. Lab. clin. Med.* **75**, 798–810.

— (1971). Abnormalities of connective tissue cells cultured from patients with rheumatoid arthritis. II. Defective regulation of hyaluronate and collagen formation. *J. Lab. clin. Med.*, **77**, 65–75.

Castor, C. W. and Dorstewitz, E. L. (1966). Abnormalities of connective tissue cells cultured from patients with rheumatoid arthritis—I. Relative unresponsiveness of rheumatoid synovial cells to hydrocortisone. *J. Lab. clin. Med.* **68**, 300–313.

Castor, C. W., Wright, D. and Buckingham, R. B. (1968). Effect of rheumatoid sera on fibroblast proliferation and hyaluronic acid synthesis. *Arthr. and Rheum.* **11**, 652–659.

Cathcart, E. S. and O'Sullivan, J. B. (1970). Rheumatoid arthritis: prevalence in a New England town. *New Engl. J. Med.* **282**, 421–424.

Cathcart, E. S., Wollheim, F. A. and Cohen, A. S. (1967). Plasma protein constituents of amyloid fibrils. *J. Immunol.* **99**, 376–385.

Cats, A. and Hazevoet, H. M. (1970). Significance of positive tests for rheumatoid factor in the prognosis of rheumatoid arthritis. A follow-up study. *Ann. rheum. Dis.*, **29**, 254–260.

Cats, A. and Pit, A. A. (1969). Clinical significance of rheumatoid vasculitis and the incidence of digital vascular lesions. *Folia Med. neerl.* **12**, 159–165.

Caughey, D. E. and Highton, T. C. (1967). Components of the fibrinolytic system in synovial joints: normal bovine compared with normal and abnormal human synovial joints. *Ann. rheum. Dis.* **26**, 297–305.

Cave, A. J. E., Griffiths, J. D. and Whiteley, M. M. (1955). Osteo-arthritis deformans of the Luschka joints. *Lancet*, **i**, 176–179.

Caygill, J. C. and Pitkeathly, D. A. (1966). A study of β-acetylglucosaminase and acid phosphatase in pathological joint fluids. *Ann. rheum. Dis.* **25**, 137–144.

Chalmers, J., Conacher, W. D. H., Gardner, D. L. and Scott, P. J. (1967). Osteomalacia; a common disease in elderly women. *J. Bone Jt Surg.* **49B**, 403–423.

Chamberlain, M. A. and Bruckner, F. E. (1970). Rheumatoid neuropathy: clinical and electrophysiological features. *Ann. rheum. Dis.* **29**, 609–616.

Champion, G. D., Robertson, M. R. and Robinson, R. G. (1968). Rheumatoid pleurisy and pericarditis. *Ann. rheum. Dis.* **27**, 521–529.

Chan, W. C. (1964). Experimental sialo-adenitis in guinea-pigs. *J. Path. Bact.* **88**, 592–595.

Chang, C. and Houck, J. C. (1970). Demonstration of the chemotactic properties of collagen. *Proc. Soc. exp. Biol.* (*N.Y.*) **134**, 22–26.

Chaplin, D., Pulkki, T., Saarimaa, A. and Vainio, K. (1969). Wrist and finger deformities in juvenile rheumatoid arthritis. *Acta rheum. scand.* **15**, 206–223.

Charcot, J. M. (1867). *Leçons sur les Maladies des Vieillards et les Maladies Chroniques.* Delahaye, Paris.

— (1889). Maladies des vieillards. Goutte et rheumatisme. In *Oeuvres complètes*, vol. 7. Lescrosnier et Babé, Paris.

Chatgidakis, C. B., and Theron, C. P. (1961) Rheumatoid pneumoconiosis (Caplan's syndrome). A discussion of the disease and a report of a case in a European Witwatersrand gold miner. *Arch. environm. Hlth* **2**, 397–408.

Chauffard, A. and Ramond, F. (1896) Des adenopathies dans le rheumatisme chronique infectieux. *Rev. Méd.* **16**, 345–359.

Chayen, J. and Bitensky, Lucille (1971). Lysosomal enzymes and inflammation with particular reference to rheumatoid disease. *Ann. rheum. Dis.* **30**, 522–536.

Chayen, J., Bitensky, L., Butcher, R. G. and Cashman, B. (1971). Evidence for altered lysosomal membranes in synovial lining cells from human rheumatoid joints. *Beitr. Path.* **142**, 137–150.

Chayen, J., Bitensky, L., Butcher, R. G. and Poulter, L. W. (1969) Redox control of lysosomes in human synovia. *Nature*, **222**, 281–282.

Chiroff, R. T. and Jowsey, J. (1970). The effect of calcitonin on immobilization osteopenia. *J. Bone Jt Surg.* **52-A**, 1138–1146.

Chisholm, D. M. and Mason, D. K. (1968) Labial salivary gland biopsy in Sjögren's disease. *J. clin. Path.* **21**, 656–660.

Chisholm, D. M., Waterhouse, J. P. and Mason, D. K. (1970). Lymphocytic sialadenitis in the major and minor glands: a correlation in postmortem subjects. *J. clin. Path.* **23**, 690–594.

Chou, S.-M. (1967). Myxovirus-like structures in a case of human chronic polymyositis. *Science*, **158**, 1453–1455.

Christian, C. L. (1965) Rheumatoid arthritis. In: *Immunological Diseases*, pp. 725–736. Edited by Samter, M. Little, Brown, Boston.

Christie, G. S. (1950). The general changes in rheumatoid arthritis. In: *Studies in Pathology presented to Peter MacCallum*, pp. 133–144. Edited by King, E. S. J., Lowe, T. E. and Cox, L. B. Melbourne University Press, Jubilee, Victoria.

— (1954). Pulmonary lesions in rheumatoid arthritis. *Aust. Ann. Med.* **3**, 49–58.

Claman, H. and Merrill, D. (1966). Serum immunoglobulins in rheumatoid arthritis. *J. Lab. clin. Med.* **67**, 850–854.

Clark, W. S. and Bauer, W. (1948). Cardiac changes in rheumatoid arthritis. *Ann. rheum. Dis.* **7**, 39–40.

Clark, W. S., Kulka, J. P. and Bauer, W. (1957). Rheumatoid arthritis with aortic regurgitation: unusual manifestation of rheumatoid arthritis (including spondylitis). *Amer. J. Med.* **22**, 580–592.

Clarke, I. C. (1971*a*). Surface characteristics of human articular cartilage—a scanning electron microscope study. *J. Anat.* **108**, 23–30.

— (1971*b*). Human articular surface contours and related surface depression frequency studies. *Ann. rheum. Dis.* **30**, 15–23.

Clasener, H. A. L. and Biersteker, P. (1969). Significance of diphtheroids isolated from synovial membranes of patients with rheumatoid arthritis. *Lancet* **ii**, 1031–1033.

Clausen, E. and Pedersen, J. (1961). Necrosis of the renal papillae in rheumatoid arthritis. *Acta med. scand.* **170**, 631–633.

Cochrane, W., Davies, D. V., Dorling, J. and Bywaters, E. G. L. (1964). Ultramicroscopic structure of the rheumatoid nodule. *Ann. rheum. Dis.* **23**, 345–363.

Cockel, R., Kendall, M. J., Becker, J. F. and Hawkins, C. F. (1971). Serum biochemical values in rheumatoid disease. *Ann. rheum. Dis.* **30**, 166–170.

Cohen, A. S. (1965). The constitution and genesis of amyloid. *Int. Rev. exp. Path.* **4**, 159–243.

— (1967). Studies on the amyloid fibril. In: *The Connective Tissue*. International Academy of Pathology Monograph. Number 7, pp. 81–94. Edited by Wagner, B. M. and Smith, D. E. Williams and Wilkins, Baltimore.

Cohen, S. M., Ducharme, C. P., Carpenter, Charlotte, A. and Deibel, R. (1968). Rubella antibody in IgG and IgM immunoglobulins detected by immunofluorescence. *J. Lab. clin. Med.* **72**, 760–766.

Coimbra, A. and Lopes-Vaz, A. (1967). Acid phosphatase-positive cytoplasmic bodies in leukocytes of rheumatoid synovial fluid. *Arthr. and Rheum.* **10**, 337–342.

Collins, D. H. (1937). The subcutaneous nodule of rheumatoid arthritis. *J. Path. Bact.* **45**, 97–115.

— (1949). *The Pathology of Articular and Spinal Diseases*. Edward Arnold, London.

Collins, D. H., Darke, C. S. and Dodge, D. G. (1958). Scleroderma with honeycomb lungs and bronchiolar carcinoma. *J. Path. Bact.* **76**, 531–540.

Collins, D. H. and McElligott, T. (1960). Sulphate ($^{35}SO_4$) uptake by chondrocytes in relation to histological changes in osteo-arthritic human articular cartilage. *Ann. rheum. Dis.* **19**, 318–330.

Collins, D. H. and Meachim, G. (1961). Sulphate ($^{35}SO_4$) fixation by human articular cartilage compared in the knee and shoulder joints. *Ann. rheum. Dis.* **20**, 117–122.

Colton, C. L. and Darby, A. J. (1970). Giant granulomatous lesions of the femoral head and neck in rheumatoid arthritis. *Ann. rheum. Dis.* **29**, 626–633.

Condemni, J. J., Barnett, E. V., Atwater, E. C., Jacox, R. F., Mongan, E. S. and Vaughan, J. H. (1965). The significance of antinuclear factors in rheumatoid arthritis. *Arthr. and Rheum.* **8**, 1080–1093.

Cook, H. P. (1958). Bilateral ankylosis of the temporomandibular joints following rheumatoid arthritis. *Proc. roy. Soc. Med.* **51**, 694–696.

Coombs, R. R. A. and Fell, Honor B. (1969). Lysosomes in tissue damage mediated by allergic reactions. In: *Lysosomes in Biology and Pathology*, vol. 2, pp. 3–18. Edited by Dingle, J. T. and Fell, Honor, B. North Holland Publishing Company. Amsterdam and London.

Coons, A. H. and Kaplan, M. H. (1950). Localization of antigen in tissue cells. II. Improvements in a method for the detection of antigen by means of fluorescent antibody. *J. exp. Med.* **91**, 1–13.

Copeman, W. S. C. (1957). Rheumatoid arthritis of the cricoarytenoid joints. *Brit. med. J.* **1**, 1398–1399.

— (1964). *A Short History of the Gout and the Rheumatic Diseases*. University of California Press, Berkeley and Los Angeles.

— (1968). Rheumatoid arthritis and the cricoarytenoid joints. *Brit. J. clin. Prac.* **22**, 421–422.

Copeman, W. S. C., Elkin, A. C. and Pearce, R. (1959). A case of rheumatoid arthritis with ankylosis of the cricoarytenoid joints. *Brit. med. J.* **1**, 1575.

Cornil, A. V. (1864). Still's disease. Mémoire sur les coincidences pathologiques du rhumatisme articulaire chronique. *C. R. Soc. Biol. (Paris), (Memoires)*, 4 sér., **1**, 3–25.

Coss, J. A. and Boots, R. H. (1946). Juvenile rheumatoid arthritis: study of 56 cases with note on skeletal changes. *J. Paediat.* **29**, 143–156.

Coste, F. and Solnica, J. (1966). La polyarthrite psoriasique. *Rev. franç. Etud. clin. biol.* **11**, 578–599.

Cotzias, G. C., Papavasiliou, P. S., Hughes, E. R., Tang, L. and Borg, D. C. (1968). Slow turnover of manganese in active rheumatoid arthritis accelerated by prednisone. *J. clin. Invest.* **47**, 992–1001.

Cracchiolo, A. and Barnett, E. V. (1969). Immunologic changes in synovial fluid following synovectomy of the knee for rheumatoid arthritis. *J. Bone Jt Surg.* **51A**, 475–486.

Cruickshank, B. (1951). Histopathology of diarthrodial joints in ankylosing spondylitis. *Ann. rheum. Dis.*, **10**, 393–404.

— (1952*a*). Interpretation of multiple biopsies of synovial tissue in rheumatic diseases. *Ann. rheum. Dis.*, **11**, 137–145.

— (1952*b*). Focal lesions in skeletal muscles and peripheral nerves in rheumatoid arthritis and other conditions. *J. Path. Bact.* **64**, 21–32.

— (1954). The arteritis of rheumatoid arthritis. *Ann. rheum. Dis.* **13**, 136–146.

— (1956). Lesions of cartilaginous joints in ankylosing spondylitis. *J. Path. Bact.* **71**, 73–84.

— (1958). Heart lesions in rheumatoid disease. *J. Path. Bact.* **76**, 223–240.

— (1959*a*). Interstitial pneumonia and its consequences in rheumatoid disease. *Brit. J. Dis. Chest* **53**, 226–240.

— (1959*b*). Lesions of joints and tendon sheaths in systemic lupus erythematosus. *Ann. rheum. Dis.* **18**, 111–119.

— (1966). The basic pattern of tissue damage and pathology of systemic lupus erythematosus. In: *Lupus Erythematosus*, pp. 10–53. Edited by Dubois, E. L. McGraw-Hill, New York and London.

Cruickshank, B., Macleod, J. G. and Shearer, W. S. (1954). Subarticular pseudocysts in rheumatoid arthritis. *J. Fac. Radiol. (Lond.)* **5**, 218–226.

Crum, R. J. and Loiselle, R. J. (1970). Incidence of temporomandibular joint symptoms in male patients with rheumatoid arthritis. *J. Amer. Dent. Assoc.* **81**, 129–133.

Cruveilhier, J. (1829–1842). *Anatomie Pathologique du corps humain.* Tome 1er, Livraison I A XX. J.-B. Baillière.

Curran, R. C. (1964). The histochemistry of the mucopolysaccharides. *Int. Rev. Cytol.* **17**, 149–212.

— (1967). Recent developments in the field of inflammation and repair. In: *Modern Trends in Pathology* (2). Edited by Crawford, T. Butterworths, London pp. 40–101.

Currey, H. L. F., Moore, C. J. and Prentice, A. I. D. (1970). Surgical synovectomy and experimental immune synovitis in the rabbit knee joint. *Ann. rheum. Dis.* **29**, 503–508.

Curtis, A. C. and Pollard, H. M. (1940). Felty's syndrome: its several features, including tissue changes, compared with other forms of rheumatoid arthritis. *Ann. intern. Med.* **13**, 2265–2284.

Curtis, P. H. Jr. and Klein, L. (1963). Destruction of articular cartilage in septic arthritis—I. *In vitro* studies. *J. Bone Jt Surg.* **45A**, 797–806.

Cutlip, R. C. (1970). Electron microscopy of cell cultures infected with a chlamydial agent causing polyarthritis of lambs. *Infect. Immun.* **1**, 499–502.

Dabrowski, W. and Jakubowski, S. (1970). Evaluation of method and technique of biopsy examination in rheumatoid arthritis. *Reumatologia*, **8**, 135–140.

Davies, D. V. (1946). The lymphatics of the synovial membrane. *J. Anat.* **80**, 21–23.

— (1969). The biology of joints. In: *Textbook of the Rheumatic Diseases.* Edited by Copeman W. S. C. Livingstone, Edinburgh and London, pp. 40–86.

Davies, D. V. and Palfrey, J. (1971). The fine structure of normal and rheumatoid synovial membrane. In: *Modern Trends in Rheumatology* (2), pp. 1–20. Edited by Hill, A. G. S. Butterworths, London.

Davies, P., Krakauer, K. and Weissman, G. (1970). Subcellular distribution of neutral protease and peptidases in rabbit polymorphonuclear leucocytes *Nature*, **228** 761–762.

Davis, J. S. and Bollet, A. J. (1964). Protection of a complement sensitive enzyme system by rheumatoid factor. *J. Immun.* **92**, 139–144.

Dawson, M. H. (1933). A comparative study of subcutaneous nodules in rheumatic fever and rheumatoid arthritis. *J. exp. Med.* **57**, 847–858.

Dazziano, L., Gagnon, J. and Laurin, C. (1969). Chemical synovectomy of an experimental arthritis. *Canad. med. Ass. J.* **101**, 24–29.

De Andrade, J. R. and Tribe, C. R. (1962). Staphylococcal septicaemia with pyoarthrosis in rheumatoid arthritis. *Brit. med. J.* **1**, 1516–1518.

Debré, R., Milhit, J. and Lamy, M. (1938). La maladie de Still. *Rev. Rhum.* **5**, 373–398.

Decker, J. L. (Editor) (1966). *Proceedings of the Conference on the Relationship of Mycoplasma to Rheumatoid Arthritis and Related Diseases.* U.S. Department of Health, Education and Welfare, Public Health Service Publication No. 1523.

de Duve, C. (1959). Lysosomes, a new group of cytoplasmic particles. In: *Subcellular Particles.* Edited by Hayashi, T. The Ronald Press, New York.

— (1963*a*). The lysosome. *Scientific Amer.* **208**, 64–72.

— (1963*b*). *The Lysosome Concept,* In *Lysosomes.* Ciba Foundation Symposium, Edited by de Reuck, A. V. S. and Cameron, M. P. Churchill, London. pp. 1–31.

de Duve, C., Pressman, B. C., Gianetto, R., Wattiaux, R. and Appelmans, F. (1955). Tissue fractionation studies. 6. Intracellular distribution patterns of enzymes in rat liver tissue. *Biochem. J.*, **60**, 604–617.

Delbarre, F., Kahan, A., Amor, B. and Krassinine, G. (1964). Le ragocyte synovial; son intérêt pour le diagnostic des maladies rhumatismales. *Presse méd.* **72**, 2129–2132.

Deller, D. J., Urban, E., Ibbotson, R. N., Horwood, J., Milazzo, S. and Robson, H. N. (1966). Folic-acid deficiency in rheumatoid arthritis: Relation of levels of serum folic-acid activity to treatment with phenylbutazone. *Brit. med. J.* **1**, 765–767.

Denko, C. W. and Old, J. W. (1969). Myopathy in the Sicca syndrome (Sjögren's syndrome). *Amer. J. clin. Path.* **51**, 631–637.

Denko, C. W. and Zumpft, C. W. (1962). Chronic arthritis with splenomegaly and leukopenia (Felty's syndrome). *Arthr. and Rheum.* **5**, 478–491.

Dequeker, J. and Rosberg, G. (1967). Digital capillaritis in rheumatoid arthritis. *Acta rheum. scand.* **13**, 299–307.

Dick, W. C., Neufeld, R. R., Prentice, A. G., Woodburn, A., Whaley, K., Nuki, G. and Buchanan. W. W. (1970). Measurement of joint inflammation: a radioisotopic method. *Ann. rheum. Dis.* **29**, 135–137.

Dick, W. C., Onge, R. A. St., Gillespie, F. C., Downie, W. W., Nuki, G., Gordon, I., Whaley, K., Boyle, J. A. and Buchanan. W. W. (1970). Derivation of knee joint synovial perfusion using the xenon (^{133}Xe) clearance technique. *Ann. rheum. Dis.* **29**, 131–134.

Diem, K. and Lentner, C. (1970) (Editors) *Documenta Geigy; Scientific Tables.* 7th Edition pp. 640–642 J. R. Geigy S. A., Basle.

DiFerrante, N. M. (1967). The measurement of urinary mucopolysaccharides. *Anal. Biochem.*, **21**, 98–106

Dimitrov, N. V., Stjernholm, R. L. and Weir, D. R. (1969). Metabolic deviations of polymorphonuclear leukocytes in rheumatoid arthritis. *Blut.* **19**, 139–145.

Dingle, J. T. (1961). Studies on the mode of action of excess of vitamin A—3. Release of a bound protease by the action of vitamin A. *Biochem J.* **79**, 509–512.

— (1962). Lysosomal enzymes and the degradation of cartilage matrix. *Proc. roy. Soc. Med.* **55**, 109–111.

— (1969a). Extracellular secretion of lysosomal enzymes. In *Lysosomes in Biology and Pathology.* Vol. 2, pp. 421–436. Ed. Dingle, J. T. and Fell, H. B.   North Holland Publishing Co., Amsterdam.

— (1969b). Some special methods for the investigation of the lysosomal system in *Lysosomes in Biology and Pathology*, vol. 2, pp. 555–566. Ed. Dingle, J. T. and Fell, H. B.   North Holland Publishing Co. Amsterdam.

Dingle, J. T. and Fell, H. B. (Editor). (1969). *Lysosomes in Biology and Pathology.* North Holland Publishing Co., Amsterdam.

Dingle, J. T., Barrett, A. J. and Weston, P. D. (1971). Cathepsin D. Characteristics of immuno-inhibition and the confirmation of a role in cartilage breakdown. *Biochem. J.* **123**, 1–13.

Dingle, J. T., Fell, Honor, B. and Coombs, R. R. A. (1967). The breakdown of embryonic cartilage and bone cultivated in the presence of complement-sufficient antiserum. 2. Biochemical changes and the role of the lysosomal system. *Int. Arch. Allerg.* **31**, 283–303.

Dingle, J. T. and Page-Thomas, D. P. (1956). *In vitro* studies on human synovial membrane. A metabolic comparison of normal and rheumatoid tissue. *Brit. J. exp. Path.* **37**, 318–323.

Dingman, R. O. (1944). Bilateral ankylosis of the temporomandibular joints with retrusion deformity: report of a case. *J. oral Surg.* **2**, 71–76.

Dixon, A. St. J. and Ball, J. (1957). Honeycomb lung and chronic rheumatoid arthritis. A case report. *Ann. rheum. Dis.* **16**, 251–245.

Dixon, A. St. J. and Grant, C. (1964). Acute synovial rupture in rheumatoid arthritis: clinical and experimental observation. *Lancet* **1**, 742–745.

Dmochowski, A. and Tyrawska-Spychal, D. (1968). Observations on the offspring of white mice experimentally infected with blood cells obtained from patients with rheumatoid arthritis. *Pol. med. J.* **7**, 399–403.

Dodson, W. H. and Hollingsworth, J. W. (1966). Pleural effusion in rheumatoid arthritis. *New Engl. J. Med.* **275**, 1337–1342.

Donald, K. J. and Kerr, J. F. R. (1968). Giant cells in the synovium in rheumatoid arthritis. *Med. J. Aust.* **55**, 761–762.

Douglas, W. (1965). The digital artery lesion of rheumatoid arthritis. *Ann. rheum. Dis.* **24**, 40–45.

Dowson, D., Wright, V. and Longfield, M. D. (1969). Human joint lubrication. *Biomed. Engng.* 160–164.

Dresner, E. (1955). Aetiology and pathogenesis of rheumatoid arthritis. *Amer. J. Med.* **18**, 74–111.

Dumonde, D. C., Bitensky, L., Cunningham, G. J. and Chayen, J. (1965). The effects of antibodies on cells —1. Biochemical and histochemical effects of antibodies and complement on ascites tumour cells. *Immunology*, **8**, 25–36.

Duncan, H., Frost, H. M., Villanueva, A. R. and Sigler, J. W. (1965). The osteoporosis of rheumatoid arthritis. *Arthr. and Rheum.* **8**, 943–954.

Dunea, G., Muehrcke, R. C., Nakamoto, S. and Schwartz, F. D. (1966). Thrombotic thrombocytopenic purpura with acute anuric renal failure. *Amer. J. Med.* **41**, 1000–1006.

Dunlop, D. M. (1969). Some dangers of drug therapy. Royal College of Physicians Symposium on *Hazards of Therapy*. R. C. P., Publication No. 36. pp. 7–22. Royal College of Physicians: Edinburgh.

Duthie, J. J. R. (1969). Rheumatoid arthritis. In: *Textbook of the Rheumatic Diseases.* 4th edition pp. 259–322. Edited by Copeman, W. S. C.   Livingstone, Edinburgh and London.

— (1971). Infection in the aetiology of rheumatoid arthritis. In: *Modern Trends in Rheumatology*, Vol. 2. pp. 78–91. Edited by Hill, A. G. S.   Butterworths, London.

Duthie, J. J. R., Brown, P. E., Knox, J. D. E. and Thompson, M. (1957). Course and prognosis in rheumatoid arthritis. *Ann. rheum. Dis.* **16**, 411–424.

Duthie, J. J. R., Stewart, S. M., Alexander, W. R. M. and Dayhoff, R. E. (1967). Isolation of diphtheroid organism from rheumatoid synovial membrane and fluid. *Lancet* **1**, 142–143.

Dykman, C. J., Galens, G. J. and Good, A. E. (1965). Linear subcutaneous bands in rheumatoid arthritis. An unusual form of rheumatoid granuloma. *Ann. intern. Med.* **63**, 134–140.

Eagles, G. H., Evans, P. R., Fisher, A. G. T. and Keith, J. D. (1937). A virus in the aetiology of rheumatic diseases. *Lancet*, **ii**, 421–428.

Ebaugh, F. G., Peterson, R. E., Rodnan, G. P. and Bunim, J. J. (1955). The anemia of rheumatoid arthritis. *Med. Clin. N. Amer.* **39**, 489–498.

Eberl, R. and Altmann, H. (1970). Characteristic differences in esterase and peroxidase isoenzymes of synovial tissue in rheumatoid arthritis. *Z. Rheumaforsch.* **29**, 98–102.

Edgcumbe, J. O. P. and Husain, O. A. N. (1952). Effects of ACTH and cortisone on the anaemia of rheumatoid arthritis. *Ann. rheum. Dis.* **11**, 257–263.

Editorial (1967). Rheumatic diseases today. *Ann. intern. Med.* **66**, 230–232.

Editorial (1968). Pleurisy and rheumatoid arthritis. *Brit. med. J.* **2**, 1–2.

Editorial (1969). Microangiopathic haemolytic anaemia. *Scot. med. J.* **14**, 187–189.

Editorial (1970*a*). Mycoplasma and Rheumatoid Arthritis. *J. Amer. med. Ass.* **214**, 583.

Editorial (1970*b*). Felty's syndrome and rheumatoid arthritis. *Brit. med. J.* **1**, 127–128.

Edstrom, G. (1945). Peritendinitens betydelse i den kroniska polyartritens klinik. *Nord. Med.* **25**, 379–385.

Ekelund, C. (1943). Om Felty's syndrom i anslutning till 2 fall. *Nord. Med.* **17**, 434–436.

Elias, H., Krishna Murphy, A. S. and Elias, P. M. (1966). Structure of the adrenal cortex in rheumatoid diseases, including some observations on the adenohypophysis. *Acta endocr. (Kbh.)* **51**, 99–113.

Elling, P., Graudal, H. and Faber, V. (1968). Granulocyte-specific antinuclear factors in serum and synovial fluid in rheumatoid arthritis. *Ann. rheum. Dis.*, **27**, 225–233.

Ellman, P. and Ball, R. E. (1948). 'Rheumatoid disease' with joint and pulmonary manifestations. *Brit. med. J.* **2**, 816–820.

Ellman, P. and Cudkowicz, L. (1954). Pulmonary manifestations in the diffuse collagen diseases. *Thorax* **9**, 46–57.

Ellman, P., Cudkowicz, L. and Elwood, J. S. (1955). Therapy of 'Felty's syndrome'. *Ann. rheum. Dis.* **14**, 84–89.

Ellman, P. and Parkes Weber, F. (1948). A case of juvenile rheumatoid arthritis with sclerodactylia and calcinosis. *Ann. rheum. Dis.* **7**, 231–234.

Ellman, P., Parkes Weber, F. and Goodier, T. E. W. (1951). A contribution to the pathology of Sjögren's disease. *Quart. J. Med.*, *N.S.* **20**, 33–42.

Empire Rheumatism Council (1960). Gold therapy in rheumatoid arthritis. Report of a multi-centre controlled trial. *Ann. rheum. Dis.* **19**, 95–119.

Engfeld, B. and Hjertquist, S.-O. (1967). The effect of various fixatives on the preservation of acid glycosaminoglycans in tissues. *Acta path. microbiol. scand.* **71**, 219–232.

— (1968). Studies on the epiphyseal growth zone—I. The preservation of acid glycosaminoglycans in tissues in some histotechnical procedures for electron microscopy. *Virchows Arch.*, *Abt. B.*, *Zellpath* **1**, 222–229.

Ennevaara, K. and Oka, M. (1964). Rheumatoid arthritis with amyloidosis. *Ann. rheum. Dis.* **23**, 131–138.

Ericson, S. (1968). The parotid gland in subjects with and without rheumatoid arthritis. *Acta Radiol (Stockh.)* **275**, 7–167.

Evanson, J. M, Jeffrey, J. J. and Krane, S. M. (1967). Human collagenase: identification and characterization of an enzyme from rheumatoid synovium in culture. *Science* **158**, 499–502.

Faber, V. and Elling, P. (1966). Leucocyte-specific anti-nuclear factors in patients with Felty's syndrome, rheumatoid arthritis, systemic lupus erythematosus and other diseases. *Acta med. scand.* **179**, 257–267.

Fagraeus, A. (1948). Antibody production in relation to the development of plasma cells. *Acta med. scand.* (*Suppl.*), 204.

Falchuk, K. H., Goetzl, E. J. and Kulka, J. P. (1970). Respiratory gases of synovial fluids. An approach to synovial tissue circulatory-metabolic imbalance in rheumatoid arthritis. *Amer. J. Med.* **49**, 223–231.

Fallet, G. H., Boussina, I. and Fellmann, N. (1968). Valeur diagnostique et rôle eventuel du ragocyte synovial en rhumatologia. *Rev. Rhum.* **35**, 590–600.

Feagler, J. R., Sorenson, G. D., Rosenfield, M. G. and Osterland, C. K. (1971). Rheumatoid pleural effusion. *Arch. Path.* **92**, 257–266.

Fearnley, G. R. and Chakrabarti, R. (1964). Pharmacological enhancement of fibrinolytic activity of blood. *J. clin. Path.* **17**, 328–332.

Federlin, K., Maini, R. N., Russell, A. S. and Dumonde, D. C. (1971). A micro-method for peripheral leucocyte migration in a study of cellular hypersensitivity to tuberculin PPD in man. *J. clin. Path.* **24**, 533–536.

Fell, H. B. (1969). Role of biological membranes in some skeletal reactions. *Ann. rheum. Dis.* **28**, 213–227.

Fell, H. B. and Dingle, J. T. (1963). Studies on the mode of action of excess of vitamin A—6. Lysosomal proteases and the degradation of cartilage matrix. *Biochem. J.* **87**, 403–408.

Fell, H. B. and Mellanby, E. (1952). Effect of hypervitaminosis A on embryonic limb bones cultivated *in vitro. J. Physiol.* **116**, 320–349.

Fell, H. B. and Thomas, L. (1960). Comparison of the effects of papain and vitamin A on cartilage. II. The effects on organ cultures of embryonic skeletal tissue. *J. exp. Med.* **iii**, 719–744.

Feltkamp, T. E. W. and Rossum, A. L. van (1968). Antibodies to salivary duct cells, and other autoantibodies, in patients with Sjögren's syndrome and other idiopathic autoimmune diseases. *Clin. exp. Immunol.* **3**, 1–16.

Felty, A. R. (1924). Chronic arthritis in the adult associated with splenomegaly and leucopenia: a report of five cases of an unusual clinical syndrome. *Bull. Johns Hopk. Hosp.* **35**, 16–20.

Fenyohazi, L., Walacher, L. and Medgyes, A. (1970). Histological investigations of the gastric mucosa in rheumatoid arthritis. *Z. Rheumaforsch.* **29**, 153–161.

Ferguson, J., Boyle, J. A. and Nuki, G. (1969). Rheological evidence for the existence of dissociated macromolecular complexes in rheumatoid synovial fluid. *Clin. Sci.* **37**, 739–750.

Fessel, J. M. and Chrisman, O. D. (1964). Enzymatic degradation of chondromucoprotein by cell-free extracts of human cartilage. *Arthr. and Rheum.* **7**, 398–405.

Finch, S. C., Crockett, C. L., Ross, J. F. and Bayles, T. B. (1951). Hematologic changes with ACTH and cortisone therapy of rheumatoid arthritis. *Blood* **6**, 1034–1050.

Fingerman, D. L. and Andrus, F. C. (1943). Visceral lesions associated with rheumatoid arthritis. *Ann. rheum. Dis.* **3**, 168–181.

Fish, A. J., Michael, A. F., Gewurz, H. and Good, R. A. (1966). Immunopathologic changes in rheumatoid arthritis synovium. *Arthr. and Rheum.* **9**, 267–280.

Fisher, A. G. T. (1929). *Chronic (Non-Tuberculous) Arthritis.* H. K. Lewis, London.

Flatt, A. E. (1962). Intraarticular thio-tepa in rheumatoid disease of the hand. *Rheumatism* **18**, 70–73.

Fleischaker, H., and Lachnit, V. (1940). Blut- und Knochenmarkbefunde bei chronischen Polyarthritiden und beim Feltychen Syndrome. *Wien klin. Wschr.* **53**, 189–193.

Flinn, J. H., Price, J. M., Yess, N. and Brown, R. R. (1964). Excretion of tryptophane metabolites by patients with rheumatoid arthritis. *Arthr. and Rheum.* **7**, 201–210.

Follis, R. H. (1961). Ionic-induced submandibular sialadenitis in the hamster. *Proc. Soc. exp. Biol. (N.Y.)* **108**, 136–140.

Font, R. L., Yanoff, M. and Zimmerman, L. E. (1967). Benign lymphoepithelial lesion of the lacrimal gland and its relationship to Sjögren's syndrome (1967). *Amer. J. clin. Path.* **48**, 365–376.

Ford, D. K. (1969). Current views on the pathogenesis and etiology of rheumatoid arthritis. *Canad. med. Ass. J.* **101**, 147–151.

Ford, D. K. and Oh, J. O. (1965). Use of 'synovial' cell cultures in the search for virus in rheumatoid arthritis. *Arthr. and Rheum.* **8**, 1047–1052.

Ford, P. M., Bell, W. R., Bluestone, R., Gumpel, J. M. and Webb, F. W. S. (1970). The effect of Arvin on experimental immune arthritis in rabbits. *Brit. J. exp. Path.* **51**, 81–86.

Franks, A. S. T. (1969). Temporomandibular joint in adult rheumatoid arthritis. A comparative evaluation of 100 cases. *Ann. rheum. Dis.* **28**, 139–145.

Fraser, J. R. E. and Catt, K. J. (1961). Human synovial cell culture. Use of a new method in a study of rheumatoid arthritis. *Lancet* **ii**, 1437–1439.

Fraser, J. R. E. and McCall, J. F. (1966). Cytoplasmic spreading of human synovial cells in culture—II. Comparison of rheumatoid and normal sera. *Ann. rheum. Dis.* **25**, 49–51.

Fraser, K. B., Shirodaria, P. V., Haire, M. and Middleton, D. (1971). Mycoplasmas in cell cultures from rheumatoid synovial membranes. *J. Hyg., Camb.*, **69**, 17–25.

Freeman, M. A. R., Little, T. D. and Swanson, S. A. V. (1970). Lubrication of synovial joints: possible significance of fat. *Proc. roy. Soc. Med.*, **63**, 579–581.

Fresco, R. (1968). Tubular (myxovirus-like) structures in glomerular deposits from a case of lupus nephritis. *Fed. Proc.* **27**, 246.

Friedberger, E. (1913). Ueber aseptisch erzeugte Gelenkschwellungen beim Kaninchen. *Berl. klin. Wschr.* **50**, 88.

Friedman, H. (1970). Intraspinal rheumatoid nodule causing nerve root compression. *J. Neurosurg.* **32**, 689–691.

Friedman, I. (1971). Personal communication.

Friis, A. J. (1968). Cell-bound rheumatoid factors in the synovial membranes in patients with rheumatoid arthritis. *Ugeskr. Laeg.* **130**, 1557–1560.

— (1969). Immunohistochemical demonstration of rheumatoid factor (RF) in alcohol-fixed synovial tissue from patients with rheumatoid arthritis (RA). *Acta path. microbiol. scand.* **75**, 71–84.

Fudenberg, H. H. (1966). Immunologic deficiency, autoimmune disease, and lymphoma: observations, implications and speculations. *Arthr. and Rheum.* **9**, 464–472.

Fujita, T., Inoue, H. and Kodama, T. (1968). Scanning electron microscopy of the normal and rheumatoid synovial membranes. *Arch. hist. jap.* **29**, 511–522.

Fujita, T., Tokunaga, J. and Inoue, H. (1971). *Atlas of scanning electron microscopy in medicine*. Elsevier Publishing Company. Amsterdam, London, New York.

Gafni, J. and Sohar, E. (1960). Rectal biopsy for the diagnosis of amyloidosis. *Amer. J. med. Sci.* **240**, 332–336.

Gardner, D. L. (1957). Observations on the pathology of rheumatoid arthritis. Ph.D. thesis, University of Edinburgh.

— (1962). Amyloidosis in rheumatoid arthritis treated with hormones. *Ann. rheum. Dis.* **21**, 298–299.

— (1964). *The Pathology of Polyarthritis*. Royal College of Physicians of Edinburgh, Publication No. 25. Royal College of Physicians, Edinburgh, pp. 47–60.

— (1965). *Pathology of the Connective Tissue Diseases*. Edward Arnold, London.

— (1966). *Problems and perspectives in the pathology of rheumatoid arthritis*. Honeyman-Gillespie Lecture, University of Edinburgh Medical School.

— (1968*a*). The lymphoreticular system and amyloidosis in rheumatoid- and in experimental arthritis. In: *Pfizer Medical Monographs No. 3*, pp. 106–121. Edited by Duthie, J. J. R. and Alexander, W. R. M. University Press, Edinburgh.

— (1968*b*). Unpublished observations. Clinicopathological Conference, Royal Postgraduate Medical School, London.

— (1969). Pathology of the Rheumatic Diseases. In: *Textbook of the Rheumatic Diseases*, pp. 87–152. Edited by Copeman, W. S. C. Livingstone, Edinburgh and London.

— (1970). General pathology of connective tissue and intercellular matrix. In: *A Companion to Medical Studies*, Vol. II, pp. 30.1–30.17. Edited by Passmore, R. and Robson, J. S. Blackwell Scientific Publications, Oxford and Edinburgh.

— (1971). Modern views on the nature of rheumatoid arthritis. *Orthopaedics. Oxford*, **4**, 1–24.

— (1972). The evolution of microscopic technology and its influence on knowledge of the connective tissues. *Ann. rheum. Dis.* in press.

Gardner, D. L., Duthie, J. J. R., Macleod, J. and Allan, W. S. A. (1957). Pulmonary hypertension in rheumatoid arthritis: report of a case with intimal sclerosis of the pulmonary and digital arteries. *Scot. med. J.* **2**, 183–188.

Gardner, D. L. and Hall, T. A. (1969). Electron-microprobe analysis of sites of silver deposition in avian bone stained by the v. Kóssa technique. *J. Path.* **98**, 105–109.

Gardner, D. L. and Holmes, F. (1961). Anaesthetic and postoperative hazards in rheumatoid arthritis. *Brit. J. Anaesth.* **33**, 258–264.

Gardner, D. L., Krieg, A. F. and Chapnick, R. (1962). Fatal systemic fungus disease in rheumatoid arthritis with cardiac and pulmonary mycotic and rheumatoid granulomata. *Interamer. Arch. Rheumatol.* **5**, 561–586.

Gardner, D. L. and Laing, Christine P. (1965). Measurement of enzyme activity of isolated small arteries in early rat hypertension. *J. Path. Bact.* **90**, 399–406.

Gardner, D. L. and McGillivray, D. C. (1971*a*). Living articular cartilage is not smooth. The structure of mammalian and avian joint surfaces demonstrated *in vivo* by immersion incident light microscopy. *Ann. rheum. Dis.* **30**, 3–9.

— (1971*b*). Surface structure of articular cartilage: historical review. *Ann. rheum. Dis.* **30**, 10–14.

Gardner, D. L. and Matthews, Margaret A. (1969). Ultrastructure of the wall of small arteries in early experimental hypertension. *J. Path.* **1**, 51–62.

Gardner, D. L. and Roy, L. M. H. (1961). Tissue iron and the reticuloendothelial system in rheumatoid arthritis. *Ann. rheum. Dis.* **20**, 258–264.

Gardner, D. L. and Woodward, D. H. (1968). Scanning electron microscopy of articular surfaces. *Lancet* ii, 1246.

— (1969). Scanning electron microscopy and replica studies of articular surfaces of guinea-pig synovial joints. *Ann. rheum. Dis.* **28**, 379–391.

Gardner, D. L. and Wyke, A. W. (1970). Influence of age and method of caging on small artery enzyme activities. *Brit. J. exp. Path.*, **51**, 518–522.

Gardner, E. and O'Rahilly, R. (1968). The early development of the knee joint in staged human embryos. *J. Anat. (Lond.)* **102**, 289–299.

Gariepy, R., Demers, R. and Laurin, Carroll A. (1966). The prophylactic effect of synovectomy of the knee in rheumatoid arthritis. *Canad. med. Ass. J.* **94**, 1349–1352.

Garrod, A. B. (1848). Quoted by Copeman, W. S. C., 1964.

— (1859). *The Nature and Treatment of Gout and Rheumatic Gout*. Walton and Maberly, London.

Gaulhofer-de Klerck, E. H. and van Dam, G. (1963). Septic complications in rheumatoid arthritis. *Acta rheum. scand.* **9**, 254–263.

Gedda, P. O. (1955). On amyloidosis and other causes of death in rheumatoid arthritis. *Acta med. scand.* **150**, 443–452.

Geens, S. (1969). Synovectomy and debridement of the knee in rheumatoid arthritis—I. Historical review. *J. Bone Jt Surg.* **51A**, 617–625.

Geens, S., Claydon, M. L., Leidholt, J. D., Smyth, C. J. and Bartholomew, B. A. (1969). Synovectomy and débridement of the knee in rheumatoid arthritis. Part II. Clinical and roentgenographic study of 31 cases. *J. Bone Jt Surg.* **51A**, 626–642.

Geidel, H. (1967). Primary chronic polyarthritis with LE cells, a link with systemic lupus erythematosus. *Münch. med. Wschr.* **109**, 2534–2539.

Gell, P. and Coombs, R. R. A. (Editors) (1968). *Clinical Aspects of Immunology.* (2nd edition). Blackwell Scientific Publications, Oxford and Edinburgh.

Gerber, D. A. (1966). Increased copper ligand reactivity in the urine of patients with rheumatoid arthritis. *Arthr. and Rheum.* **9**, 975–803.

Gerber, D. A. and Gerber, M. G. (1967). Decreased concentration of histidine in the serum of patients with rheumatoid arthritis. A new diagnostic aid. *Clin. Res.*, **15**, 294.

Gerber, D. A., Sakamoto, A., Carmody, S. E. and Perry, H. M. (1969). Hypohistidinemia in patients with a history of hydralazine-induced arthritis. *Arthr. and Rheum.* **12**, 295–296.

Germuth, F. G., Maumenee, A. E., Senterfit, L. D. and Pollack, A. D. (1962). Immunohistologic studies on antigen–antibody reactions in the avascular cornea. *J. exp. Med.* **115**, 919–928.

Germuth, F. G. and Pollack, A. D. (1967). Immune complex disease—III. The granulomatous manifestations. *Hopkins Med. J.* **120**, 254–262.

Ghadially, F. N. and Roy, S. (1967). Ultrastructure of synovial membrane in rheumatoid arthritis. *Ann. rheum. Dis.* **26**, 426–443.

— (1969). *Ultrastructure of Synovial Joints in Health and Disease.* Butterworths, London.

Gibberd, F. B. (1965). A survey of four hundred and six cases of rheumatoid arthritis. *Acta rheum. Scand.* **11**, 62–70.

Gibberd, F. B., Gilbertson, C. and Jepson. E. M. (1965). Felty's syndrome. Radioactive isotope studies and splenectomy. *Ann. rheum. Dis.* **24**, 46–51.

Gieseking, R. (1969). Das feinmikroskopische Bild des Rheumatismus nodosus. *Beitr. path. Anat.* **138**, 292–320.

Gieseking, R., Baümer, A. and Backmann, L. (1969). Elektronenoptische Untersuchungen an Granulomen des Rheumatismus nodosus. *Z. Rheumaforsch.* **28**, 163–175.

Gilliland, B. C. and Turner, Elizabeth (1969). Mechanism of complement binding by the red cell in rheumatoid arthritis. *Arthr. and Rheum.* **12**, 498–503.

Gitlin, D. and Craig, J. M. (1957). Variations in the staining characteristics of human fibrin. *Amer. J. Path.* **33**, 267–283.

Glass, D. (1971). Corticosteroid and growth hormone response to hypoglycaemia in patients on longterm treatment with corticotrophin. *Lancet* **i**, 476–477.

Glenner, G., Harada, M., Isersky, C., Cuatrecasas, P., Page, D. and Keiser, H. (1970). Human amyloid protein: diversity and uniformity. *Biochem. Biophys. Res. Commun.* **41**, 1013–1019.

Glenner, G. G., Harbaugh, J., Ohms, J. I., Harada, M. and Cuatrecasas, P. (1970). An amyloid protein: the amino-terminal variable fragment of an immunoglobulin light chain. *Biochem. biophys. Res. Commun.* **41**, 1287–1289.

Glenner, G. G., Page, D., Isersky, C., Harada, M., Cuatrecasas, P., Eanes, E. D., DeLellis, R. A., Bladen, H. A. and Keiser, H. R. (1971). Murine amyloid fibril protein: isolation, purification and characterization. *J. Histochem. Cytochem.* **19**, 16–28.

Glynn, L. E. (1968). The chronicity of inflammation and its significance in rheumatoid arthritis. *Ann. rheum. Dis.* **27**, 105–121.

Glynn, L. E. and Holborow, E. J. (1960). Immunological aspects of rheumatoid arthritis: a review. *Ann. rheum. Dis.* **19**, 197–208.

— (1965). *Autoimmunity and Disease*, pp. 132–157. Blackwell Scientific Publications, Oxford.

Godwin, J. T. (1952). Benign lymphepithelial lesion of the parotid gland (adenolymphoma, chronic inflammation, lymphoepithelioma, lymphocytic tumour, Mikulicz disease): report of 11 cases. *Cancer* **5**, 1089–1103.

Goehrs, H. R., Baggenstoss, A. H. and Slocumb, C. H. (1960). Cardiac lesions in rheumatoid arthritis. *Arthr. and Rheum.* **3**, 298–308.

Goldenberg, G. J., Paraskevas, F. and Israels, L. G. (1969). The association of rheumatoid arthritis with plasma cell and lymphocytic neoplasms. *Arthr. and Rheum.* **12**, 569–579.

Goldfischer, S., Smith, Carol and Hamerman, D. (1968). Altered acid hydrolase activities in rheumatoid synovial cells in culture. *Amer. J. Path.* **52**, 569–578.

Goldie, I. (1969). The synovial microvascular derangement in rheumatoid arthritis and osteoarthritis. *Acta orthop. scand.* **40**, 751–764.

— (1970). On the presence of rheumatoid factor in joints before and after synovectomy. *Acta rheum. scand.* **16**, 114–120.

Golding, P. L., Bown, R., Mason, A. M. S. and Taylor, E. (1970). 'Sicca complex' in liver disease. *Brit. med. J.* **2**, 340–342.

Goldthwait, J. E. (1904). The differential diagnosis and treatment of the so-called rheumatoid disease. *Boston med. surg. J.* **151**, 529–534.

Good, A. E., Lang, K., Olson, J. R. and Frishette, W. A. (1970). Cardiac necrobiotic (rheumatoid?) granulomas without arthritis. Report of two cases. *Arthr. and Rheum.* **13**, 166–174.

Good, R. A. and Rotstein, J. (1960). Rheumatoid arthritis and agammaglobulinemia. *Bull. Rheum. Dis.* **10**, 203–206.

Goodsir, J. (1868). *The Anatomical Memoirs of John Goodsir* (*The process of ulceration in articular cartilages*). Vol. 2, pp. 408–411. Edited by W. Turner. Black, Edinburgh.

Goodwill, C. J. and Steggles, B. G. (1966). Destruction of the temporomandibular joints in rheumatoid arthritis. *Ann. rheum. Dis.* **25**, 133–136.

Gospodinoff, A., Gospodinoff, L. and Fiore, L. (1965a). Histological findings of pathogenetic considerations on rheumatoid myositis—I. *Policlinico, Sez. med.* **72**, 251–266.

— (1965b). Histological remarks and pathogenetic considerations on rheumatoid myositis. II. *Policlinico, Sez. med.* **72**, 311–319.

Gough, J. (1959). Occupational pulmonary diseases. In: *Modern Trends in Pathology*, pp. 276–281. Edited by Collins, D. H.   Paul B. Hoeber, New York.

Gough, J., Rivers, D. and Seal, R. M. E. (1955). Pathological studies of modified pneumoconiosis in coalminers with rheumatoid arthritis (Caplan's syndrome). *Thorax* **10**, 9–18.

Gough, K. R., McCarthy, C., Read, A. E., Mollin, D. L. and Waters, A. H. (1964). Folic-acid deficiency in rheumatoid arthritis. *Brit. med. J.* **1**, 212–217.

Gough, W. W. and Davis, J. S. (1966). Effects of rheumatoid factor on complement levels *in vivo*. *Arthr. and Rheum.* **9**, 555–565.

Gould, B. S. (Editor) (1968). *Treatise on Collagen*, Vol. 2, Biology of collagen, parts A and B. Academic Press, London and New York.

Gowans, J. D. C. (1960). Complete heart block with Stokes–Adams syndrome due to rheumatoid heart disease, report of a case with autopsy findings. *New Engl. J. Med.* **262**, 1012–1014.

Graef, I., Hickey, D. V. and Altman, V. (1949). Cardiac lesions in rheumatoid arthritis. *Amer. Heart J.* **37**, 635.

Granda, J. L., Ranawat, C. S. and Posner, A. S. (1971). Levels of three hydrolases in rheumatoid and regenerated synovium. *Arthr. and Rheum.* **14**, 223–230.

Grayzel, A. I. and Beck, C. (1970). Rubella infection of synovial cells and the resistance of cells derived from patients with rheumatoid arthritis. *J. exp. Med.* **131**, 367–376.

Greenwood, B. M. (1969a). Polyarthritis in Western Nigeria—I. Rheumatoid arthritis. *Ann. rheum. Dis.* **28**, 488–496.

— (1969b). Polyarthritis in Western Nigeria—II. Still's disease. *Ann. rheum. Dis.* **28**, 617–623.

— (1969c). Acute tropical polyarthritis. *Quart. J. Med.* **38**, 295–306.

Greiling, H., Kisters, R. and Vojtisek, O. (1970). The inhibition of DNA and RNA synthesis in synovial cells by immunosuppressive substances. *Z. Rheumaforsch.* **29**, 146–152.

Gresham, G. A. and Kellaway, T. D. (1958). Rheumatoid disease in the larynx and lung. *Ann. rheum. Dis.* **17**, 286–292.

Grimley, P. M. (1967). Rheumatoid arthritis: ultrastructure of the synovium. *Ann. intern. Med.* **66**, 623–624.

Grimley, P. M. and Sokoloff, L. (1966). Synovial giant cells in rheumatoid arthritis. *Amer. J. Path.* **49**, 931–954.

Gritsman, N. N. and Rogov, A. A. (1965). A comparison of tissue changes of the synovial membrane in patients suffering from infectious arthritis (rheumatoid arthritis) and systemic lupus erythematosus according to puncture biopsy data. *Arkh. Patol.* **27**, No. 6, 67–75.

Gross, D. (1963). Chemische Synovektomie mit Senfgas bei primär chronischer Polyarthritis. *Z. Rheumaforsch.* **22**, 456–459.

Gruenwald, P. (1948). Visceral lesions in a case of rheumatoid arthritis. *Arch. Path.* **46**, 59–67.

Gryfe, A., Sanders, Philippa M. and Gardner, D. L. (1971). The mast cell in early rat adjuvant arthritis. *Ann. rheum. Dis.* **30**, 24–30.

Gryfe, A., Woodward, D. H. and Gardner, D. L. (1969). Scanning electron microscopy of normal and inflamed synovial tissue from a rheumatoid patient. *Lancet* **ii**, 156–157.

Gschwend, N. (1970). The value of synovectomy. *Z. Rheumaforsch.* **29**, 129–137.

Guicciardi, E. and Little, K. (1967). Some observations on the effects of blood and a fibrinolytic enzyme on articular cartilage in the rabbit. *J. Bone Jt Surg.* **49B**, 342–350.

Gupta, J. D. and Peterson, V. (1970). Rubella and rheumatoid arthritis. *Lancet,* **ii**, 781.

Gürich, H. G. (1968). Three further cases of unusual rheumatic tissue changes in rheumatoid arthritis treated with cortisone. *Verh. Deutsch. Ges. Path.* **52**, 519–525.

Gusev, A. V. and Elizarova, N. A. (1969). The status of bone marrow hematopoiesis and peripheral blood in patients with psoriasis. *Vestn. Derm. Vener.* **43**, 33–38.

Györkey, F., Min, K. W., Sincovics, J. G. and Györkey, P. (1968). Systemic lupus erythematosus and myxovirus. *New Engl. J. Med.* **280**, 333.

Haas, J. E. and Yunis, E. J. (1970). Tubular inclusions of systemic lupus erythematosus. Ultrastructural observations regarding their possible viral nature. *Exp. Molec. Path.* **12**, 257–263.

Hadden, W. B. (1888). On 'dry mouth', or suppression of the salivary and buccal secretions. *Trans. clin. Soc. Lond.* **21**, 176–179.

Hahn, B. H., Yardley, J. H. and Stevens, M. B. (1970). 'Rheumatoid' nodules in systemic lupus erythematosus. *Ann. intern. Med.* **72**, 49–58.

Hamerman, D. (1966). New thoughts on the pathogenesis of rheumatoid arthritis. (Editorial.) *Amer. J. Med.*, **40**, 1–9.

— (1969). Cartilage changes in the rheumatoid joint. *Clin. Orthop.* **64**, 91–97.

Hamerman, D., Barland, P. and Janis, Rosamund (1969). The structure and chemistry of the synovial membrane in health and disease. In: *The Biological Basis of Medicine*, Vol. 3, pp. 269–309. Edited by Bittar, E. E. and Bittar, N. Academic Press, London and New York.

Hamerman, D., Janis, R. and Smith, C. (1967). Cartilage matrix depletion by rheumatoid synovial cells in tissue culture. *J. exp. Med.* **126**, 1005–1012.

Hamerman, D., Rosenberg, L. C. and Schubert, M. (1970). Diarthrodial joints revisited. *J. Bone Jt Surg.* **52**A, 725–774.

Hamerman, D. and Sandson, J. (1963). Unusual properties of hyaluronate protein isolated from pathological synovial fluids. *J. clin. Invest.* **42**, 1882–1889.

Hamerman, D. and Sandson, J. (1970). Antigenicity of connective tissue components. *Mount Sinai J. Med.* **37**, 453–465.

Hamerman, D., Stephens, M. and Barland, P. (1961). Comparative histology and metabolism of synovial tissue in normal and arthritic joints. In: *Inflammation and Diseases of Connective Tissue*, pp. 158–168. Edited by Mills, L. C. and Moyer, J. H. Saunders, Philadelphia and London.

Hammar, J. A. (1894). Ueber den feineren Bau der Gelenke. Abth. II. Der Gelenkknorpel. *Arch. mikros. Anat.* **43**, 813–885.

Hannestad, K. and Mellbye, O. J. (1967). Rheumatoid factor in synovial effusions: local production and consumption. *Clin. exp. Immunol.* **2**, 501–509.

Harada, M., Isersky, C., Cuatrecasas, P., Page, D., Bladen, H. A., Eanes, E. D., Keiser, H. R. and Glenner G. G. (1971). Human amyloid protein: chemical variability and homogeneity. *J. Histochem. Cytochem.* **19**, 1–15.

Harris, E. D., DiBona, D. R. and Krane, S. M. (1969). Collagenases in human synovial fluid. *J. clin. Invest.* **48**, 2104–2113.

Harris, E. D., Evanson, J. M., DiBona, D. R. and Krane, S. M. (1970). Collagenase and rheumatoid arthritis (a review). *Arthr. and Rheum.* **13**, 83–94.

Harris, M. (1970). Rheumatoid heart disease with complete heart block. *J. clin. Path.* **23**, 623–626.

Harrold, B. P. (1968). Non-tuberculous constrictive peri-carditis. *Brit. med. J.* **1**, 290–292.

Hart, F. D. (1969). Extraarticular manifestations of rheumatoid arthritis. *Brit. med. J.* **3**, 131–136.

— (1970). Rheumatoid arthritis: extraarticular manifestations. Part II. *Brit. med. J.* **2**, 747–752.

Hashimoto, H. (1912). Zur Kenntniss der lymphomatösen Veränderung der Schildrüse (Struma lymphomatosa). *Arch. klin. Chir. Berl.* **97**, 219–248.

Hashimoto, K. (1969). Paramyxovirus-like structures in lupus and dermatomyositis. In: *Proceedings of the 27th Annual Meeting of the Electron Microscopy Society of America*, p. 222. Claitor's Publishing Division, Baton Rouge, La.

Haslock, D. I., Wright, V. and Harriman, D. G. F. (1970). Neuromuscular disorders in rheumatoid arthritis: A motor-point muscle biopsy study. *Quart. J. Med.* **39**, 335–358.

Haygarth, J. (1805). *A Clinical History of Diseases*. Cadell and Davies, London.

Hayhoe, F. G. J. and Smith, D. R. (1951). Plasmacytosis in the bone marrow in rheumatoid arthritis. *J. clin. Path.* **4**, 47–54.

Healey, L. A., Wilske, K. R. and Sagebiel, R. W. (1967). Rheumatoid nodules simulating basal-cell carcinoma. *New Engl. J. Med.* **277**, 7–9.

Heaton, J. M. (1959). Sjögren's syndrome and systemic lupus erythematosus. *Brit. med. J.* **1**, 466–469.

Hedberg, H. and Moritz, U. (1959). Intrinsic viscosity of hyaluronic acid synthesized in tissue culture in the presence of normal and rheumatoid arthritic serum respectively. *Acta rheum. scand.* **5**, 169–178.

Hedberg, H., Nordén, Å. Lundquist, A. and Afzelius, B. (1964). Depression of haemolytic complement of synovial fluid in adult rheumatoid arthritis. *Acta med. scand.* **175**, 347–351.

Heller, P., Kellow, W. F. and Chomet, B. (1956). Needle biopsy of the parietal pleura. *New Engl. J. Med.* **255**, 684–690.

Hendry, N. G. C. and Carr, A. J. (1963). A glycosidase abnormality in synovial membrane in joint disease. *Nature* **199**, 392.

Heppleston, A. G. (1951). Chronic diffuse interstitial fibrosis of the lungs. *Thorax* **6**, 426–432.

— (1956). The pathology of honeycomb lung. *Thorax* **11**, 77–93.

Heptinstall, R. H. and Joekes, A. M. (1960). Renal amyloid. *Ann. rheum. Dis.* **19**, 126–134.

Herp, A., Fabianek, J., Calick, A. and Pigman, W. (1966). Dermal connective tissue permeability in rheumatoid arthritis. *Ann. rheum. Dis.* **25**, 345–352.

Highton, T. C., Caughey, D. E. and Rayns, D. G. (1966). A new inclusion body in rheumatoid synovia. *Ann. rheum. Dis.* **25**, 149–155.

Highton, T. C. and Donaldson, L. A. (1970). Scanning electron microscopy of synovial joints with preservation of mucopolysaccharides. *Proc. Univ. Otago med. Sch.* **48**, 64–65.

Hijmans, W., Doniach, D., Roitt, I. M. and Holborow, E. J. (1961). Serological overlap between lupus erythematosus, rheumatoid arthritis, and thyroid autoimmune disease. *Brit. med. J.* **2**, 909–914.

Hill, A. G. S., McCormick, J. N., Greenbury, G. L., Morris, C. J. and Keningale, J. (1967). *Ann. rheum. Dis.* **26**, 566 (abstract).

Hindle, W. and Yates, D. A. H. (1965). Pyopneumothorax complicating rheumatoid lung disease. *Ann. rheum. Dis.* **24**, 57–60.

Hinzpeter, E. N., Naumann, G. and Bartelheimer, H. K. (1971). Ocular histopathology in Still's Disease. *Ophthal. Res.* **2**, 16–24.

Hirohata, K. and Kobayashi, I. (1964). Fine structure of the synovial tissues in rheumatoid arthritis. *Kobe J. Med. Sci.* **10**, 195–225.

Hirohata, K., Mizuhara, K., Fujiwara, A., Sato, T., Imura, S. and Kobayashi, I. (1963a). Electron microscopic studies on the joint tissues under the normal and pathologic conditions—1. Normal joint tissues (1st report). *J. Jap. orthop. Ass.* **36**, 15–19.

— (1963b). Electron microscope studies on the joint tissues under the normal and pathologic conditions— 2. Normal joint tissues (2nd report). *J. Jap. Orthop. Ass.* **37**, 291–301.

Hoaglund, F. T. and Lord, G. P. (1967). Haemophilus influenzal septic arthritis in adults. Two case reports with review of previous cases. *Arch. intern. Med.* **119**, 648–652.

Hoffa, A. and Wollenberg, G. A. (1908). *Arthritis deformans und sogenannter chronischer Gelenkrheumatismus.* Stuttgart.

Hollander, J. L., Fudenberg, H., Rawson, A. J., Anelson, Neva M. and Torralba, T. P. (1966). Further studies on the pathogenesis of rheumatoid joint inflammation. *Arthr. and Rheum.* **9**, 675–681.

Hollander, J. L., McCarty, D. J., Astorga, G. and Castro-Murillo, E. (1965). Studies on the pathogenesis of rheumatoid joint inflammation—I. The 'R.A.' cell and a working hypothesis. *Ann. intern. Med.* **62**, 271–280.

Hollingsworth, J. W. H. (1968). Laboratory tests. In: *Local and Systemic Complications of Rheumatoid Arthritis*, pp. 13–17. Saunders, Philadelphia and London.

Holt, P. J. L., Holloway, V., Raghupati, N. and Calnan, J. S. (1969). The effect of a fibrinolytic agent (Arvin) on wound healing and collagen formation. *Clin. Sci.* **38**, 9.

Hopkins, J. S. (1967). Lower cervical rheumatoid subluxation with tetraplegia. *J. Bone Jt Surg.* **49B**, 46–51.

Horler, A. R. and Thomson, M. (1959). The pleural and pulmonary complications of rheumatoid arthritis. *Ann. Intern. Med.* **51**, 1179–1203.

Hosford, J. P. (1937). Arthrogram to show extent of synovial cavity after synovectomy. *Proc. roy. Soc. Med.* **30**, 1264.

Houli, J. and Monteiro Marinho, H. (1954). Bone marrow in rheumatoid arthritis. *Ann. rheum. Dis.* **13**, 327–330.

Howes, R. G. and Jarvis, B. (1965). The effects of intraarticular thiotepa on synovial fluids. *Arthr. and Rheum.* **8**, 495–500.

Hume, R., Dagg, J. H., Fraser, T. N. and Goldberg, A. (1964). Anaemia of Felty's syndrome. *Ann. rheum. Dis.* **23**, 267–271.

Humphrey, J. H. and Dourmashkin, R. R. (1969). The lesions in cell membranes caused by complement. *Advanc. Immunol.* **11**, 75–115.

Hunder, G. G., Ward, L. E. and Ivins, J. C. (1965). Rheumatoid granulomatous lesion simulating malignancy in the head and neck of the femur. *Mayo Clinic Proc.* **40**, 766–770.

Hunter, W. (1742–43). Of the structure and diseases of articulating cartilages. *Phil. Trans.* **42**, 514–521.

Hurd, E. R., Eigenbrodt, E., Ziff, M. and Strunk, S. W. (1969). Cytoplasmic tubular structures in kidney biopsies in systemic lupus erythematosus. *Arthr. and Rheum.* **12**, 541–542.

Hurd, E. R., LoSpalluto, J. and Ziff, M. (1970). Formation of leukocyte inclusions in normal polymorphonuclear cells incubated with synovial fluid. *Arthr. and Rheum.* **13**, 724–733.

Hurd, E. R., Snyder, W. B. and Ziff, M. (1970). Choroidal nodules and retinal detachments in rheumatoid arthritis. Improvement with fall in immunoglobulin levels following prednisolone and cyclophosphamide therapy. *Amer. J. Med.* **48**, 273–278.

Hurri, L., Sievers, K. and Oka, M. (1963). Intraarticular osmic acid in rheumatoid arthritis. *Acta rheum. scand.* **9**, 20–27.

Hutt, M. S. R., Richardson, J. S. and Staffurth, J. S. (1951). Felty's syndrome. A report of four cases treated by splenectomy. *Quart. J. Med.* **20**, 57–71.

Igari, T., Tsuchizawa, M., Obara, K. and Ono, S. (1968). Hydroxyproline metabolism in serum synovial fluid, and synovial membrane in joint diseases. *Arch. Jap. Chir.* **37**, 836–840.

Inoue, H. and Gardner, D. L. (1971). Unpublished observations.

Inoue, H., Julkunen, H., Oka, M. and Vainio, K. (1970). Scanning electron microscopic studies of extensor tendon degeneration in rheumatoid arthritis. *Acta rheum. Scand.* **16**, 311–318.

Inoue, H., Kodama, T. and Fujita, T. (1969). Scanning electron microscopy of normal and rheumatoid articular cartilages. *Arch. hist. jap.* **30**, 425–435.

Ishikawa, A. (1967). Fine-structures of the normal and rheumatoid synovial membrane—with special reference to the acid mucopolysaccharide localization in the living cells. *Arch. jap. Chir.* **36**, 107–117.

Jacox, R. F. and Feldmahn, A. (1955). Variations of β-glucuronidase concentration in abnormal human synovial fluid. *J. clin. Invest.* **34**, 263–267.

Janeway, C. A., Gitlin, D., Craig, J. M. and Grice, D. S. (1956). 'Collagen Disease' in patients with congenital agammaglobulinemia. *Trans. Assoc. Amer. Physcns.* **69**, 93–97.

Janis, R. and Hamerman, D. (1969). Articular cartilage changes in early arthritis. *Bull. Hosp. Jt Dis. (N.Y.)* **30**, 136–152.

Janis, R., Sandson, J., Smith, C. and Hamerman, D. (1967). Synovial cell synthesis of a substance immunologically like cartilage protein-polysaccharide. *Science, N.Y.* **158**, 1464–1467.

Janoff, A. and Scherer, J. (1968). Mediators of inflammation in leucocyte lysosomes. IX. Elastinolytic activity in granules of human polymorphonuclear leucocytes. *J. exp. Med.* **128**, 1137–1155.

Janoff, A. and Zweifach, B. W. (1964). Production of inflammatory changes in the microcirculation by cationic proteins extracted from lysosomes. *J. exp. Med.* **120**, 747–764.

Jansson, E., Vainio, U., Snellman, O. and Tuuri, S. (1971). Search for mycoplasma in rheumatoid arthritis. *Ann. rheum. Dis.* **30**, 413–418.

Jasani, M. K., Katori, M. and Lewis, G. P. (1969). Intracellular enzymes and kinin enzymes in synovial fluid in joints. *Ann. rheum. Dis.* **28**, 497–512.

Jasin, H. E., LoSpalluto, J. and Ziff, M. (1970). Rheumatoid hyperviscosity syndrome. *Amer. J. Med.* **49**, 484–493.

Jasiński, B. and Staehelin, A. (1951). Über die Beteiligung des Knockenmarkes bei der Polyarthritis chronica rheumatica und ihre Beeinflussung durch Cortison. *Schweiz. med. Wschr.* **81**, 619–623.

Jayson, M. I. V. and Jones, D. E. P. (1971). Scleritis and rheumatoid arthritis. *Ann. rheum. Dis.* **30**, 343–347.

Jayson, M. I. V. and Dixon, A. St. J. (1970a). Intraarticular pressure in rheumatoid arthritis of the knee—1. Pressure changes during passive joint distension. *Ann. rheum. Dis.* **29**, 261–265.

— (1970b). Intraarticular pressure in rheumatoid arthritis of the knee.—2. Effect of intraarticular pressure on blood circulation to the synovium. *Ann. rheum. Dis.* **29**, 266–268.

— (1970c). Intraarticular pressure in rheumatoid arthritis of the knee. *Ann. rheum. Dis.* **29**, 401–408.

Jayson, M. I. V., Rubinstein, D. and Dixon, A. St. J. (1970). Intraarticular pressure and rheumatoid geodes (bone 'cysts'). *Ann. rheum. Dis.* **29**, 496–502.

Jeffrey, M. R. (1953). Some observations on anemia in rheumatoid arthritis. *Blood* **8**, 502–518.

Jennings, J. F. (1971). Lymphocyte responsiveness in rheumatoid arthritis. *Lancet* **i**, 1239.

Jeremy, R., Schaller, J., Arkless, R., Wedgwood, R. J. and Healey, L. A. (1968). Juvenile rheumatoid arthritis persisting into adulthood. *Amer. J. Med.* **45**, 419–434.

Julkunen, H. (1966). Synovial inflammatory cell reaction in chronic arthritis. *Acta rheum. scand.* **12**, 188–196.

Kacaki, J. N., Balduzzi, P. C. and Vaughan, J. H. (1970). A study of rubella haemagglutination inhibition antibodies in rheumatoid arthritis. *Clin. Exp. Immun.* **6**, 885–889.

Kadar, Anna, Bush, Valerie and Gardner, D. L. (1971). Direct elastase treatment of ultrathin sections embedded in water-soluble Durcupan. *J. Path.* **103**, 64–67.

Kadar, Anna and Gardner, D. L. (1970). An experimental study of elastic-tissue formation in the chick and rat aortas. *J. Path.* **100**, P ii.

Kadar, Anna, Gardner, D. L. and Bush, Valerie (1971a). The relation between the fine structure of smooth muscle cells and elastogenesis in the chick-embryo aorta. *J. Path.*, **104**, 253–260.

— (1971b). Susceptibility of the chick-embryo aorta to elastase. An electron microscopic study. *J. Path.*, **104**, 261–266.

Kaether, H. (1938). Sternalpunctionen bei rheumatischen Erkrankungen. *Z. Rheumaforsch.* **1**, 473–481.

Kaplan, M. H. (1963). The site of formation of rheumatoid factor. *Arthr. and Rheum.* **6**, 475–478.

Kaplan, M. H. and Vaughan, J. (1962). The site of formation of rheumatoid factor. Conference on Host Response Mechanisms in Rheumatoid Arthritis. *Arthritis and Rheumatism Foundation Conference Series* **6**, 57.

Karten, I. (1969a). Septic arthritis complicating rheumatoid arthritis. *Ann. intern. Med.* **70**, 1147–1158.

— (1969b). Arteritis, myocardial infarction and rheumatoid arthritis. *J. Amer. med. Ass.* **210**, 1717–1720.

Kawano, K., Miller, L. and Kimmelstiel, P. (1969). Virus-like structures in lupus erythematosus. *New Engl. J. Med.* **281**, 1228–1229.

Kayanjian, V. H. (1938). Ankylosis of the temporomandibular joint. *Surg. Gynec. Obstet.* **67**, 333–348.

Kazakova, I. S., Orlovskaya, G. V. and Pavlov, V. P. (1967). The localization of the rheumatoid factor in the synovial tissue in rheumatoid arthritis. *Vop. Revm.* **7**, 67–73.

Keele, C. A. (1969). Clinical and pathological aspects of kinins in man. *Proc. Roy. Soc., Ser. B.* **173**, 361–369.

Keil, H. (1938). Rheumatic subcutaneous nodules and simulating lesions. *Medicine* **17**, 261–380.

Kellgren, J. H. (Editor) (1963). *The Epidemiology of Chronic Rheumatism.* Blackwell Scientific Publications, Oxford (2 Vols.).

— (1966). Epidemiology of rheumatoid arthritis (Joseph J. Bunim Memorial Lecture). *Arthr. and Rheum.* **9**, 658–674.

Kellgren, J. H. and Ball, J. (1950). Tendon lesions in rheumatoid arthritis. *Ann. rheum. Dis.* **9**, 48–65.

— (1959). Clinical significance of the rheumatoid serum factor. *Brit. med. J.* **1**, 523–531.

Kellgren, J. H., Ball, J., Astbury, W. T., Reed, R. and Beighton, E. (1951). Biophysical studies of rheumatoid connective tissue. *Nature* **168**, 493–494.

Kellgren, J. H., Ball, J., Fairbrother, R. W. and Barnes, K. L. (1958). Suppurative arthritis complicating rheumatoid arthritis. *Brit. med. J.* **1**, 1193–1200.

Kemper, J. W., Baggenstoss, A. H. and Slocumb, C. H. (1957). The relationship of therapy with cortisone to the incidence of vascular lesions in rheumatoid arthritis. *Ann. intern. Med.* **46**, 831–851.

Kennedy, J. S. (1962). ^{35}Sulphur in experimental amyloidosis. *J. Path. Bact.* **83**, 165–181.

Kennedy, W. P. U., Partridge, R. E. H. and Matthews, M. B. (1966). Rheumatoid pericarditis with cardiac failure treated by pericardiectomy. *Brit. Heart J.* **28**, 602–608.

Kerby, G. P. and Taylor, S. M. (1967). Enzymatic activity in human synovial fluid from rheumatoid and non-rheumatoid patients. *Proc. Soc. exp. Biol. Med. (N.Y.)* **126**, 865–868.

Kessler, H. S. (1968). A laboratory model for Sjögren's syndrome. *Amer. J. Path.* **52**, 671–685.

Key, J. A. (1925). The reformation of synovial membrane in the knees of rabbits after synovectomy. *J. Bone Jt Surg.* **7**, 793.

Kibrick, A. C., Hashiro, C. Q. and Safier, L. B. (1962). Hydroxyproline peptides of urine in arthritic patients and controls on a collagen-free diet. *Proc. Soc. exp. Biol. Med.* **109**, 473–478.

Kilroy, A. W., Schaffner, W., Fleet Jr., W. F., Lefkowitz, Jr., L. B., Karzon, D. T. and Fenichel, G. M. (1970). Two syndromes following rubella immunization. *J. Amer. med. Ass.* **214**, 2287–2293.

Kinsella, T. D., Baum, J. and Ziff, M. (1969). Immunofluorescent demonstration of an IgG–β_1C complex in synovial lining cells of rheumatoid synovial membrane. *Clin. exp. Immunol.* **4**, 265–271.

Kinsella, T. D., Baum, J. and Ziff, M. (1970). Studies of isolated synovial lining cells of rheumatoid and nonrheumatoid synovial membranes. *Arthr. and Rheum.* **13**, 734–75£.

Kirk, J. and Cosh, J. (1969). The pericarditis of rheumatoid arthritis. *Quart. J. Med.* **38**, 297–423.

Kissane, J. M. (1964). Sjögren's syndrome. *Amer. J. Med.* **37**, 578–591.

Kitridou, R., McCarty, D. J., Prockop, D. J. and Hummeler, K. (1969). Identification of collagen in synovial fluid. *Arthr. and Rheum.* **12**, 580–588.

Klein, H. and Block, M. (1953). Bone marrow plasmacytosis: a review of 60 cases. *Blood* **8** (2), 1034–1041.

Klemperer, P. (1955). The significance of the intermediate substances of the connective tissue in human disease. *The Harvey Lectures, Series 49*, pp. 100–123. Academic Press, New York.

Klemperer, P., Gueft, B., Lee, S. L., Leuchtenberger, C. and Pollister, A. W. (1950). Cytochemical changes of acute lupus erythematosus. *Arch. Path.* **49**, 503–516.

Klemperer, P., Pollack, A. D. and Baehr, G. (1942). Diffuse collagen disease; acute disseminated lupus erythematosus and diffuse scleroderma. *J. Amer. med. Ass.* **119**, 331–332.

Klinge, F. (1929). Die Eiweissüberempfindlichkeit (Gewebs anaphylaxie) der Gelenke. Experimentelle pathologisch-anatomische Studie zur Pathogenese des Gelenkrheumatismus. *Beitr. path. Anat.* **83**, 185–189.

— (1930a). Das Gewebsbild des fieberhaften Rheumatismus: das rheumatische Fruhinfiltrat. (Akutes degenerativexsudatives Stadium). *Virchows Arch. path. Anat.* **278**, 438–461.

— (1930b). Das Gewebsbild des fieberhaften Rheumatismus: das subakut-chronische Stadium des Zellnotschens. *Virchows Arch. path. Anat.* **279**, 1–15.

— (1930c). Das Gewebsbild des fieberhaften Rheumatismus: Narbe und Rezidiv. *Virchows Arch. path. Anat.* **279**, 16–29.

Klinge, F. (1933). *Der Rheumatismus: pathologisch-anatomische und experimentell-pathologische Tatsachen und ihre Auswertung für das ärztliche-rheumaproblem.* Bergman, Munich. pp. 163–176.

— (1934). Die rheumatischen Erkrankungen der Knochen und Gelenke und der Rheumatismus. In: *Handbuch der Speziellen Pathologischen Anatomie und Histologie.* Vol. 9, part III, pp. 107–251. Edited by Lubarsch, O. and Henke, F., Springer, Berlin.

Kodama, T., Takatori, M. and Inoue, H. (1968). A study of rheumatoid joint with the use of scanning electron microscopy. *J. Jap. orthop. Ass.* (n.a.) **36**, 871–883.

Kodama, T., Narasaki, K., Ogino, T., Takatori, M., Oka, Y., Hiramatsu, H., Miyoshi, K., Hiraba, K., Yamamoto, S., Tomita, S., Tsuji, H., Inoue, H., Senoo, T., Yamamoto, A., Miwa, Y. and Oobuchi, S. (1966). Dynamics of rheumatoid joint. *Acta Med. Okayama* **20**, 53–89.

Kormano, M. (1970). A microradiographic and histological study of the manubriosternal joint in rheumatoid arthritis. *Acta rheum. scand.* **16**, 47–59.

Koskelo, P., Kekki, M., Nikkilä, E. A. and Virkkunen, M. (1967). Turnover of ^{131}I-labelled ceruloplasmin in rheumatoid arthritis. *Scand. J. clin. Lab. Invest.* **19**, 259–262.

Koskelo, P., Kekki, M., Virkkunen, M., Lassus, A. and Somer, T. (1966). Serum ceruloplasm concentration in rheumatoid arthritis, ankylosing spondylitis, psoriasis and sarcoidosis. *Acta rheum. scand.* **12**, 261–266.

Kozicka-Polak, I., Kblebanowski, J., Szymańska-Jagiello, W., Zabokrzycki, J. and Zdrojewska, M. (1970). Monoarticular reactions of nonspecific aetiology in children. *Pol. Tyg. lek.* **25**, 605–607.

Krassinine, G., Kahan, Alice, Amon, B. and Delbarre, F. (1966). Study, by immunofluorescence, of characteristic inclusions of the synovial ragocyte. *C.R. Acad. Sci. (Paris)* (D) **263**, 801–803.

Kriegel, W., Langness, U. and Jahn, P. (1970). 'Collagen-like' protein (CLP) and anticollagen antibodies in the serum of patients with rheumatoid arthritis and patients with non-rheumatoid connective tissue disorders. *Klin. Wschr.* **48**, 368–370.

Kriegel, W., Langness, U., Jahn, P. and Muller, W. (1970). 'Collagen-like protein' and collagen antibodies in rheumatoid arthritis. *Z. Rheumaforsch.* **29**, 173–178.

Kulka, J. P. (1959). The pathogenesis of rheumatoid arthritis. *J. chron. Dis.* **10**, 388–402.

— (1966). Vascular derangement in rheumatoid arthritis. In: *Modern Trends in Rheumatology* (1st Edition) pp. 49–69. Edited by Hill, A. G. S. Butterworth, London.

Kulka, J. P., Bocking, D., Ropes, M. W. and Bauer, W. (1955). Early joint lesions of rheumatoid arthritis: report of eight cases, with knee biopsies of lesions of less than one year's duration. *Arch. Path.* **59**, 129–150.

Lachmann, P. J., Coombs, R. R. A., Fell, Honor B. and Dingle, J. T. (1969). The breakdown of embryonic (chick) cartilage and bone cultivated in the presence of complement-sufficient antiserum. III. Immunological analysis. *Int. Arch. Allerg.* **36**, 469–485.

Lack, C. H. (1959). Chondryolysis in arthritis. *J. Bone Jt Surg.* **41**B, 384–387.

— (1966). The role of lysosomes in experimental arthritis. *Proc. roy. Soc. Med.* **59**, 875–877.

— (1969). Lysosomes in relation to arthritis. In: *Lysosomes in Biology and Pathology*, Vol. 1, pp. 493–508. Edited by Dingle, J. T. and Fell, H. B. North-Holland Publishing Co., Amsterdam and London.

Lackington, C. (1959). Tissue culture of fibroblasts and round cells from arthritic synovial fluid. *Arthr. and Rheum.* **2**, 42 (abstract).

Laine, V. A. (1967). Early synovectomy in rheumatoid arthritis. *Ann. Rev. Med.* **18**, 173–184.

Laing, Christine P. and Gardner, D. L. (1964). Cardiac metabolism in early rat hypertension: quantitative enzyme histochemistry in the prenecrotic phase. *Brit. J. exp. Path.* **45**, 502–513.

Laitinen, H., Saksanen, S. and Suoranta, H. (1970). Involvement of the manubrio-sternal articulation in rheumatoid arthritis. *Acta rheum. scand.* **16**, 40–46.

Lamas Da Silva, J. M. and Adler, H. E. (1969). Pathogenesis of arthritis induced in chickens by *Mycoplasma gallisepticum*. *Path. Vet.* **6**, 385–395.

Lamvik, J. (1963). Rheumatoid pneumoconiosis. A case of Caplan's syndrome in a chalk-mine worker. *Acta path. microbiol. scand.* **57**, 169–174.

Landré-Beauvais, A. J. (1800). Doit-on admettre une nouvelle espèce de goutte, sous la dénomination de goutte asthénique primitive? Paris, J. A. Brosson.

Lange, R. K., Weiss, T. E. and Ochsner, J. L. (1965). Rheumatoid arthritis and constrictive pericarditis. A patient benefited by pericardectomy. *Arthr. and Rheum.* **8**, 403–417.

Laskin, D. M., Engel, M. B., Joseph, N. R. and Pollack, V. E. (1961). A test of connective tissue state and reactivity in collagen diseases. *J. clin. Invest.* **40**, 2153–2161.

Lassiter, G. S. and Tassy, F. T. (1965). Malignant rheumatoid disease with aortic stenosis. *Arch. intern. Med.* **116**, 930–936.

Latvalahti, J. (1953). Experimental studies on the influence of certain hormones on the development of amyloidosis. Acta Endocrinol. (Kbh) (Suppl.), 16.

Lawrence, J. S. (1966). Epidemiology of the rheumatic diseases. In: *Modern Trends in Rheumatology–I*, pp. 1–17. Edited by Hill, A. G. S. Butterworths, London.

— (1969). The epidemiology of rheumatic diseases. In: *Textbook of the Rheumatic Diseases*, pp. 163–181, Edited by Copeman, W. S. C. Livingstone, Edinburgh and London.

— (1970). Rheumatoid arthritis—nature or nurture? *Ann. rheum. Dis.* **29**, 357–379.

Lawrence, J. S., Sharp, J., Ball, J. and Bier, Frida (1964). Rheumatoid arthritis of the lumbar spine. *Ann. rheum. Dis.* **23**, 205–217.

Lawson, A. A. H. and Maclean, N. (1966). Renal disease and drug therapy in rheumatoid arthritis. *Ann. rheum. Dis.* **25**, 441–449.

Lawson, A. A. H., Owen, E. T. and Mowat, A. G. (1967). Nature of anaemia in rheumatoid arthritis—VII. Storage of iron in rheumatoid disease. *Ann. rheum. Dis.* **26**, 552–559.

Lazarus, G. S., Decker, J. L. Oliver, H. C., Daniels, J. R., Multz, C. V. and Fullmer, H. M. (1968). Collagenolytic activity of synovium in rheumatoid arthritis. *New Engl. J. Med.* **279**, 914–919.

Lebowitz, W. B. (1963). Heart in rheumatoid arthritis (rheumatoid disease): clinical and pathological study of sixty-two cases. *Ann. intern. Med.* **58**, 102–123.

Lee, F. I. and Brain, A. T. (1962). Chronic diffuse interstitial pulmonary fibrosis and rheumatoid arthritis. *Lancet* **ii**, 693–695.

Lefkovits, A. M. and Farrow, I. J. (1955). The liver in rheumatoid arthritis. *Ann. rheum. Dis.* **14**, 162–169.

Lehman, M. A., Kream, J. and Brogna, D. (1964). Acid and alkaline phosphatase activity in the serum and synovial fluid of patients with arthritis. *J. Bone Jt Surg.* **46**A, 1732–1738.

Leichentritt, B. (1943). American Rheumatism Association meeting, discussion on perineural rheumatoid nodules. *Ann. intern. Med.* **43**, 116–117.

Leitner, S. J. (1949). *Die intravitale Knockenmarkesuntersuchung*. English translation by Britton, C. W. C. and Neumark, E. Churchill, London. pp. 288–289.

Lendrum, A. C. (1969). The validation of fibrin, and its significance in the story of hyalin. In: *Trends in Clinical Pathology: Essays in Honour of Gordon Signy*, pp. 159–188. British Medical Association, London.

LeRoy, E. C. and Sjoerdsma, A. (1965). Clinical significance of a hydroxyproline-containing protein in human plasma. *J. clin. Invest.* **44**, 914–919.

Lever, J. D. and Ford, E. H. R. (1958). Histological, histochemical and electronic microscopic observations on synovial membrane. *Anat. Rec.* **132**, 525–539.

Levin, M. H., Kaplan, L., Marans, S., Weinberger, H. J. and Pattersson, J., Jr. (1955). Heart in rheumatoid arthritis: clinical-pathologic correlation of 43 autopsied patients. *Ann. rheum. Dis.* **14**, 430–431.

Lewis, D. C. and Ziff, M. (1966). Intraarticular administration of gold salts. *Arthr. and Rheum.* **9**, 682–692.

Lightfoot, R. W. and Christian, C. L. (1969). Rheumatoid Arthritis. In: *Textbook of Immunopathology*, Vol. II, pp. 733–744. Edited by Miescher, P. A. and Muller-Eberhard, H. J. New York, Grune and Stratton.

Linder, E. and Pasternack, A. (1970). Immunofluorescence studies on kidney biopsies in ankylosing spondylitis. *Acta path. microbiol. scand.* **78**, 517–525.

Lindner, J. (1968). Rheumatic connective tissue metabolism and pathological structure of the connective tissue in rheumatoid arthritis. *Verh. Deutsch. Ges. Inn. Med.* **74**, 1315–1349.

Lindström, J. (1966). Studies in experimental synovectomy. *Acta rheum. scand.* **12**, 175–187.

Linquist, P. R. and McDonnell, D. E. (1970). Rheumatoid cyst causing extradural compression. A case report. *J. Bone Jt Surg.* **52**A, 1235–1240.

Lipscomb, P. R. (1965). Synovectomy of the wrist for rheumatoid arthritis. *J. Amer. med. Ass.* **194**, 655–659.

Liso, V., Gillardi, U. and Trizio, D. (1968). Giant cells in rheumatoid synovial membrane. *Reumatismo* **20**, 638–640.

Litwin, S. D., Allen, J. C. and Kunkel, H. G. (1966). Disappearance of the clinical and serologic manifestations of rheumatoid arthritis following a thoracotomy for a lung tumour. *Arthr. and Rheum.* **9**, 865.

Longfield, M. D., Dowson, D., Walker, P. S. and Wright, V. (1969). 'Boosted lubrication' of human joints by fluid enrichment and entrapment. *Biomed. Engineering* **4**, 517–522.

Lopes-Vaz, A. and Coimbra, A. (1967). Cytochemical and ultra-microscopic study of RA cells in rheumatic diseases. *Presse méd*, **75**, 2221–2222.

Lorber, A. (1966). Penicillamine therapy for rheumatoid lung disease: effects on protein sulphhydryl groups. *Nature* **210**, 1235–1237.

Lorber, A., Pearson, C. M., Meredith, W. L. and Gautz-Mandell, L. E. (1964). Serum sulfydryl determinations and significance in connective tissue disease. *Ann. intern. Med.* **61**, 423–434.

Lorber, A., Pearson, C. M. and Rene, R. M. (1961). Osteolytic vertebral lesions as a manifestation of rheumatoid arthritis and related disorders. *Arthr. and Rheum.* **4**, 514–532.

Louyot, P., Legras, B., Montet, Y., Diebold, P., Pourel, J. and Bertrand, A. (1970). Use of intraarticular injection of radium 224 (Thorium X) for rheumatoid arthritis. *Ann. Méd. Nancy* **9**, 423–430.

Lövgren, O. (1945). Plasma proteins in rheumatoid disease. *Acta med. scand.* **163**, 60–66.

Lowney, E. D., and Simons, H. M. (1963). Rheumatoid nodules of the skin. *Arch. Derm.* **88**, 853–858.

Lowry, O. H., Roberts, N. R., Wu, M-L., Hixon, W. S. and Crawford, E. J. (1954). The quantitative histochemistry of brain II. Enzyme measurements. *J. biol. Chem.* **207**, 19–49.

Lucchesi, M., Lucchesi, O. and Da Silva, M. P. (1946). O mielograma na artrite reumatoide. *Rev. argent. Reum.* **10**, 294–296.

Lucy, J. A., Dingle, J. T. and Fell, H. B. (1961). Studies on the mode of action of excess of vitamin A. 2. A possible role of intracellular proteases in the degradation of cartilage matrix. *Biochem. J.* **79**, 500–508.

Luft, J. H. (1966). Fine structure of capillary and endocapillary layer as revealed by ruthenium red. *Fed. Proc.* **25**, 1773–1783.

Lundberg, M. and Ericson, S. (1967). Changes in the temporo-mandibular joint in psoriasis arthropathica. *Acta derm.-venereol.* (*Stockholm*) **47**, 354–358.

Lund-Olsen, K. (1970). Oxygen tension in synovial fluids. *Arthr. and Rheum.* **13**, 769–776.

Luscombe, M. (1963). Acid phosphatase and catheptic activity in rheumatoid synovial tissue. *Nature* **197**, 1010.

Lycette, R. R. and Pearmain, G. E. (1965). Lymphocyte cultures in rheumatoid arthritis and thyroid diseases. *New Zealand Med. J.* **64**, 81.

McCall, J. G. (1968). The microarchitecture of articular cartilage and its load deformation response. M. Sc. thesis. University of Strathclyde.

McCarty, D. J., Polcyn, R. E. and Collins, P. A. (1970). ^{99m}Technetium scintiphotography in arthritis—II. Its nonspecificity and clinical and roentgenographic correlations in rheumatoid arthritis. *Arthr. and Rheum.* **13**, 21–32.

McCarty, D. J., Polcyn, R. E., Collins, P. A., and Gottschalk, A. (1970). ^{99m}Technetium scintiphotography in arthritis—I. Technic and interpretation. *Arthr. and Rheum.* **13**, 11–20.

McConkey, E., Fraser, G. M. and Bligh, A. S. (1962). Osteoporosis and purpura in rheumatoid disease: prevalence and relation to treatment with corticosteroids. *Quart. J. Med.* **31**, 419–427.

McCormick, J. N. (1963). An immunofluorescence study of rheumatoid factor. *Ann. rheum. Dis.*, **22**, 1–10.

— (1967). Autoimmunity and the rheumatic diseases. *Practitioner* **199**, 150–156.

McCormick, J. N., Day, J., Morris, C. J. and Hill, A. G. S. (1969). The potentiating effect of rheumatoid arthritis serum in the immediate phase of nephrotoxic nephritis. *Clin. exp. Immunol.* **4**, 17–28.

McDevitt, C. A. and Muir, Helen, (1971). Gel electrophoresis of proteoglycans and glycosaminoglycans on large pore composite polyacrylamide-agarose gels. *Analyt. Biochem.* (in press).

Mackenzie, G. H. (1894). Rheumatism of the larynx. *Edinb. med. J.* **40**, 507–509.

McKusick, Anne B., Sherwin, R. W., Jones, L. G. and Hsu, J. M. (1964). Urinary excretion of pyridoxine and 4-pyridoxic acid in rheumatoid arthritis. *Arthr. and Rheum.* **7**, 636–653.

McMillan, M. (1960). The identification of a fluorescent reducing substance in the urine of patients with rheumatoid arthritis. *J. clin. Path.* **13**, 140–148.

MacSween, R. N. M., Dalakos, T. G., Jasani, M. K., Boyle, J. A., Buchanan, W. W. and Goudie, R. B. (1968). A clinico-immunological study of serum and synovial fluid antinuclear factors in rheumatoid arthritis and other arthritides. *Clin. exp. Immunol.* **3**, 17–24.

Mahallaway, M. N. El. and Sabour, M. S. (1959). Renal lesions in rheumatoid disease. *Lancet* **ii**, 852–853.

Maher, J. A. (1954). Dural nodules in rheumatoid arthritis. *Arch. Path.* **58**, 354–359.

Maini, R. N., Bryceson, A. D. M., Wolstencroft, R. A. and Dumonde, D. C. (1969). Lymphocyte mitogenic factor in man. *Nature* **224**, 43–44.

Maini, R. N., Stewart, Sheila M. and Dumonde, D. C. (1970). Peripheral leucocyte migration inhibited by diphtheroid organisms isolated from patients with rheumatoid arthritis. *Ann. rheum. Dis.* **29**, 541–545.

Maldyk, E. (1969a). Histopathological-histochemical comparative studies on fibrinoid necrosis. *Rheumatologia* (*Warsz.*) **7**, 101–109.

— (1969b). Periarticular changes in bone in rheumatoid arthritis. *Reumatologia* (*Warsz.*) **7**, 281–289.

Maldyk, E. and Kalczak, M. (1968). Histopathological and histochemical picture of the rheumatoid nodule. *Reumatologia* (*Warsz.*) **6**, 85–91.

Maldyk, E., Piotrowska, D., Drecka, K. and Maldyk, H. (1967). Diagnosis of amyloidosis in patients with rheumatoid arthritis and ankylosing spondylitis by biopsy of gingival and rectal mucosa. *Reumatologia* (*Warsz.*) **5**, 153–160.

Malinin, T. I., Pekin, T. J. and Zvaifler, N. J. (1967). Cytology of synovial fluid in rheumatoid arthritis. *Amer. J. clin. Path.* **47**, 203–208.

Mandema, E., Ruinen, L., Scholten, J. H. and Cohen. A. S. (Editors) (1968). Amyloidosis. *Proceedings of the Symposium on Amyloidosis, University of Groningen, The Netherlands.* Excerpta Medica Foundation, Amsterdam.

Marcolongo, R. Jr., Carcassi, A., Bianco, G., Bravi, A., Di Paolo, N. and Lunghetti, R. (1969). Isolation of mycoplasma and antibody studies from patients with rheumatoid arthritis. *Boll. 1st sieroter, milan.* **48**, 363–377.

Marin, D., Negoescu, M., Stoia, I., Pierette, A., Petrescu, A. and Constantinescu, S. (1969). The morphology of the synovial tissue and articular fluid cells in rheumatoid polyarthritis—studied with the optical and electron microscope. *Acta rheum. scand.* **15**, 126–134.

Marin, D., Stoia, I., Athanasiu, P. and Petrescu, A. (1969). Viral infections, factors with an allergic potential in the pathogenic complex of some chronic rheumatic diseases. *Rev. Roum. Inframicrobiol.* **6**, 277–290.

Marmont, A. (1948). Il sangue ed il midollo osseo nella poliartrite cronica primaria. *Arch. 'Maragliano' Pat. Clin.* **3**, 1289–1360.

Maroudas, Alice (1970). Electron probe microanalysis of uncalcified articular cartilage. *Proc. Roy. micro. Soc.* **6**, 21–22.

Maroudas, Alice and Muir, Helen, (1970). The distribution of collagen and glycosaminoglycans in human articular cartilage and the influence of hydraulic permeability. In: *Molecular Biology of the Intercellular Matrix*. Edited by Balazs, E. A., Proceedings NATO Advanced Study Institute, Academic Press, London. In press.

Marshall, A. H. E. (1956). *An Outline of the Cytology and Pathology of the Reticular Tissue*, pp. 122–124. Oliver and Boyd, Edinburgh.

Martel, W. (1968). Cervical spondylitis in rheumatoid disease. A comment on neurologic significance and pathogenesis. *Amer. J. Med.* **44**, 441–446.

Martel, W. and Bole, G. G. (1968). Pathological fracture of the odontoid process in rheumatoid arthritis. *Radiology* **90**, 948–952.

Massell, B. F., Coen, W. B. and Jones, T. D. (1952). *Rheumatic Diseases, VIIth International Congress Proceedings*. pp. 27–42. W. B. Saunders, Philadelphia and London.

Matthews, J. A. (1969). Atlanto-axial subluxation in rheumatoid arthritis. *Ann. rheum. Dis.* **28**, 260–266.

Matsura, Y. (1967). Arthroscopic, optical and electron microscope observations of the synovial membrane of the knee joint, with reference to electron microscopic changes of the synovial membrane in chronic articular rheumatism, deformative arthropathy and osteoarticular tuberculosis. *J. Jap. orthop. Ass.* (n.a.) **40**, 1281–1298.

Mattingley, S. (1964). The lungs and rheumatoid arthritis. *Ann. phys. Med.* **7**, 185–202.

Medical Research Council Annual Report, (1968). *Immunological Aspects of Rheumatoid Arthritis*, pp. 51–56. H.M.S.O., London.

Mellors, R. C., Heimer, R., Corcos, J. and Korngold, L. (1959). Cellular origin of rheumatoid factor. *J. exp. Med.* **110**, 875–886.

Mellors, R. C., Nowoslawski, A. and Korngold L. (1961). Rheumatoid arthritis and the cellular origin of rheumatoid factors. *Amer. J. Path.* **39**, 533–546.

Mellors, R. C., Nowoslawski, A., Korngold, L. and Sengson, B. C. (1961). Rheumatoid factor and the pathogenesis of rheumatoid arthritis. *J. exp. Med.* **113**, 475–484.

Meltzer, M., Franklin, F. C., Elias, K., McCluskey, R. T. and Cooper, N. (1966). Cryoglobulinaemia: a clinical and laboratory study. II. Cryoglobulins with rheumatoid factor activity. *Amer. J. Med.* **40**, 837–856.

Merlo, P. and Tortori-Donati, B. (1945). Il quadro ematologico periferico e midollare nelle artropatie croniche. *Rass. Fisiopat. clin. ter.* **17**, Suppl. 2, 37–80.

Mesara, B. W., Brody, G. L. and Oberman, H. A. (1966). 'Pseudo-rheumatoid' subcutaneous nodules. *Amer. J. clin. Path.* **45**, 684–691.

Messner, R. P., Caperton, E. M., King, R. A. and Williams, R. C., Jr. (1969). Interactions among rheumatoid factors, γG antibodies, lymphocytes and phagocytes. *Ann. N. Y. Acad. Sci.* **168**, 93–104.

Messner, R. P., Laxdal, T., Quie, P. G. and Williams, R. C. (1968). Rheumatoid factors in subacute bacterial endocarditis—bacterium, duration of disease or genetic predisposition? *Ann. intern. Med.* **68**, 746–756.

Mester, A. (1938). Morphologische und bacteriologische Untersuchungen des Knockenmarkpunktates bei rheumatischen gelenkerkrankungen und nicht-rheumatischen Gelenkentzundungen. *Z. Rheumaforsch.* **1**, 534–543.

Meyer, A. W. (1931). The minuter anatomy of attrition lesions. *J. Bone Jt Surg.* **13**, 341–360.

Michelazzi, A. M. (1937). Osservazioni sulla ghiandola linfatica nel reumatismo cronico primativo. *Minerva Med.* **28**, 609–613 (quoted by *J. Amer. med. Ass.* **404**, 110, 1938).

Miller, B., Markheim, H. R. and Towbin, M. N. (1967). Multiple stress fractures in rheumatoid arthritis. A case report. *J. Bone Jt Surg.* **49A**, 1408–1414.

Mills, D. M., Salky, N. K. and Diluzio, N. R. (1964). Activity of the reticuloendothelial system in rheumatoid arthritis. *Arthr. and Rheum.* **7**, 331.

Milne, J. A., Anderson, J. R., MacSween, R. N., Fraser, K., Short, I., Steven, J., Shaw, G. B. and Tankel H. I. (1967). Thymectomy in acute systemic lupus erythematosus and rheumatoid arthritis. *Brit. med. J.* **1**, 461–464.

Milstoc, M. (1970). Cholinesterase activity in patients with rheumatoid arthritis. *Amer. J. clin. Path.* **53**, 452–457.

Missen, G. A. K. and Taylor, J. D. (1956). Amyloidosis in rheumatoid arthritis. *J. Path. Bact.* **71**, 179–192.

Mitchell, N. and Shepard, N. (1970). The ultrastructure of articular cartilage in rheumatoid arthritis: a preliminary report. *J. Bone Jt Surg.* **52A**, 1405–1423.

Mitchinson, M. J. (1970). The pathology of idiopathic retroperitoneal fibrosis. *J. clin. Path.* **23**, 681–689.

Mitchison N. A. (1967). The concept of autoimmunity. *Practitioner* **199**, 143–149.

Moberg, E., Wassen, E., Kjellberg, S. R., Zettergren, L., Scheller, S. and Aschan, W. (1966). The early pathological changes in rheumatoid arthritis. *Acta. chir. scand.* (Suppl.) **357**, 142–147.

Moesmann, G. (1969). Malignancy and mortality in subacute rheumatoid arthritis in old age. *Acta rheum. scand.* **15**, 193–199.

Mohing, W. (1967). Synovectomie und Arthroplastik bei primar chronischer polyarthritis. *Dtsch. med. Wschr.* **92**, 863–864.

Mohos, S. C. and Wagner, B. M. (1969). Damage to collagen in corneal immune injury; observations of connective tissue structure. *Arch. Path.* **88**, 3–20.

Montgomery, W. W. (1963). Crycoarytenoid arthritis. *Laryngoscope* **73**, 801–836.

Montgomery, W. W., Perone, P. M. and Schall, L. A. (1955). Arthritis of the crycoarytenoid joint. *Ann. Otol (St. Louis)* **64**, 1025–1033.

Morelli, A. and Arciello, G. (1952). Sui rapporti tra protidemia frazionata e composizione citologica del midollo osseo nelle artropatie croniche. *Rif. med.* **66**, 620–622.

Morgagni, G. B. (1761). *De Sedidus et Causis Morborum per Anatomen Indigatis libri quinque.* 2 Volumes, typeg. Remondiniana, Venice.

Morgan, W. S. and Castleman, B. (1953). A clinicopathologic study of 'Mikulicz's Disease'. *Amer. J. Path.* **29**, 471–503.

Morton, H. E. (1970). Mycoplasmas from man with undetermined specific relationships to their human host. In: *The role of mycoplasmas and L forms of bacteria on disease*, pp. 147–711. Ed. Sharp, J. T. Charles C Thomas, Springfield, Illinois.

Moschowitz, E. (1936–1937). The clinical apects of amyloidosis. *Ann. intern. Med.* **10**, 73–88.

Motulsky, A. G., Weinberg, S., Saphir, O. and Rosenberg, E. (1952). Lymph nodes in rheumatoid arthritis. *Arch. intern. Med.* **90**, 660–676.

Movat, H. Z., Fernando, N. P. V., Urinhara, T. and Weiser, W. J. (1963). Allergic inflammation: III. The fine structure of collagen fibrils at sites of antigen–antibody interaction in Arthus-type lesions. *J. exp. Med.* **118**, 557–564.

Movat, H. Z. and More, R. H. (1957). The nature and origin of fibrinoid. *Amer. J. clin. Path.* **28**, 331–353.

Movitt, E. R. and Davis, A. E. (1953). Liver biopsy in rheumatoid arthritis. *Amer. J. med. Sci.* **226**, 516–520.

Mowat, A. D. (1971). Anaemia in rheumatoid arthritis. In: *Modern Trends in Rheumatology—II*, pp. 106–116. Edited by Hill. A. G. S. Butterworths, London.

Mowat, A. G. and Hothersall, T. E. (1968). Nature of anaemia in rheumatoid arthritis—VIII. Iron content of synovial tissue in patients with rheumatoid arthritis and in normal individuals. *Ann. rheum. Dis.* **27** 345–351.

Mowat, A. G., Hothersall, T. E. and Aitchison, W. R. C. (1969). Nature of anaemia in rheumatoid arthritis —XI. Changes in iron metabolism induced by the administration of corticotrophin. *Ann. rheum. Dis.* **28**, 303–309.

Mowat, A. G., Hothersall, T. E. and Gould, J. C. (1970). Urinary tract infection in patients with rheumatoid arthritis. *Ann. rheum. Dis.* **29**, 143–148.

Muir, H. M. (1969). The structure and metabolism of mucopolysaccharides (glycosaminoglycans) and the problem of the mucopolysaccharidoses. *Amer. J. Med.* **47**, 673–690.

— (1971). In *Structure and metabolism of proteoglycans and glycosaminoglycans in relation to rheumatoid arthritis.* Academic Press, New York and London. (in press).

Muirden, K. D. (1966). Ferritin in synovial cells in patients with rheumatoid arthritis. *Ann. rheum. Dis.* **25**, 387–401.

— (1969). Clearance of Fe^{59} labelled erythrocytes from normal and inflamed rabbit knee joints—I. Relationship to the anaemia of rheumatoid arthritis. *Ann. rheum. Dis.* **28**, 548–551.

— (1970a). Lymph node iron in rheumatoid arthritis. Histology, ultrastructure and chemical concentration. *Ann. rheum. Dis.* **29**, 81–88.

— (1970b). Giant cells, cartilage and bone fragments within rheumatoid synovial membrane: clinico-pathological correlations. *Aust. Ann. Med.* **19**, 105–110.

— (1970c). The anaemia of rheumatoid arthritis: the significance of iron deposits in the synovial membrane. *Aust. Ann. Med.* **19**, 97–104.

Muirden, K. D. and Mills, K. W. (1971). Do lymphocytes protect the rheumatoid joint? *Brit. med. J.*, **4**, 219–221.

Muirden, K. D. and Senator, G. B. (1968). Iron in the synovial membrane in rheumatoid arthritis and other joint diseases. *Ann. rheum. Dis.* **27**, 38–48.

Müller, W., Kluthe, R. and Muller, H. (1963). On the diagnosis of the activity of chronic rheumatic diseases, with special reference to the quantitative determination of haptoglobins and caeruloplasmin. *Z. Rheumaforsch.* **22**, 1–10.

Nairn, R. C. (1969). *Fluorescent Protein Tracing* (3rd Edition). Livingstone, Edinburgh and London.

Namba, T. and Grob, D. (1970). Familial concurrence of myasthenia gravis and rheumatoid arthritis. *Arch. int. Med.* **125**, 1056–1058.

Nettlebladt, E. and Sandell, B.-M. (1963). Amino-acid content of serum in rheumatoid arthritis. *Ann. rheum. Dis.* **22**, 269–272.

Neumann, E. (1880). Die Picrocarminfärbung und ihre Anwendung auf die Entzündungslehre. *Arch. mikr. Anat.* **18**, 130–150.

Newcombe, D. S. and Cohen, A. S. (1965). Chylous synovial effusion in rheumatoid arthritis. Clinical and pathogenetic significance. *Amer. J. Med.* **38**, 156–164.

Nichols, E. H. and Richardson, F. L. (1909). Arthritis deformans. *J. med. Res.* **21**, 149–222.

— (1915). Quoted by Copeman.

Niedermeier, W. (1965). Concentration and chemical state of copper in synovial fluid and blood serum of patients with rheumatoid arthritis. *Ann. rheum. Dis.* **24**, 544–548.

— (1967). Inhibition of ascorbic acid-induced depolymerization of hyaluronic acid by ceruloplasmin in synovial fluid. *Ann. rheum. Dis.* **27**, 71–76.

Niedermeier, W., Creitz, E. E. and Holley, H. L. (1962). Trace metal composition of synovial fluid from patients with rheumatoid arthritis. *Arthr. and Rheum.* **5**, 439–444.

Niedobitek, F. (1969). Zur Morphologie und Pathogenese des Caplan-Syndroms. *Z. Rheumaforsch.* **28**, 175–190.

Nilsson, F. (1948). Anaemia problems in rheumatoid arthritis. *Acta med. scand. (Suppl.)* **210**.

Norden, C. W. and Sellers, T. F. (1964). *Haemophilus influenzae* pyoarthrosis in an adult. *J. Amer. med. Ass.* **189**, 693–695.

Norton, W. L. (1969). Endothelial inclusions in active lesions of systemic lupus erythematosus. *J. Lab. clin. Med.* **74**, 369–379.

Norton, W. L., Velayos, E. and Robison, L. (1970). Endothelial inclusions in dermatomyositis. *Ann. rheum. Dis.* **29**, 67–72.

Norton, W. L. and Ziff, M. (1964). The ultrastructure of rheumatoid synovium and subcutaneous nodule. *Arthr. and Rheum.* **7**, 335.

— (1966). Electron microscopic observations on the rheumatoid synovial membrane. *Arthr. and Rheum.* **9**, 589–610.

Nosanchuk, J. S. and Naylor, B. (1968). A unique cytologic picture in pleural fluid from patients with rheumatoid arthritis. *Amer. J. clin. Path.* **50**, 330–335.

Nosanchuk, J. S. and Schnitzer, B. (1969). Follicular hyperplasia in lymph nodes from patients with rheumatoid arthritis. A clinicopathologic study. *Cancer (Philad.)* **24**, 343–354.

Novikoff, A. B., Beaufay, H. and de Duve, C. (1956). Electron microscopy of lysosome-rich fractions from rat liver. *J. Biophys.-Biochem. Cytol.*, 2 suppt. 179–184.

Nowoslawski, A. and Brzosko, W. J. (1966). Immunolopatologia gośćca przewlekego postępującego (Immunopathology of rheumatoid arthritis). *Reumatologia, Warsz.* **4**, 439–448.

Nowoslawski, A. and Brzosko, W. J. (1967a). Immunopathology of rheumatoid arthritis—I. The rheumatoid synovitis. *Path. europ. (Brux.)* **2**, 198–219.

— (1967b). Immunopathology of rheumatoid arthritis—II. The rheumatoid nodule. *Path. europ. (Brux.)* **2**, 302–321.

Omer, A. and Mowat, A. G. (1968). Nature of anaemia in rheumatoid arthritis. IX. Folate metabolism in patients with rheumatoid arthritis. *Ann. rheum. Dis.* **27**, 414–424.

— (1969). Nature of anaemia in rheumatoid arthritis—X. Folate-releasing properties of plasma in health and disease, with special reference to rheumatoid arthritis. *Ann. rheum. Dis.* **28**, 24–27.

O'Quinn, S. E., Barrett, K. C. and Baker, D. T. (1965). Peripheral vascular lesions in rheumatoid arthritis. *Arch. Derm.* **92**, 489–494.

Orabona, M. L. and Semeraro, V. (1961). Behaviour of the synovial tissue in systemic lupus erythematosus (S.L.E.). Study conducted on 5 patients by means of needle-biopsy of the knee. *Reumatismo* **13**, 196–208.

Orlovskaya, G. V., Muldiyarov, P. Y. and Kazakova, I. S. (1970). Synovial plasma cells in rheumatoid arthritis: electron microscopic and immunofluorescence studies. *Ann. rheum. Dis.* **29**, 524–532.

Owen, D. S., Toone, E. and Irby, R. (1966). Coexistent rheumatoid arthritis and chronic tophaceous gout. *J. Amer. med. Ass.* **197**, 953–956.

Owen, D. S., Waller, M. and Toone, E. C. (1970). Rheumatoid arthritis and malignancy. *Med. Coll. Va. Quart.* **6**, 8–10.

Owen, E. T. and Lawson, A. A. H. (1966). Nature of anaemia in rheumatoid arthritis—VI. Metabolism of endogenous iron. *Ann. rheum. Dis.* **25**, 547–552.

Page, J. W. (1961). Spontaneous tendon rupture and cervical vertebral subluxation in patients with rheumatoid arthritis. *J. Mich. med. Soc.* **60**, 888–892.

Page Thomas, D. P. (1967). The role of lysosomes in rheumatoid disease. In: *Rheumatology, An Annual Review*, Vol. 1, Ed. Rotstein, J. pp. 29–50. Karger, Basel.

— (1969). Lysosomal enzymes in experimental and rheumatoid arthritis. In: *Lysosomes in Biology and Pathology*. Vol. 2, pp. 87–110. Edited by Dingle, J. T. and Fell, H. B. North Holland Publishing Company, Amsterdam and London.

Page Thomas, D. P. and Dingle, J. T. (1955). *In vitro* studies of rheumatoid synovium. Preliminary metabolic comparison between synovial membrane and villi. *Brit. J. exp. Path.* **36**, 195–198.

— (1958). Studies on human synovial membrane *in vitro*. The metabolism of normal and rheumatoid synovia and the effect of hydrocortisone. *Biochem. J.* **68**, 231–238.

Pagel, W. and Treip, C. S. (1955). Viscero-cutaneous collagenosis. A study of the intermediate forms of dermatomyositis, scleroderma and disseminated lupus erythematosus. *J. clin. Path.* **8**, 1–18.

Pakuła, A. and Artiucha, Z. (1965). Rzadki przypadek wspołistnienia zespołu feltyégo i łuszczycy (A rare case of concurrence of Felty's syndrome and psoriasis). *Reum. pol.* **3**, 297–298.

Pal, S. B. (1967). The determination of the urinary excretion of 11-oxy-17-ketosteroids in normal human individuals and in patients with rheumatoid arthritis. *Folia Endocr. (Roma)* **20**, 1–12.

Palmer, D. G. (1970). Dispersed cell cultures of rheumatoid synovial membrane. *Acta rheum. scand.* **16**, 261–270.

Palmer, D. G. (1971). The differentiation of cells cultured from synovial effusions. *Proc. Univ. Otago Med. Sch.* **49**, 18–19.

Parker, F., Jr. and Keefer, C. S. (1935). Gross and histologic changes in the knee joint in rheumatoid arthritis. *Arch. Path.* **20**, 507–522.

Parker, M. T. (1965). Infection acquired in medical wards. (Public Health Laboratory Service Report). *J. Hyg. (Lond.)* **63**, 457–477.

Parker, R. A. and Thomas, P. M. (1959). Intestinal perforation and widespread arteritis in rheumatoid arthritis during treatment with cortisone. *Brit. Med. J.* **1**, 540–542.

Parker, R. L. and Schmid, F. R. (1962). Phagocytosis of particulate complexes of gamma globulin and rheumatoid factor. *J. Immunol.* **88**, 519–525.

Parkins, R. A. and Bywaters, E. G. L. (1959). Regression of amyloidosis secondary to rheumatoid arthritis. *Brit. med. J.* **1**, 536–540.

Paronetto, F. (1969). Systemic nonsuppurative necrotizing angiitis. In: *Textbook of Immunopathology*, Vol. I, pp. 722–732. Edited by Miescher, P. A. and Muller-Eberhard, H. J. Grune and Stratton, New York and London.

Partridge, R. E. H. and Duthie, J. J. R. (1963a). Incidence of macrocytic anaemia in rheumatoid arthritis. *Brit. med. J.* **1**, 88–91.

— (1963b). Controlled trial of the effect of complete immobilization of the joints in rheumatoid arthritis. *Ann. rheum. Dis.* **22**, 91–99.

Pasternack, A., Wegelius, O. and Mäkisara, P. (1967). Renal biopsy in rheumatoid arthritis. *Acta med. scand.* **182**, 591–595.

Patterson, C. D., Harville, W. E. and Pierce, J. A. (1965). Rheumatoid lung disease. *Ann. intern. Med.* **62**, 685–697.

Paul, W. D. (1967). Synovectomy of the digital joint of the hand. *Symposium on the Early Synovectomy in Rheumatoid Arthritis*. I.S.R.A.: Amsterdam.

Pazderka, V. and Středa, A. (1965). Bone lesions and the activity of the process in progressive polyarthritis. *Acta Univ. Carol. Med. (Praha)* **11**, 521–527.

Pearse, A. D. and Gardner, D. L. (1972). Preparation of unfixed undemineralised bone sections: the Bright bone cryostat. *J. clin. Path.* **25**, 26–29.

Pearse, A. G. E. (1953). Cytological and cytochemical investigations on the foetal and adult hypophysis in various physiological and pathological states. *J. Path. Bact.* **65**, 355–370.

Pearson, C., Barnett, E., Kroening, R., Marmor, L., Murray, J., Peter, J. and Salick, A. (1966). Rheumatoid arthritis and its systemic manifestations. *Ann. intern. Med.* **65**, 1101–1130.

Pease, D. C. (1964). *Histological techniques for electron microscopy*. Academic Press, New York and London.

Pease, Phyllis E. (1969). Bacterial L-forms in the blood and joint fluids of arthritic subjects. *Ann. rheum. Dis.*, **28**, 270–274.

Pekin, T. J., Jr., and Zvaifler, N. J. (1964). Haemolytic complement in synovial fluid. *J. clin. Invest.* **43**, 1372–1382.

Perez-Tamayo, R. (1961). General pathology of connective tissue. In: *Mechanisms of Disease: an Introduction to Pathology*, pp. 251–302. Saunders, Philadelphia and London.

Perri, J. A., Rodnan, G. P. and Mankin, H. J. (1968). Giant synovial cysts of the calf in patients with rheumatoid arthritis. *J. Bone Jt Surg.* **50A**, 709–719.

Petrescu, A., Athanasiu, P., Marin, D., Negoescu. M. and Stoia, I. (1970). Morphology of the synovial tissue and articular fluid cells in patients with rheumatoid polyarthritis, studied in the light and electron microscope. *Rom. Med. Rev.* **14**, 24–31.

Philips, J. M., Kaklamanis, P. and Glynn, L. E. (1966). Experimental arthritis associated with autoimmunization to inflammatory exudate. *Ann. rheum. Dis.* **25**, 165–174.

Piercy, D. W. (1970). Synovitis induced by intraarticular inoculation of inactivated *mycoplasma mycoides* in valves. *J. Comp. Path.* **80**, 549–558.

Pinals, R. S. (1966). Rheumatoid arthritis presenting with laryngeal obstruction. *Brit. med. J.* **1**, 842.

Pirani, C. L. and Bennett, G. A. (1951). Rheumatoid arthritis. A report of 3 cases progressing from childhood and emphasizing certain systematic manifestations. *Bull. Hosp. Joint Dis.*, **12**, 335–367.

Pirani, C. L. and Manaligod, J. R. (1966). The kidney in collagen diseases. In: *The Kidney: International Academy of Pathology Monograph No. 6*, pp. 147–203. Edited by Mostofi, F. K. and Smith, D. E. Williams and Wilkins, Baltimore.

Pitcher, C. S. (1966). Anaemia in rheumatoid arthritis. In: *Modern Trends in Rheumatology*, pp. 139–152. Edited by Hill, A. G. S. Butterworths, London.

Polisar, I. A. (1959). The cricoarytenoid joint: a diarthrodial articulation subject to rheumatoid arthritic involvement. *Laryngoscope* **69**, 1129–1164.

Pollak, V. E., Pirani, C. L., Steek, I. E. and Kark, R. M. (1962). The kidney in rheumatoid arthritis: studies by renal biopsies. *Arthr. and Rheum.* **5**, 1–9.

Pompidou, Alain and Schramm, Berthold (1971). Identification of thymic-dependent lymphocytes. *Lancet*, **ii**, 245.

Poole, A. R. (1970). The degradation of cartilage matrix by a lysosomal preparation, isolated from a malignant tumour, and its inhibition by an antiserum to this preparation. *Histochem. J.*, **2**, 431–439.

Poppius, H. and Tani, P. (1964). Non-tuberculous pleurisy. *Acta tuberc. scand.* **44**, 310–315.

Portner, M. M. and Gracie, W. A. (1966). Rheumatoid lung disease with cavitary nodules, pneumothorax and eosinophilia. *New Engl. J. Med.* **275**, 697–700.

Posner, E. (1960). Pneumoconiosis in makers of artificial grinding wheels, including a case of Caplan's syndrome. *Brit. J. Indust. Med.* **17**, 109–113.

Potter, J. L. and Duthie, J. J. R. (1961). Effects of environmental temperature upon capillary resistance in patients with rheumatoid arthritis and other individuals. *Ann. rheum. Dis.* **20**, 144–148.

Potter, J. L., Duthie, J. J. R. and Alexander, W. R. M. (1961). Aetiological factors in the collagen diseases: impairment of enzyme-binding capacity of serum in rheumatoid disease. *Proc. roy. Soc. Med.* **55**, 109–116.

Potter, T. A., Barkin, R. and Stillman, J. S. (1946). Occurrence of spondylitis in juvenile rheumatoid arthritis. *Ann. rheum. Dis.* **13**, 364–365.

Poynton, F. J. and Paine, A. (1913). *Researches on Rheumatism*. Churchill, London.

Price, A. E. and Schoenfeld, J. B. (1934). Felty's syndrome: Report of a case with complete postmortem findings. *Ann. intern. Med.* **7**, 1230–1239.

Price, T. M. L. and Skelton, M. O. (1956). Rheumatoid arthritis with lung lesions. *Thorax* **11**, 234–240.

Pruzanski, W., Saito, S. and Ogryzlo, M. A. (1970). The significance of lysozyme (muramidase) in rheumatoid arthritis. *Arthr. and Rheum.* **13**, 389–399.

Pugh, D. and Walker, P. G. (1961). The localization of N-acetyl-β-glucosaminidase in tissue. *J. Histochem. Cytochem.* **9**, 242–250.

Quintarelli, G., Scott, J. E. and Dellovo, M. C. (1964). The chemical and histochemical properties of alcian blue—II. Dye binding of tissue polyanions. *Histochemie* **4**, 86–98.

Rademakers, J. M., Eulderink, F. and Cats, A. (1969). Scleral lesions in rheumatoid arthritis. *Folia Med. Neerl.* **12**, 166–172.

Radin, E. L., Swann, D. A. and Weisser, P. A. 1970). Separation of a hyaluronate-free lubricating fraction from synovial fluid. *Nature (Lond.)* **228**, 377–378.

Radnai, B. (1953). Vascular changes in peripheral nerves and skeletal muscles in rheumatoid arthritis. *Acta morph. Acad. Sci. hung.* **3**, 87–100.

— (1969). Comparative morphology of small vessel lesions in rheumatoid arthritis and periarteritis nodosa. *Acta morph. Acad. Sci. hung.* **17**, 69–79.

Ragan, C. (1966). The clinical picture of rheumatoid arthritis. In: *Arthritis and Allied Conditions* (7th Edition). pp. 211–219. Edited by Hollander, J. L. Henry Kimpton, London.

Ramachandran, G. N. (Editor) (1968). *Treatise on Collagen*, Vol. 1: Chemistry. Academic Press, London and New York.

Raven, R. W., Parkes Weber, F. and Price, L. W. (1948). The necrobiotic nodules of rheumatoid arthritis. *Ann. rheum. Dis.* **7**, 63–75.

Rawson, A. J., Abelson, N. M. and Hollander, J. L. (1965). Studies on the pathogenesis of rheumatoid joint inflammation—II. Intracytoplasmic particulate complexes in rheumatoid synovial fluids. *Ann. intern. Med.* **62**, 281–284.

Redler, I. and Zimmy, Marilyn, L. (1970). Scanning electron microscopy of normal and abnormal articular cartilage and synovium. *J. Bone Jt Surg.* **52A**, 1395–1404.

Reed, W. B. and Wright, V. (1966). Psoriatic arthritis. In: *Modern Trends in Rheumatology*, pp. 375–383. Edited by Hill, A. G. S. Butterworths, London.

Reid, M. McC. (1968). Extensive vascular calcification in association with juvenile rheumatoid arthritis and amyloidosis. *Arch. Dis. Child.* **43**, 607–610.

Reimann, H. A. and Eklund, C. M. (1935). Long-continued vaccine therapy as a cause of amyloidosis. *Amer. J. med. Sci.* **190**, 88–92.

Reiter, H. (1916). Ueber eine bisher unerkannte Spirochäten Infektion (*Spirochaetosis arthritica*). *Dtsch. med. Wschr.* **42**, 1535–1536.

Restifo, R. A., Lussier, A. J., Rawson, A. J., Rockey, J. H. and Hollander, J. L. (1965). Studies on the pathogenesis of rheumatoid joint inflammation—III. The experimental production of arthritis by the intra-articular injection of purified 7S gamma globulin. *Ann. intern. Med.* **62**, 285–291.

Reynolds, J. J. (1970). Degradation Processes in Bone and Cartilage. *Calc. Tiss. Res. Suppl.* 52–56.

Rich, A. R. (1947). Hypersensitivity in disease: with especial reference to perarteritis nodosa, rheumatic fever, disseminated lupus erythematosus and rheumatoid arthritis. *The Harvey Lectures, Series XLII.* The Science Press Printing Company, Lancaster, Pennsylvania.

Rich, A. R., Voisin, G. A. and Bang, F. B. (1953). Electron microscopic studies of the alteration of collagen fibrils in the Arthus phenomenon. *Bull. Johns Hopk. Hosp.* **92**, 222–232.

Richards, A. G. and Barrett, G. M. (1958). Rheumatoid lung changes associated with pneumoconiosis. *Thorax* **13**, 185–193.

Richmond, J., Alexander, W. R. M., Potter, J. L. and Duthie, J. J. R. (1961). Nature of anaemia in rheumatoid arthritis—V. Red cell survival measured by radioactive chromium. *Ann. rheum. Dis.* **20**, 133–137.

Richmond, J., Gardner, D. L., Roy, L. M. H. and Duthie, J. J. R. (1956). Nature of anaemia in rheumatoid arthritis—III. Changes in the bone marrow and their relation to other features of the disease. *Ann. rheum. Dis.* **15**, 217–226.

Richmond, J., Roy, L. M. H., Gardner, D. L., Alexander, W. R. M. and Duthie, J. J. R. (1958). Nature of anaemia in rheumatoid arthritis—IV. Effects of the intravenous administration of saccharated oxide of iron. *Ann. rheum. Dis.* **17**, 406–415.

Riddle, J. M. and Barnhart, M. I. (1964). Ultrastructural study of fibrin dissolution via emigrated polymorphonuclear neutrophils. *Amer. J. Path.* **45**, 805–823.

Riddle, J. M., Bluhm, G. B. and Barnhart, M. I. (1965). Interrelationships between fibrin, neutrophils and rheumatoid synovitis. *J. Reticuloendothel. Soc.* **2**, 420–436.

Riese, H. (1895). Die Reiskörperchen in tuberculös erkrankten Synovalsäcken. *Dtsch. Z. Chir.* **42**, 1–99.

Riley, M. and Harrison, S. H. (1968). Interosseous muscle biopsy during hand surgery for rheumatoid arthritis. *Brit. J. Plast. Surg.* **21**, 342–346.

Roberts, A. D. (1971). Role of electrical repulsive forces in synovial fluid. *Nature* (Lond.) **231**, 434–436.

Roberts, J. E., McLees, B. D. and Kerby, G. P. (1967). Pathways of glucose metabolism in rheumatoid and nonrheumatoid synovial membrane. *J. Lab. clin. Med.* **70**, 503–511.

Roberts, W. C., Kehoe, J. A., Carpenter, D. F. and Golden, A. (1968). Cardiac valvular lesions in rheumatoid arthritis. *Arch. intern. Med.* **122**, 141–146.

Robertson, M. D. J., Hart, F. D., White, W. F., Nuki, G. and Boardman, P. L. (1968). Rheumatoid lymphadenopathy. *Ann. rheum. Dis.* **27**, 253–260.

Robinson, H. S. (1966). Rheumatoid arthritis—atlanto-axial subluxation and its clinical presentation. *Canad. med. Ass. J.* **94**, 470–477.

Rodman, W. S., Williams, R. C., Jr., Bilka, P. J. and Muller-Eberhard, H. J. (1967). Immunofluorescent localization of the third and the fourth component of complement in synovial tissue from patients with rheumatoid arthritis. *J. Lab. clin. Med.* **69**, 141–150.

Rodman, G. P. (1965). *Progressive systemic sclerosis* in *Immunological Diseases*. pp. 769–783. Edited by Samter, M. and Alexander, H. L. Little, Brown, Boston.

Rodnan, G. P., Yunis, E. J. and Totten, R. S. (1960). Experience with punch biopsy of synovium in the study of joint disease. *Ann. intern. Med.* **53**, 319–331.

Roegel, E., Weitzenblum, E., Lenz, D., Stoebner, P. and Oudet, P. (1969). Diffuse fibrotic rheumatoid lung disease associated with a carcinoma of the right lower lung lobe. *Rev. Tuberc. (Paris)* **33**, 543–554.

Roitt, I. M., Greaves, M. F., Torrigiani, G., Brostoff, J. and Playfair, J. H. L. (1969). The cellular basis of immunological responses. *Lancet*, **ii**, 367–370.

Rokitansky, C. von (1842–1846). *Handbuch der pathologischen Anatomie.* Braumüller und Seidel, Wien.

Ropes, Marian, W. and Bauer, W. (1953). *Synovial Fluid Changes in Joint Disease.* Harvard University Press, Cambridge, Mass.

Rose, H. M., Ragan, C., Pearce, E. and Lipman, M. O. (1948). Differential agglutination of normal and sensitized sheep erythrocytes by sera of patients with rheumatoid arthritis. *Proc. Soc. exp. Biol. (N. Y.)* **68**, 1–16.

Rosenberg, E. F., Baggenstoss, A. H. and Hench, P. S. (1943). The cause of death in 30 cases of rheumatoid arthritis. *Ann. intern. Med.* **19**, 114–115.

Rosenow, E. C. (1914). Etiology of arthritis deformans. *J. Amer. med. Ass.* **62**, 1146–1147.

Rössle, R. (1933). Zum Formenkreis der rheumatischen Gewebsveranderungen, mit besonderer Berücksichtigung der rheumatischen Gefässentzündungen. *Virchows Arch.* **288**, 780–832.

Rostropowicz-Denisiewicz, K. and Holub, Ada (1969). Amyloidosis in the rectoscopic examination in children with rheumatoid arthritis. *Pediat. pol.* **44**, 823–828.

Rothenberger, W. and Thiele, H. G. (1970). *In vitro* study on the pathogenesis of primary rheumatoid arthritis by means of migration inhibition tests. *Klin. Wschr.* **48**, 1308–1311.

Rotstein, J. and Good, R. A. (1962). Significance of the simultaneous occurrence of connective tissue disease and agammaglobulinaemia. *Ann. rheum. Dis.* **21**, 202–206.

Roujeau, J. and Amouroux, J. (1968). Rheumatoid lung. An anatomical study. *Rev. Tuberc. (Paris)* **32**, 717–728.

Roy, L. M. H., Alexander, W. R. M. and Duthie, J. J. R. (1955). Nature of anaemia in rheumatoid arthritis. 1. Metabolism of iron. *Ann. rheum. Dis.* **14**, 63–72.

Roy, L. M. H., Wigzell, F. W., Demers, R., Sinclair, R. J. G., Duthie, J. J. R., Atherden, S. M. and Marrian, G. F. (1955). Liver function in relation to possible abnormalities of steroid metabolism in rheumatoid arthritis. *Ann. rheum. Dis.* **14**, 183–190.

Roy, S. (1970). Ultrastructure of articular cartilage in experimental immobilization. *Ann. rheum. Dis.* **29**, 634–642.

Roy, S. and Ghadially, F. N. (1967). Aetiological significance of rod-shaped bodies in rheumatoid synovia. *Nature (Lond.)* **213**, 1139–1140.

Rubens-Duval, A., Villiaumey, J. and Kaplan, G. (1966). Aspects histologiques de la synoviale dans les arthrites subaiguës du genou. *Sem. Hôp. Paris* **42**, 3271–3275.

Rubin, E. H., Gordon, M. and Thelmo, W. L. (1967). Nodular pleuropulmonary rheumatoid disease: report of 2 cases and review of literature. *Amer. J. Med.* **42**, 567–581.

Ruderman, M., Miller, L. M. and Pinals, R. S. (1968). Clinical and serologic observations on 27 patients with Felty's syndrome. *Arthr. and Rheum.* **11**, 377–384.

Rylance, H. J. (1969). Hypertaurinuria in rheumatoid arthritis. *Ann. rheum. Dis.* **28**, 41–44.

Sanerkin, N. G. and Weaver, C. M. (1964). Chronic phenacetin nephropathy ('chronic interstitial nephritis') with papillary necrosis. *Brit. med. J.* **1**, 288.

Saville, P. D. and Kharmosh, O. (1967). Osteoporosis of rheumatoid arthritis: influence of age, sex and corticosteroids. *Arthr. and Rheum.* **10**, 423–430.

Saxton, H. M., Kilpatrick, F. R., Kinder, C. H., Lessof, M. H., McHardy-Young, S. and Wardle, D. F. H. (1969). Retroperitoneal fibrosis: a radiological and follow-up study of fourteen cases. *Quart. J. Med.* **38**, 159–181.

Scadding, J. G. (1969). The lungs in rheumatoid arthritis. *Proc. roy. Soc. Med.* **62**, 227–238.

Scapinelli, R. and Little, K. (1970). Observations on the mechanically induced differentiation of cartilage from fibrous connective tissue. *J. Path.* **101**, 85–91.

Scherbel, A. L., Schuchter, S. L. and Harrison, J. W. (1957). V. Chemotherapy in rheumatoid arthritis; a concept. *Cleveland Clin. Quart.* **24**, 105–115.

Scherbel, A. L., Schuchter, S. L. and Weyman, S. J. (1957). II. Intraarticular administration of nitrogen mustard alone and combined with a corticosteroid for rheumatoid arthritis. *Cleveland Clin. Quart.* **24**, 78–89.

Schleiden, M. J. (1838). Beiträge zur Phytogenesis. *Arch. Anat. Physiol. u. Wiss. Med. (Berl.)* **2**, 137–174.

Schlesinger, S., and Cathie, I. A. B. (1951). Effect of Still's disease on the haemopoietic system. *Ann. rheum. Dis.* **10**, 412–417.

Schmid, F. R., Cooper, N. S., Ziff, M. and McEwan, C. (1961). Arteritis in rheumatoid arthritis. *Amer. J. Med.* **30**, 56–83.

Schneider, R. E. and Dobbins III, W. O. (1968). Suction biopsy of the rectal mucosa for the diagnosis of arteritis in rheumatoid arthritis and related diseases. *Ann. intern. Med.* **68**, 561–568.

Schoen, R. (1969). Chronic progressive polyarthritis. *Rheumatismus* **41**, 1–147.

Schools, G. S. and Davey, W. N. (1960). Needle biopsy of the parietal pleura. *Univ. Mich. med. Bull.* **26**, 1–5.

Schools, G. S. and Mikkelsen, W. M. (1962). Rheumatoid pleuritis. *Arthr. and Rheum.* **5**, 369–377.

Schourup, K. (1957). Necrosis of the renal papillae. *Acta path. microbiol. scand.* **41**, 462–477.

Schubert, M. and Hamerman, D. (1968). *A Primer on Connective Tissue Biochemistry*. Lea and Febiger, Philadelphia.

Schueller, M. (1906). The relations of chronic villous polyarthritis to the dumb-bell shaped bacilli. *Amer. J. med. Sci.* **132**, 231–237.

Schull, W. J. and Cobb, S. (1969). The intrafamilial transmission of rheumatoid arthritis—III. The lack of support for a genetic hypothesis. *J. Chronic Dis.* **22**, 217–222.

Schüller, M. (1887). *Die Pathologie und Therapie der Gelenkentzundungen.* Urban und Schwarzenberg, Vienna.

Schumacher, H. R., Jr. (1970). Tubular paramyxovirus-like structures in synovial vascular endothelium. *Ann. rheum. Dis.* **29**, 445–447.

Schwann, T. (1839). *Mikroskopische Untersuchungen über die Übereinstimmung unter Struktur und dem Wachstum der Tiere und Pflanzen.* Sander, Berlin.

Schwartz, S. (1967). Rheumatoid carditis. *J. Amer. med. Ass.* **201**, 556–558.

Scott, J. E., Quintarelli, G. and Dellovo, M. C. (1964). The chemical and histochemical properties of alcian blue—I. The mechanism of alcian blue staining. *Histochemie* **4**, 73–85.

Scott, J. T. (1969). Neurological aspects of the rheumatic diseases. In: *Textbook of the Rheumatic Diseases,* pp. 643–700. Edited by Copeman, W. S. C. Livingstone, Edinburgh and London.

Scott, J. T., Hourihane, D. O., Doyle, F. H., Steiner, R. E., Laws, J. W., Dixon, A. St. J. and Bywaters, E. G. L. (1961). Digital arteritis in rheumatoid disease. *Ann. rheum. Dis.* **20**, 224–234.

Scudamore, C. (1816). *A Treatise on the Nature and Cure of Gout.* London.

— (1827). *A Treatise on the Nature and Cure of Rheumatism, with Observations on Rheumatic Neuralgia and on Spasmodic Neuralgia or Tic Douloureux,* p. 348. Longman, London.

Selye, H. (1950). *The Physiology and Pathology of Exposure to Stress,* pp. 393–402. Acta Inc., Montreal.

Senator, G. B. and Muirden, K. D. (1968). Concentrations of iron in synovial membrane, synovial fluid, and serum in rheumatoid arthritis and other joint diseases. *Ann. rheum. Dis.* **27**, 49–54.

Shannon, S. L. and Graham, R. C. Jr. (1971). Protein uptake by synovial cells. I. Ultrastructural study of the fate of intraarticularly injected peroxidases. *J. Histochem. Cytochem.* **19**, 29–42.

Sharp, J. T. (1957). Differential diagnosis of ankylosing spondylitis. *Brit. med. J.* **1**, 975–978.

Sharp, J. T., Calkins, E. and Cohen, A. S. (1964). Observations on the clinical, chemical and serological manifestations of rheumatoid arthritis, based on the course of 154 cases. *Medicine (Baltimore)* **43**, 41–58.

Sharp, J. T. and Purser, D. W. (1961). Spontaneous atlanto-axial dislocation in ankylosing spondylitis and rheumatoid arthritis. *Ann. rheum. Dis.* **20**, 47–77.

Shearn, M. A., Tu, W. H., Stephens, B. G. and Lee, J. C. (1970). Virus like structures in Sjögren's syndrome. *Lancet* **i**, 568–569.

Sherman, M. S. (1952). Psoriatic arthropathy. *J. Bone Jt Surg.* **34A**, 831–851.

Shirahama, T. and Cohen, A. S. (1967). High resolution electron microscopic analysis of the amyloid fibril. *J. Cell. Biol.* **33**, 679–708.

Shmueli, U., Gafni, J., Sohar, E. and Ashkenazi, Y. (1969). An X-ray study of amyloid. *J. Molec. Biol.* **41**, 309–311.

Short, C. L., Bauer, W. and Reynolds, W. E. (1957). *Rheumatoid Arthritis.* Harvard University Press, Cambridge, Mass.

Sievers, K., Aho, K., Hurri, L. and Perttala, Y. (1964). Studies of rheumatoid pulmonary disease. *Acta tuberc. scand.* **45**, 21–34.

Sinclair, R. J. G. and Cruickshank, B. (1956). A clinical and pathological study of sixteen cases of rheumatoid arthritis with extensive visceral involvement ('rheumatoid disease'). *Quart. J. Med.* **25**, 313–332.

Singer, H. A. and Levy, H. A. (1936). Relationship of Felty's and allied syndromes to sepsis lenta. *Arch. intern. Med.* **57**, 576–600.

Singer, C. and Underwood, E. A. (1962). *A Short History of Medicine.* Oxford, Clarendon Press.

Sjögren, H. (1933). A new conception of keratoconjunctivitis sicca. *Acta ophthal. (Kbh.)* Suppl. **2**, 1–151.

— (1943). *A New Conception of Keratoconjunctivitis Sicca (Keratitis Filiformis in Hyperfunction of the Lachrymal Glands),* translated by Hamilton, J. B. Australasian Medical Publishing Company, Sydney.

— (1951). Some problems concerning keratoconjunctivitis sicca and the sicca-syndrome. *Acta ophthal. (Kbh.)* **29**, 33–47.

Sjöstrand, F. S. (1967). *Electron microscopy of cells and tissues.* Academic Press, New York and London.

Skrifvars, B., Laine, V. and Wegelius, O. (1969). Sclerosis of the arteries of the extremities in rheumatoid arthritis. *Acta med. scand.* **186**, 145–147.

Sledge, C. B. and Dingle, J. T. (1965). Activation of lysosomes by oxygen. *Nature,* **205**, 140–141.

Sliwinski, A. J. and Zvaifler, N. H. (1970). *In vivo* synthesis of IgG by rheumatoid synovium. *J. Lab. clin. Med.* **76**, 304–310.

Smith, Carol, and Hamerman, D. (1962). Acid phosphatase in human synovial fluid. *Arthr. and Rheum.* **5**, 411–414.

— (1969). Significance of persistent differences between normal and rheumatoid synovial membrane cells in culture. *Arthr. and Rheum.* **12**, 639–645.

Smith, C., Janis, R., Haberman, E. and Hamerman, D. (1970). Changes in rabbit joints injected with rheumatoid synovial membrane cells (abstract). *Arthr. and Rheum.* **13**, 349.

Smith, E. M., Juvinall, R. C., Bender, L. F. and Pearson, R. (1966). Flexor forces and rheumatoid metacarpophalangeal deformity. *J. Amer. med. Ass.* **198**, 130–134.

Smith, R. F. and Shine, K. I. (1964). Rheumatoid arthritis of the cricoarytenoid joint with ankylosis. A report of a case presenting as a serious medical emergency. *Ann. intern. Med.* **60**, 473–475.

Smith, R. J. and Kaplan, E. B. (1967). Rheumatoid deformities at the metacarpophalangeal joints of the fingers. *J. Bone Jt Surg.* **49A**, 31–47.

Sobin, L. H. and Hagstrom, J. W. C. (1962). Lesions of cardiac conduction tissue in rheumatoid aortitis. *J. Amer. med. Ass.* **180**, 1–5.

Sokoloff, L. (1953). The heart in rheumatoid arthritis. *Amer. Heart J.*, **45**, 635–643.

— (1961). The pathogeneis of rheumatoid arthritis. In: *Inflammation and Diseases of Connective Tissue: a Hahnemann Symposium*, pp. 146–152. Edited by Mills, L. C. and Moyer, J. H. Saunders, Philadelphia and London.

— (1963). The pathophysiology of peripheral blood vessels in collagen diseases. In: *The Peripheral Blood Vessels*, pp. 297–325. Edited by Orbison, J. H. and Smith, D. E. Williams and Wilkins, Baltimore.

— (1964). Cardiac involvement in rheumatoid arthritis and allied disorders: current concepts. *Mod. Conc. cardiov. Dis.* **33**, 847–850.

— (1966). The pathology of rheumatoid arthritis and allied disorders. In *Arthritis and Allied Conditions* (7th Edition), pp. 187–210. Edited by Hollander, J. L. Lea and Febiger, Philadelphia.

Sokoloff, L. and Bunim, J. J. (1957). Vascular lesions in rheumatoid arthritis. *J. Chron. Dis.* **5**, 668–685.

Sokoloff, L., McCluskey, R. T. and Bunim, J. J. (1953). Vascularity of the early subcutaneous nodule of rheumatoid arthritis. *Arch. Path.* **55**, 475–495.

Sokoloff, L., Wilens, S. L. and Bunim, J. J. (1951). Arteritis of striated muscle in rheumatoid arthritis. *Amer. J. Path.* **27**, 157–173.

Solomon, W. M. (1943). Amyloidosis in chronic atrophic arthritis. *Ann. intern. Med.* **18**, 846–850.

Sood, S. C. (1971). A study of the effects of experimental immobilisation on rabbit articular cartilage. *J. Anat.* **108**, 497–507.

Sorenson, A. W. (1967). A method for quantitative evaluation of the nuclear distribution in the glomeruli of renal biopsy specimens. *Acta path. microbiol. scand.* **69**, 71–76.

Sorenson, G. D., Heefner, W. A. and Kirkpatrick, J. B. (1966). Experimental amyloidosis. *Meth. Achiev. exp. Path.*, Volume **1**, pp. 514–543. Edited by Bajusz, E. and Jasmin, G. Karger, Basel and New York.

Soria-Herrera, C., Morley, J., Inoue, H. and Gardner, D. L. (1971a). Experimental turpentine arthritis: measurement of treated and untreated inflammatory response by the accumulation of ^{125}I-albumin. *J. Path.*, **104**, iii.

— (1971b). Three-dimensional structure of normal rat articular surfaces and of surfaces in early turpentine arthritis. *J. Path.*, **104**, xv.

Spector, W. G. (1964). (Ed.) The acute inflammatory response. *Ann. N.Y. Acad. Sci.* **116**, 747–1084.

Spector, W. G. and Heesom, Nicolette (1969). The production of granulomata by antigen–antibody complexes. *J. Path.* **98**, 31–39.

Spence, M. P. (1955). Rheumatoid disease of the lungs and pleura. *Arch. Middx. Hosp.* **5**, 95–106.

Spencer, H. (1968). Pulmonary changes in rheumatoid arthritis. In: *Pathology of the Lung* (2nd Edition). Pergamon Press, Oxford.

Spicer, S. S. and Bryant, J. H. (1958). Cartilage changes in papain-treated rabbits. *Amer. J. Path.* **33**, 1237–1245.

Spiera, H. (1963). Excretion of a tryptophan metabolite in rheumatoid arthritis. *Arthr. and Rheum.* **6**, 364–371.

Spiera, H. and Vallarino, R. (1969). Serum kynurenine in rheumatoid arthritis. *J. clin. Invest.* **48**, 856–859.

Spitzy, H. (1903). Zur chronischen Arthritis des Kindes. *Z. orthopäed. Chir.* **11**, 699–795.

Stanfield, A. B. (1966). Cells with filopodia cultured from human synovialis. *Anat. Rec.* **154**, 73–79.

Stanfield, A. B. and Stephens, C. A. L., Jr. (1963). Studies of cells cultured from 188 rheumatoid and non-rheumatoid synovial tissues. *Texas Rep. Biol. Med.* **21**, 400–411.

Statistical Appendix prepared by A. R. C. Field Unit (1969). Digest of morbidity and mortality data on the rheumatic diseases. *Ann. rheum. Dis.* **28**, 443–446.

Steffen, C. (1970). Consideration of pathogenesis of rheumatoid arthritis as collagen autoimmunity. *Z. Immun.-Forsch.* **139**, 219–227.

Stengel, B. F., Watson, R. R. and Darling, R. J. (1966). Pulmonary rheumatoid nodule with cavitation and chronic lipid effusion. *J. Amer. med. Ass.* **198**, 1263–1266.

Steples, T. C., Toome, E. C., Kirby, P. and Kag, S. (1962). Fatal glomerulonephritis with nephrosis developing during a course of chrysotherapy for rheumatoid arthritis. *Arthr. and Rheum.* **5**, 123.

Sternlieb, I., Sandson, J. I., Morell, A. G., Korotkin, E. and Scheinberg, I. H. (1969). Nonceruloplasmin copper in rheumatoid arthritis. *Arthr. and Rheum.* **12**, 458.

Stewart, Sheila M., Alexander, W. R. M. and Duthie, J. J. R. (1969). Isolation of diphtheroid bacilli from synovial membrane and fluid in rheumatoid arthritis. *Ann. rheum. Dis.* **28**, 477–487.

Stewart, T. G. (1860–1861). On the waxy or amyloid form of Bright's disease. *Edin. med. J.* **6**, 710–728.

Still, G. F. (1896–1897). On a form of chronic joint disease in children. *Med.-chir. Trans.* **80**, 47–59.

Stinchfield, F. E. (1962). Current concepts of bone formation. *Trans. Amer. surg. Assoc.* **80**, 185–186.

Stockman, R. (1904). The causes, pathology and treatment of chronic rheumatism. *Edin. med. J.* **15**, 107–116 and 223–235.

— (1920). *Rheumatism and Arthritis.* Green and Sons, Edinburgh.

Strangeways, T. S. P. and Burt, J. B. (1905). A study of skiagrams from the hands of 100 cases of so-called rheumatoid arthritis and chronic gout. *Rep. Comm. Study Spec. Dis.* Vol. 1. Edinburgh, pp. 145–164.

Straub, L. R. (1960). The etiology of finger deformities in the hand affected by rheumatoid arthritis. *Bull. Hosp. Jt Dis (N.Y.)* **21**, 322–329.

Středa, A., Králová, M. and Brémová, A. (1966). Osteonekrózy velkých kloubů při progresívní polyartritide (Osteonecrosis of the large joints in polyarthritis). *Čas. Lék. čes.* **105**, 370–372.

Stroescu, O. and Leahu, S. (1969). Punch biopsy of the knee synovial membrane and its value in the study of rheumatoid arthritis. *Rev. roum. Méd. interne* **6**, 349–357.

Stroescu, O. and Mihailescu, E. (1970). Contribution to the study of the lymphocyte in patients with rheumatoid arthritis. I. Cytologic and cytochemical investigations in the blood and synovial fluid. *Rev. roum. Méd. interne.* **7**, 203–208.

Stuart, A. E., Davidson, A. E. and Cuming, R. A. (1967). Sensitivity and methodology of erythrophagocytosis for the detection of heteroantibodies and natural isoantibodies to human red cells. *J. Reticuloendothel. Soc.* **4**, 109–121.

Stůdnička, F. K. (1934). The symplasmic state of the tissues of the animal body. *Biol. Rev.* **9**, 263–298.

Sundberg, J. and Brattström, M. (1965). Juvenile rheumatoid gonarthritis. II. Disturbance of ossification and growth. *Acta rheum. scand.* **11**, 279–290.

Sutro, C. J. (1961). Changes in the synovial tissues of the knees of rabbits following intraarticular injection of thorium (thorotrast). *Bull. Hosp. Jt Dis.* **22**, 39–42.

Sutton, R. A. L. (1967). Rheumatoid pericarditis. *Proc. roy. Soc. Med.* **60**, 339–341.

Svartz, N. (1969). The affinity of the rheumatoid factor for different tissues and the production in animals of a rheumatoid factor-like macroglobulin, simultaneously with arthritis. *J. belge Rhum. Med. phys.* **24**, 200–208.

— (1971). Macroglobulins provoking haemagglutination in rheumatoid arthritis and other diseases. Almqvist and Wiksell, Stockholm.

Szasz, G., Kovacs, L., Takacs, B. and Lux, A. (1968). Hinweise auf immunologische Bedingungen in der Pathogenese der Polyarthritis chronica progressiva auf Grund von Untersuchungen des Knochenmarks. *Folia Haematologica* **89**, 28–41.

Szpilmanowa, H. and Stachurska, J. (1968). Hageman factor (Factor XII) activity in synovial fluid of rheumatoid arthritis patients and its possible pathogenic significance. *Experientia* **24**, 784–785.

Szpunar, J. and Miszke, A. (1970). Fibrous ankylosis of the incudostapedial joint. *Arch. Otolaryng.* **92**, 138–141.

Takagi, K. (1933). Practical experiences using Takagi's arthroscope. *J. Jap. Orthop. Ass.* **8**, 132.

Takeda, Y. (1967). Studies of the metabolism and distribution of fibrinogen in patients with rheumatoid arthritis. *J. Lab. clin. Med.* **69**, 624–633.

Talal, N. (1971). Sjögren's syndrome, lymphoproliferation and renal tubular acidosis. *Ann. intern. Med.* **74**, 633–634.

Talal, N., Asofysky, R. and Lightbody, P. (1970). Immunoglobulin synthesis by salivary gland lymphoid cells in Sjögren's syndrome. *J. clin. Invest.* **49**, 49–54.

Talal, N., Zisman, E. and Schur, P. H. (1968). Renal tubular acidosis, glomerulonephritis and immunologic factors in Sjögren's syndrome. *Arthr. and Rheum.* **11**, 774–786.

Talbott, J. A. and Calkins, E. (1964). Pulmonary involvement in rheumatoid arthritis. *J. Amer. med. Ass.* **189**, 911–913.

Tanner, E., Neumann, W., Ebner, E., Unverricht, A. and Correns, H.-J. (1970). Erythrocytic blood picture during the active phase of rheumatoid arthritis—I. The red blood picture and serum iron levels in relation to degree of activity. *Dtsch. Gesundh.-Wes.* **25**, 144–147.

Taylor, A. G. (1971). The mechanism of experimental arthritis produced by streptolysin S. *Proc. roy. Soc. Med.* **64**, 644–645.

Teilum, G. (1952). Cortisone-ascorbic acid interaction and the pathogenesis of amyloidosis. Mechanism of action of cortisone on mesenchymal tissue. *Ann. rheum. Dis.* **11**, 119–136.

Teilum, G. and Lindahl, A. (1954). Frequency and significance of amyloid changes in rheumatoid arthritis. *Acta med. scand.* **149**, 449–455.

Teleszyński, Z., and Patroś, J. (1970). Regeneration of synovial membrane previously removed because of rheumatoid arthritis. *Chir. Narzad. Ruchu Ortop. Pol.* **35**, 211–212.

Tellesson, W. G. (1961). Rheumatoid pneumoconiosis (Caplan's syndrome) in an asbestos worker. *Thorax* **16**, 372–377.

Thoma, K. H. (1946). Ankylosis of the mandibular joint. *Amer. J. Orthodont.* **32**, 259–272.

Thomas, L. (1956). Reversible collapse of rabbit ears after intravenous papain, and prevention of recovery by cortisone. *J. exp. Med.* **104**, 245–252.

Thompson, G. R. and Castor, C. W. (1966). The excretion of non-dialyzable urinary mucopolysaccharide in rheumatic and other systemic disease states. *J. Lab. clin. Med.* **68**, 617–627.

Thompson, G. R., Ferreyra, A. and Brackett, R. G. (1971). Acute arthritis complicating rubella vaccination. *Arthr. and Rheum.* **14**, 19–26.

Thompson, M. and Eadie, Stella (1956). Kerato-conjunctivitis sicca and rheumatoid arthritis. *Ann. rheum. Dis.* **15**, 21–25.

Thomson, D. and Gardner, D. L. (1969). Thrombotic microangiopathy in rheumatoid arthritis. *Scot. med. J.* **14**, 190–193.

Thomson, M. (1966). Non-articular features of rheumatoid disease. In: *Modern Trends in Rheumatology*, pp. 32–48. Edited by Hill, A. G. S. Butterworths, London.

Tonietti, G., Oldstone, B. A. and Dixon, F. J. (1970). The effect of induced chronic viral infections on the immunologic diseases of New Zealand mice. *J. exp. Med.* **132**, 89–109.

Topp, J. R. and Hart, G. D. (1967). Widespread necrotizing arteritis in rheumatoid arthritis: report of a patient who survived. *Canad. med. Ass. J.* **97**, 412–415.

Townes, A. S. and Sowa, J. M. (1970). Complement in synovial fluid. *Johns Hopkins Med. J.* **127**, 23–37.

Trnvská, Z. and Sitaj, S. (1960). The changes of free amino acids in the serum and urine of patients with primary chronic polyarthritis. *Z. Rheumaforsch.* **19**, 125–130.

Tu, W. H., Shearn, M. A., Lee, J. C. and Hopper, J. (1968). Interstitial nephritis in Sjögren's syndrome. *Ann. intern. Med.* **69**, 1163–1170.

Turner-Warwick, M. and Doniach, D. (1965). Autoantibody studies in interstitial pulmonary fibrosis. *Brit. med. J.* **1**, 886–891.

Uddin, J., Kraus, A. S. and Kelly, H. G. (1970). Survivorship and death in rheumatoid arthritis. *Arthr. and Rheum.* **13**, 125–131.

Unger, P. N., Zuckerbrod, M., Beck, G. J. and Steele, J. M. (1948). Amyloidosis in rheumatoid arthritis: report of ten cases. *Amer. J. med. Sci.* **216**, 51–56.

Vainio, K. and Julkunen, H. (1960). Intraarticular nitrogen mustard treatment of rheumatoid arthritis. *Acta rheum. scand.* **6**, 25–30.

Vainio, U. (1966). A histochemical study on leucineaminopeptidase activity in the synovial membrane of patients with rheumatoid arthritis. *Ann. rheum. Dis.* **25**, 253–258.

— (1970). Leucineaminopeptidase in rheumatoid arthritis: localization in subchondral bone and in synovial fluid cells. *Ann. rheum. Dis.* **29**, 434–438.

Van Swaay, H. (1950). Spondylosis ankylopoietica. Een pathogenetische studie. Thesis, University of Leiden.

Vassallo, C. L. (1966). Rheumatoid arthritis of the crico-arytenoid joints. *Arch. intern. Med.* **117**, 273–275.

Vaubel, E. (1933). The form and function of synovial cells in tissue cultures—II. The production of mucin. *J. exp. Med.* **58**, 85–95.

Vaughan, Janet M. (1970). *The Physiology of Bone.* Clarendon Press, Oxford.

Vaughan, J. H. (1969). Rheumatoid factors and their biological significance. *Ann. N.Y. Acad. Sci.* **168**, 204–207.

Vaughan, J. H., Barnett, E. V., Sobel, M. V. and Jacox, R. F. (1968). Intracytoplasmic inclusions of immunoglobulins in rheumatoid arthritis and other diseases. *Arthr. and Rheum.* **11**, 125–134.

Vaughan, J. H., Jacox, G. A. and Clark, R. (1969). Relation of rheumatoid factor to intracellular inclusions. *Ann. N.Y. Acad. Sci.* **168**, 111–121.

Vaughan-Jackson, O. J. (1966). The rheumatoid hand. In: *Clinical Surgery, The Hand*, pp. 173–196. Edited by Pulvertaft, R. G. Butterworths, London.

Vazquez, J. J. and Dixon, F. J. (1957). Immunohistochemical study of lesions in rheumatic fever, systemic lupus erythematosus and rheumatoid arthritis. *Lab. Invest.* **6**, 205–217.

Velican, C. and Stroescu, O. (1969). Studies on macromolecular complexes of rheumatoid synovial tissue. *Rev. roum. Méd. interne* **6**, 385–395.

Virchow, R. (1858). Die Cellularpathologie in ihrer Begründung auf physiologische und pathologisches Gewebelehre. A. Hirschwald, Berlin. (Engl. translation by Chance, 1860).

Vojtisek, O., Freund, U. and Greiling, H. (1970). Cytologic and biochemical changes in synovial fluid after intraarticular treatment with immunosuppressive substances. *Z. Rheumaforsch.* **29**, 138–146.

Waaler, E. (1940). On the occurrence of a factor in human serum activating the specific agglutination of sheep blood corpuscles. *Acta path. microbiol. scand.* **17**, 172–188.

— (1967). The visceral lesions in rheumatoid arthritis. *Acta rheum. scand.* **13**, 20–41.

Wagner, B. M. (1967). Hyalin and fibrinoid: current status. In: *The Connective Tissue*, pp. 68–80. Edited by Wagner, B. M. and Smith, D. E.   Williams and Wilkins, Baltimore.

Wagner, T. and Abgarowicz, T. (1970). Microscopic appearance of Baker's cyst in cases of rheumatoid arthritis. *Reumatologia* **8**, 21–26.

Walker, P. S. (1969). Lubrication and Wear in Human Joints. Ph.D. thesis, Univ. Leeds.

Walker, P. S., Dowson, D., Longfield, M. D. and Wright, V. (1968). 'Boosted lubrication' in synovial joints by fluid entrapment and enrichment. *Ann. rheum. Dis.* **27**, 512–520.

Walker, P. S., Sikorski, J., Dowson, D., Longfield, M. D., Wright, V. and Buckley, T. (1969). Behaviour of synovial fluid on surfaces of articular cartilage: a scanning electron microscope study. *Ann. rheum. Dis.* **28**, 1–14.

Walker, W. C. (1967). Pulmonary infections and rheumatoid arthritis. *Quart. J. Med.* **36**, 239–251.

Walker, W. C. and Wright, V. (1967). Rheumatoid pleuritis. *Ann. rheum. Dis.* **26**, 467–474.

— (1968). Pulmonary lesions and rheumatoid arthritis. *Medicine* **47**, 501–520.

— (1969). Diffuse interstitial pulmonary fibrosis and rheumatoid arthritis. *Ann. rheum. Dis.* **28**, 252–259.

Waller, M., Irby, R., Mullinax, F. and Toone, E. C. (1965). Connective tissue disease and rheumatoid factors in patients with renal transplants. *New Engl. J. Med.* **273**, 12–18.

Walton, K. W. (1968a). Hypersensitivity and infection in the pathogenesis of rheumatic diseases. *Int. Rev. exp. Path.* **6**, 285–374.

— (1968b). Rheumatoid factor: The immunochemistry of rheumatoid factor reactivity. In: *Rheumatic Diseases, Pfizer Medical Monographs No. 3*, pp. 132–142. Edited by Duthie, J. J. R. and Alexander, W. R. M.   University Press, Edinburgh.

Ward, R. (1961). Pleural effusion and rheumatoid disease. *Lancet* **ii**, 1336–1338.

Warren, S. L., Marmor, L., Liebes, D. M. and Hollins, R. L. (1969a). Congenital transmission in mice of an active agent from human rheumatoid arthritis. *Nature* **223**, 646–647.

Warren, S. L., Marmor, L., Liebes, D. M. and Hollins, R. (1969b). An active agent from human rheumatoid arthritis which is transmissible in mice: Preliminary Report. *Arch. intern. Med.* **124**, 629–634.

Warren, S. L., Marmor, L., Liebes, D. M. and Hollins, R. L. (1970). Congenital deformities of mice transmitted by an agent from rheumatoid synovium. *Clin. Orthop.* **70**, 217–219.

Wassilev, W. (1971). Uber die Ultrastruktur der regenerierten Synovialmembran beim Menschen. *Arch. orthop. Unfall-Chir.*, **69**, 197–205.

Watanabe, M., Takeda, S. and Ikeuchi, H. (1969). *Atlas of Arthroscopy*. Igaku Shoin, Tokyo. Springer-Verlag, Berlin.

Waterhouse, J. P. (1963). Focal adenitis in salivary and lacrimal glands. *Proc. roy. Soc. Med.* **56**, 911–918.

Waterhouse, J. P. and Doniach, I. (1966). Postmortem prevalence of focal lymphocytic adenitis of the submandibular salivary gland. *J. Path. Bact.* **91**, 53–64.

Watt, T. L. and Baumann, R. R. (1967). Pseudoxanthomatous rheumatoid nodules. *Arch. Derm.* **95**, 156–160.

Webb, F. W. S., Hickman, J. A. and Brew, D. St. J. (1968). Death from vertebral artery thrombosis in rheumatoid arthritis. *Brit. med. J.* **2**, 537–538.

Webb, F. W. S., Lowe, J. and Bluestone, R. (1969). Uptake of colloidal radioactive yttrium by synovial membrane. *Ann. rheum. Dis.* **28**, 300–302.

Webb, J. and Payne, W. H. (1970). Abdominal apoplexy in rheumatoid arthritis. *Aust. Ann. Med.* **19**, 168–170.

Wegelius, O., Klockars, M. and Vainio, K. (1970). Collagenolytic activity in synovial fluid cells in rheumatoid arthritis. *Ann. Clin. Res.* **2**, 171–174.

Wegelius, O., Pasternack, A. and Kuhlbäck, B. (1969). Muscular involvement in rheumatoid arthritis. *Acta rheum. scand.* **15**, 257–261.

Wegelius, O., Skrifvars, B. and Andersson, L. (1970). Rheumatoid arthritis terminating in plasmacytoma. *Acta med. scand.* **187**, 133–138.

Weibel, E. R. and Palade, G. E. (1964). New cytoplasmic components in arterial endothelia. *J. cell. Biol.* **23**, 101–112.

Weichselbaum, A. (1887). Die senilen Veränderungen der Gelenke und deren Zusammenhang mit der Arthritis deformans. *S. B. Akad. Wiss. Wien (math.-nat. Klasse).* **75**, Abt. 3, p. 193.

Weiss, T. E. and Keller, K. E. (1967). Uncommon manifestations of rheumatoid arthritis. *Med. Clin. N. Amer.* **51**, 1019–1026.

Weissman, G. (1964). Lysosomes, autoimmune phenomena and diseases of connective tissue. *Lancet*, **ii**, 1373–1375.

— (1965). Lysosomes. *New Eng. J. Med.* **273**, 1084–1090, 1143–1149.

— (1967). The role of lysosomes in inflammation and disease. *Ann. rev. Med.* **18**, 97–112.

— (1967). Structure and function of lysosomes. *Rheumatology, An Annual Review* **1**, 1–28.

Weissman, G., Dukor, P. and Zurier, R. B. (1971). Effect of cyclic AMP on release of lysosomal enzymes from phagocytes. *Nature (New Biology)*, **231**, 131–135.

Weissman, G. and Spilberg, I. (1968). Breakdown of cartilage proteinpolysaccharide by lysosomes. *Arthr. and Rheum.* **11**, 162–169.

Weissman, G. and Thomas, L. (1963). Studies on lysosomes. II. The effect of cortisone on the release of acid hydrolases from a large granule fraction of rabbit liver induced by an excess of vitamin A. *J. clin. Invest.* **42**, 661–669.

— (1964). The effects of corticosteroids upon connective tissue and lysosomes. *Recent Progr. Hormone Res.* **20**, 215–245.

Wenley, W. G. and Glick, E. N. (1964). Medical synovectomy with thiotepa. *Ann. Phys. Med.* **7**, 287–293.

West, H. F. (1970). *The Chemical Pathology of Rheumatoid Arthritis*. Springfield, Illinois: Charles C Thomas.

Weston, P. D., Barrett, A. J. and Dingle, J. T. (1969). Specific inhibition of cartilage breakdown. *Nature (Lond.)*, **222**, 285–286.

Whaley, K. (1970). Liver disease in Sjögren's syndrome and rheumatoid arthritis. *Lancet*, **i**, 861–863.

Whaley, K. and Buchanan, W. W. (1971). Recent advances in Sjögren's syndrome. In: *Modern Trends in Rheumatology*, Vol. 2, pp. 139–157. Edited by Hill, A. G. S. Butterworths, London.

Whaley, K., Chisholm, D. M., Goudie, R. B., Downie, W. W., Dick, W. C., Boyle, J. A. and Williamson, J. (1969). Salivary duct autoantibody in Sjögren's syndrome: correlation with focal sialadenitis in the labial mucosa. *Clin. exp. Immunol.* **4**, 273–282.

Whaley, K. and Dick, W. C. (1968). Fatal subaxial dislocation of cervical spine in rheumatoid arthritis. *Brit. med. J.* **2**, 31.

— (1969). Rheumatoid arthritis. Aetiological and pathogenic considerations. *Hosp. Med.* **2**, 1916–1930.

Whaley, K., Pack, A. I., Boyle, J. A., Dick, W. C., Downie, W. W., Buchanan, W. W. and Gillespie, F. C. (1968). The articular scan in patients with rheumatoid arthritis: a possible method of quantitating joint inflammation using radiotechnetium. *Clin. Sci.* **35**, 547–552.

White, R. G. and Gordon, J. (1970). Adjuvant-activity of 'diphtheroid' organisms isolated from the joints of cases of rheumatoid arthritis. *Clin. exp. Immun.* **7**, 139–145.

Whitman, R. (1903). A report of final results in two cases of polyarthritis in children of the type first described by Still, together with remarks on rheumatoid arthritis. *Med. Rec. (N.Y.)* **63**, 601–605.

Wichman, G. (1893). Die Amyloiderkrankung. *Beitr. path. Anat.* **13**, 487–628.

Wilkinson, M. (1962). Rheumatoid pericarditis: a report of four cases. *Brit. med. J.* **2**, 1723–1726.

Wilkinson, M. and Jones, B. S. (1963). Evaluation of needle biopsy of synovial membrane. *Ann. rheum. Dis.* **22**, 100–105.

Wilkinson, M. C. and Lowry, J. H. (1965). Synovectomy for rheumatoid arthritis. *J. Bone Jt Surg.* **47B**, 482–488.

Wilkinson, P., Jeremy, R., Brooks, F. P. and Hollander, J. L. (1965). The mechanism of hypoalbuminemia in rheumatoid arthritis. *Ann. intern. Med.* **63**, 109–114.

Wilkoszewski, E., Małdyk, E. and Roztropowicz-Denisiewicz, K. (1965). Kliniczny i bioptyczny obraz nerek w przebiegu gośćca prewlekłego postępującego u dzieci. (Clinical and biopsy picture of the kidneys in rheumatoid arthritis in children. (Report I.)) *Reumatologia* **3**, 333–342.

Williams, M. H. (1968). Recovery of mycoplasma from rheumatoid synovial fluid. In: *Rheumatic Diseases: Pfizer Medical Monograph, No. 3*, pp. 172–181. Edited by Duthie, J. J. R. and Alexander, W. R. M. University Press, Edinburgh.

Williams, M. H., Brostoff, J. and Roitt, I. M. (1970). Possible role of *Mycoplasma fermentans* in pathogenesis of rheumatoid arthritis. *Lancet* **ii**, 277–280.

Williams, M. H. and Bruckner, F. E. (1971). Immunological reactivity to Mycoplasma fermentans in patients with rheumatoid arthritis. *Ann. rheum. Dis.* **30**, 271–273.

Williams, R. H. (1936). Felty's syndrome: report of a case with necropsy findings. *Ann. intern. Med.* **9**, 1247–1255.

Williamson, J., Cant, J., Stanley, J., Mason, D. K., Greig, W. R. and Boyle, J. A. (1967). Sjögren's syndrome and thyroid disease. *Brit. J. Ophthal.* **51**, 721–726.

Williamson, N. and Ling, N. R. (1965). Cellular reaction to complexes formed between rheumatoid factor and aggregated human gamma globulin. *Ann. rheum. Dis.* **24**, 513–521.

Willmer, E. N. (1965). (Ed.) Cells and Tissues in Culture. Academic Press, London and New York.

— (1970). Cells in tissue culture: mechanocytes. In *Cytology and Evolution* (2nd Edition), pp. 20–63. Academic Press, New York and London.

Willoughby, D. A. and Ryan, G. B. (1970). Evidence for a possible endogenous antigen in chronic inflammation. *J. Path.* **101**, 233–239.

Wilson, J. T. and Sokoloff, L. (1970). Epidermoid cysts simulating rheumatoid nodules in the olecranon region. *J. Amer. med. Ass.* **214**, 593–595.

Winchester, R. J., Agnello, V. and Kunkel, H. G. (1969). The joint-fluid gamma G-globulin complexes and their relation to intraarticular complement diminution. *Ann. N.Y. Acad. Sci.* **168**, 195–203.

Wirostko, E. and Johnson, L. A. (1970). Cytology of inflamed aqueous humour in patients with rheumatoid arthritis. *Amer. J. clin. Path.* **54**, 369–373.

Woessner, J. F. (1965). Acid hydrolases of connective tissue. *Int. Rev. Connect. Tissue. Res.* **3**, 201–260.

Wolf, E. (1970). Amyloidosis in rheumatoid arthritis. *Harefuah* **78**, 549–550.

Wolman, L., Darke, C. S. and Young, A. (1965). The larynx in rheumatoid arthritis. *J. Laryng.* **79**, 403–434.

Woodward, D. H., Gryfe, A. and Gardner, D. L. (1969). Comparative study by scanning electron microscopy of synovial surfaces of four mammalian species. *Experientia.* **25**, 1301–1303.

Wright, J. R., Calkins, E., Breen, W. J., Stolte, G. and Schultz, R. T. (1969). Relationship of amyloid to ageing. *Medicine* **48**, 39–60.

Wright, V. (1969). Psoriatic arthritis. In: *Textbook of the Rheumatic Diseases*, pp. 632–642. Edited by Copeman, W. S. C. Livingstone, Edinburgh.

Wyke, A. W. and Gardner, D. L. (1970). Microchemical determination of enzyme activities in small arteries of rats with early adrenal-regeneration hypertension. *Brit. J. exp. Path.* **51**, 512–517.

Wyllie, J. C., Haust, M. D. and More, R. H. (1966). The fine structure of synovial lining cells in rheumatoid arthritis. *Lab. invest.* **15**, 519–529.

Young, D. and Schwedel, J. B. (1944). The heart in rheumatoid arthritis. *Amer. Heart J.* **28**, 1–33.

Zawadzki, Z. A. and Benedek, T. C. (1969). Rheumatoid arthritis, dysproteinemic arthropathy and paraproteinemia. *Arthr. and Rheum.* **12**, 555–568.

Zawadzki, Z. A., Benedek, T. G., Ein, D. and Easton, J. M. (1969). Rheumatoid arthritis terminating in heavy-chain disease. *Ann. intern. Med.* **70**, 335–347.

Zevely, H. A., French, A. J., Mikkelsen, W. M. and Duff, I. F. (1956). Synovial specimens obtained by knee joint punch biopsy: histologic study in joint diseases. *Amer. J. Med.* **20**, 510–519.

Ziff, M. (1968). Immunological aspects of rheumatoid arthritis. In: *Rheumatic Diseases: Pfizer Medical Monograph No. 3*, pp. 90–94. University Press, Edinburgh.

Ziff, M., Brown, P., Badin, J. and McEwen, C. (1954). Hemagglutination test for rheumatoid arthritis with enhanced sensitivity using euglobulin factor. *Bull. rheum. Dis.* **5**, 75–76.

Ziff, M., Gribetz, H. J. and LoSpalluto, J. (1960). Effect of leucocyte and synovial membrane extracts on cartilage mucoprotein. *J. clin. Invest.* **39**, 405–412.

Ziff, M. and Scully, R. E. (1967). Pulmonary and cardiac disease complicating rheumatoid arthritis. *New Engl. J. Med.* **277**, 1079–1089.

Zucker-Franklin, D. (1966). The phagosomes in rheumatoid synovial fluid leukocytes: A light, fluoresence, and electron microscope study. *Arthr. and Rheum.* **9**, 24–36.

Zucker-Franklin, D. (1968). Electron microscopic studies of human leucocytes: structural variations related to function. *Seminars Hemat.* **5**, 109–113.

Zvaifler, N. J. (1965). A speculation on the pathogenesis of joint inflammation in rheumatoid arthritis. *Arthr. and Rheum.* **8**, 289–293.

— (1969). Rheumatoid factor and the fixation of complement. *Ann. N.Y. Acad. Sci.* **168**, 146–160.

Zweifach, B. W. (1955). Structural make-up of capillary walls. *Ann. N.Y. Acad. Sci.* **61**, 670–677.

Index

Bold figures indicate a main reference

253